CLINICAL MICROBIOLOGY AND INFECTIOUS DISEASE

VOLUME 1

FUNDAMENTALS OF MICROBIAL SCIENCE AND INFECTIOUS PATHOGENESIS

Yevhen Tarasov and
Hanna Shevchuk

ALLIED
HEALTH
PRESS

Clinical Microbiology and Infectious Disease

Volume 1: Fundamentals of Microbial Science and Infectious Pathogenesis

Authors: **Yevhen Tarasov and Hanna Shevchuk**

Allied Health Press
4164 Lakeshore Road
Burlington ON L7L 1A4
Canada
www.alliedhealthpress.com
Email: orders@arclereducation.com

ISBN: 978-1-77956-810-6

Allied Health Press publishes wide variety of books and eBooks. For more information about Allied Health Press and its products, visit our website at www.alliedhealthpress.com

ABOUT THE AUTHORS

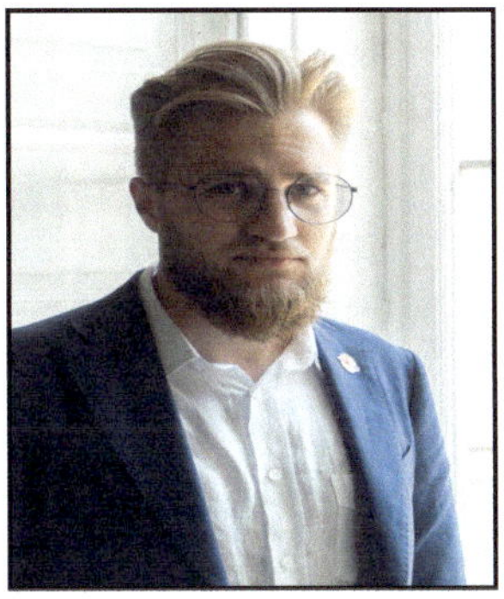

Yevhen Tarasov, MD, EuSpLM is a Senior Lecturer at the Department of General and Clinical Epidemiology and Biosafety with a course on Microbiology and Virology at Odesa National Medical University. Yevhen Tarasov received his MD in 2018 and got specialization in Medical Laboratory Science in 2019 with residency at The Filatov Institute of Eye Diseases and Tissue Therapy of the National Academy if Medical Science of Ukraine. He then joined the Department of General and Clinical Epidemiology and Biosafety with a course on Microbiology and Virology at Odesa National Medical University, Odesa, Ukraine as an assistant professor. His research interests include epidemiology and diagnostics of autoimmune diseases and allergy. He is a group leader of work group on Ukrainian adaptation of the the International Consensus on Antinuclear Antibody (ANA) Patterns (ICAP).

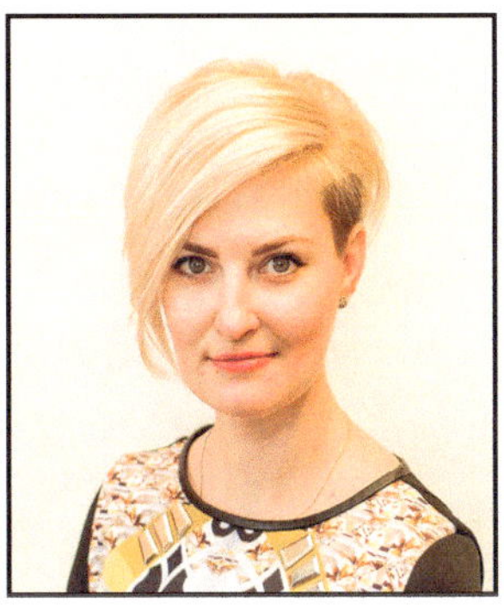

Hanna Shevchuk, PhD, is an Associate Professor and Head of Study at the Department of General and Clinical Epidemiology and Biosafety with a course in Microbiology and Virology at Odessa National Medical University (ONMedU), Ukraine. She also serves as a visiting lecturer at the International European University, Malta Campus. As. Prof. Shevchuk received her Master's degree in Microbiology and Virology from Odessa I.I. Mechnikov National University in 2005 and earned her PhD in Biological Sciences (specialty: molecular genetics) from the Institute of Food Biotechnology and Genomics of the National Academy of Sciences of Ukraine in 2012. Her academic journey includes positions ranging from laboratory assistant to researcher and faculty member at leading Ukrainian research institutes and universities. Her research interests focus on molecular genetics, microbiology, immunology, virology, epidemiology and innovative pedagogical practices in medical education. As. Prof. Shevchuk is an active member of the Society of Microbiologists of Ukraine named after S.M. Vynogradskyi, the Vavilov Society of Geneticists and Breeders of Ukraine and the Association of Clinical Chemistry and Laboratory Medicine of Ukraine. She has participated in international internships and seminars dedicated to modern challenges in higher medical education and is the author and co-author of scientific publications in microbiology, immunology, and pedagogy.

As. Prof. Shevchuk is recognized for her contributions to the development of educational programs and the implementation of advanced teaching methods, aiming to enhance the quality of training for specialists in medicine. In 2024, she was awarded the academic title of Associate Professor at Odessa National Medical University.

Brief Table of Contents

Detailed Table of Contents

CHAPTER 5

Microbiological of Infectious Diseases 137

CHAPTER 6

Bacterial Structure and Genetics 167

CHAPTER 7

Gram-negative Bacterial Infections 203

CHAPTER 8

Gram-positive Bacterial Infections 233

CHAPTER 9

Mycobacterial Infections 265

LIST OF FIGURES

PREFACE

Clinical microbiology occupies a pivotal position at the intersection of laboratory science and patient care, offering essential tools to detect, identify, and comprehend microorganisms responsible for disease. Across hospitals, clinics, and research centres globally, clinical microbiologists employ a range of techniques—from traditional culture methodologies to molecular diagnostics—to identify pathogens, monitor outbreaks, and inform treatment strategies. Their expertise underpins infection control protocols, antimicrobial stewardship programmes, and public health initiatives, thereby empowering healthcare providers to respond effectively to bacterial, viral, fungal, or parasitic threats.

Advancements in microbial genetics, next-generation sequencing, and immunological assay technology have significantly enhanced our comprehension of pathogen biology and host responses. Processes previously concealed regarding antibiotic resistance, virulence factor production, and microbial adaptation to environmental stresses are now elucidated with remarkable detail. This expanding knowledge base not only improves diagnostic accuracy but also encourages the development of novel therapeutics and vaccines, thereby influencing the future strategies for infectious disease management and global health security.

Clinical Microbiology and Infectious Disease: Volume 1 consolidates fundamental concepts and contemporary advances to direct readers through the core principles of pathogen biology, laboratory diagnosis, and disease management. This volume is designed to support students, clinicians, and laboratory personnel by offering lucid explanations, practical applications, and current examples drawn from real clinical environments.

Chapter 1 delineates the historical milestones and contemporary scope of clinical microbiology, illustrating the evolution from initial observations of pathogenic microorganisms to the sophisticated diagnostic laboratories of the present day. It acknowledges key pioneers and landmark discoveries that have influenced the development of our knowledge base and emphasises the transition from microscopy to automated and molecular diagnostic platforms.

Chapter 2 addresses the organisation and nomenclature of microorganisms, concluding with an overview of the hierarchical taxonomic system and methodologies for classifying bacteria, fungi, viruses, and parasites. Topics discussed include binomial nomenclature, phylogenetic relationships, and the practical applications of taxonomic revisions in laboratory reporting and public health surveillance.

Chapter 3 covers microbial physiology and genetics, elucidating the mechanisms by which microorganisms grow, reproduce, and adapt to their environments. The chapter encompasses metabolic pathways, genetic regulation, horizontal gene transfer, and the mechanisms underlying antibiotic resistance. Emphasis is placed on the influence of these biological traits on pathogenicity and laboratory diagnostics.

Chapter 4 examines host-microorganism interactions, including factors influencing susceptibility, immune responses, and disease progression. It discusses innate and adaptive immunity, microbial strategies for evading immune defences, and the equilibrium between commensal and pathogenic microorganisms within the human microbiome.

Chapter 5 discusses various laboratory tests employed to diagnose infectious diseases. It provides an overview of specimen collection, culture techniques, biochemical assays, serology tests, molecular diagnostics, and emerging point-of-care technologies. Practical advice is included on interpreting results, understanding test limitations, and incorporating laboratory data into clinical decisions.

Chapter 6 provides a comprehensive examination of bacterial cell structure and genetic organisation, including detailed discussions on cell wall composition, membrane systems, plasmids, transposons, and bacteriophages. A thorough understanding of these components is essential for interpreting staining outcomes, selecting appropriate antibiotic targets, and elucidating the molecular foundations of pathogen identification.

Chapter 7 discusses Gram-positive bacterial infections, encompassing staphylococci, streptococci, enterococci, and related genera. It addresses clinical syndromes, virulence factors, diagnostic criteria, and treatment protocols for both prevalent and emerging pathogens. Additionally, it emphasises antibiotic resistance patterns and infection control measures.

Chapter 8 covers *Enterobacteriaceae* and nonfermenter Gram-negative bacterial infections. It includes urinary tract infections, gastrointestinal illnesses, respiratory illnesses, and sepsis, alongside laboratory detection, antimicrobial susceptibility patterns, and the public health impact of multidrug-resistant strains.

Chapter 9 covers mycobacterial infections, including tuberculosis and nontuberculous mycobacterial disease. The chapter discusses culture techniques, molecular assays, drug sensitivity testing, and the challenges of outbreak control. It also examines global efforts to control tuberculosis through diagnostic innovation and treatment guidelines.

Chapter 10 discusses spirochetal and rickettsial diseases, including pathogens such as *Treponema, Borrelia, Leptospira, Ricketts*ia, and *Orientia* species. It covers clinical features, vector associations, serology and molecular diagnostic tests, as well as treatment, epidemiological surveillance, and prevention measures.

Written for medical students, pathology and microbiology trainees, clinical laboratory scientists, and infectious disease clinicians, this book provides readers with a solid understanding of the science and practice of diagnosing and treating microbial diseases. Researchers and public health practitioners alike will appreciate information on new methodologies and antimicrobial resistance issues.

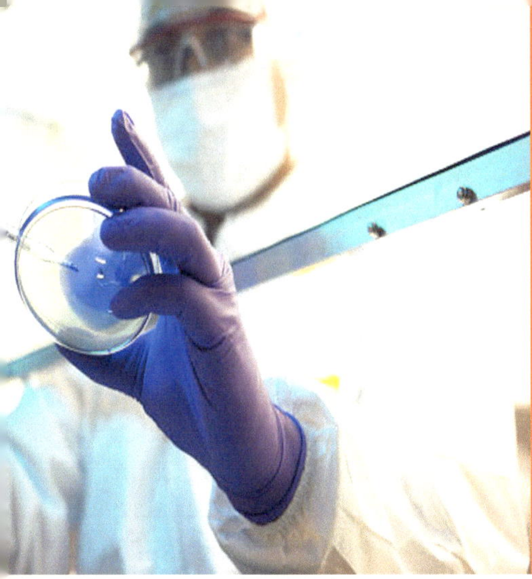

Chapter 1

INTRODUCTION TO CLINICAL MICROBIOLOGY

Contents

Introduction

Clinical microbiology constitutes a highly specialized branch of microbiology dedicated to the diagnosis, treatment, and prevention of microbial infections in humans, including bacteria, viruses, fungi, and parasites. It involves various activities, including specimen collection, microbial identification, susceptibility testing, and the interpretation of laboratory results to ensure optimal patient management. Furthermore, clinical microbiologists collaborate closely with clinicians, thereby establishing a vital link between microbiology and clinical practice. As infectious diseases continue to pose significant public health challenges globally, the significance of clinical microbiology has escalated, particularly in the study of emerging pathogens and antimicrobial resistance, emphasising the necessity for expert knowledge and advanced laboratory technology (Dar et al., 2016). The scope of clinical microbiology extends beyond individual diagnosis and treatment, influencing broader health initiatives and policies. A core function of clinical microbiologists involves monitoring microbial resistance patterns, providing crucial data to inform public health policy and infection control strategies. For instance, understanding the burden of antimicrobial resistance (AMR) is indispensable for guiding policies aimed at reducing infections and antibiotic consumption. The integration of microbiological data with epidemiological research enhances comprehension of disease transmission and evolution, thereby supporting public health interventions. Consequently, clinical microbiology is fundamental in the development of effective strategies to combat infectious diseases, with an emphasis on education and prevention at national and community levels (Dar et al., 2016). Recent technological advancements have expanded the capabilities of clinical microbiology. Innovations such as molecular diagnostics, high-throughput sequencing, and bioinformatics have revolutionised the field by enabling rapid and precise pathogen detection and resistance profiling. These technologies augment the capacity of clinical microbiologists to investigate outbreaks and improve patient outcomes through early, targeted therapies. Additionally, increasing interest in the microbiome — the microbial community residing within the human body — has opened new research avenues. As our understanding of host-microbe interactions deepens, clinical microbiology is broadening its scope, underscoring the importance of microbial ecology in health and disease. With ongoing advancements, clinical microbiology continues to be an essential tool for addressing current and future public health challenges, offering a comprehensive approach to infectious disease control.

Overview of Microbiology as a Science

Microbiology, as a science, forms a foundation within life at the microscopic level. It investigates a range of organisms such as bacteria, viruses, fungi, and protozoa, which not only play crucial roles in ecosystems but are also central to human health. Using various methods, microbiologists can study these microorganisms' genetics, physiology, and interactions with their environment. Advances in microbiology have significantly benefited the development of clinical practices, especially in the diagnosis and treatment of infectious diseases. This mutual reliance between clinical science and microbiology underpins the importance of understanding these microorganisms so that health professionals can formulate effective treatment plans.

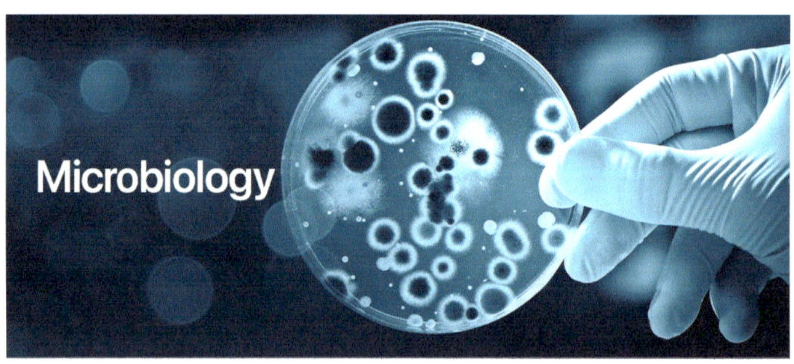

Figure 1.1. Overview of microbiology.

Source: https://www.yodadiagnostics.com/playground_assets/inner-pages/departments/yoda_daignostics_microbiology.webp.

A key area of microbiology is the study of pathogenic microorganisms, which infect humans, animals, and plants. This is especially relevant in clinical settings, where microbial actions influence treatment strategies. The emerging threat of antibiotic resistance fuels ongoing research and development in microbiology. Recently, innovative approaches such as phage therapy have gained prominence for combating resistant bacteria, representing a potential paradigm shift in clinical microbiology (Maimaiti et al., 2023) (Figure 1.1).

Therefore, integrating microbiological science into healthcare is essential for controlling infectious agents and safeguarding patient safety. In addition to uncovering new treatments, microbiology also significantly contributes to public health through research on microbial contamination risks within the environment. For instance, studies have shown that oral surgeries can emit considerable amounts of aerosolised bacteria, thereby increasing the risk of infection for both patients and healthcare personnel (Jennifer et al., 2020). This underscores the importance of microbiological research in the formulation of infection control guidelines across various medical disciplines. Through meticulous examination of microbial contamination, healthcare professionals can implement effective safety protocols and best practices, thereby promoting health within clinical settings. Collectively and individually, these insights serve to reinforce our appreciation of microbiology as a vital instrument for continuous advancement in clinical procedures and the protection of public health.

Importance of Clinical Microbiology in Healthcare

The role of clinical microbiology in patient care is of paramount importance, particularly in diagnosing infectious diseases. Clinical microbiologists facilitate strategies for targeted treatment, thereby improving patient outcomes through the identification of causative infectious agents. The discipline employs various laboratory methodologies to detect and characterise microorganisms, which are crucial in selecting appropriate antimicrobial therapies. As data-driven practice becomes increasingly reliant on healthcare practitioners, the integration of clinical microbiology into routine hospital operations is widely regarded as best practice. For example, electronic health records now contain comprehensive patient data accessible for research purposes, enhancing practitioners' ability to understand disease patterns and resistance trends (Alistair et al., 2023). These insights are vital not only for individual patient care but also for implementing public health interventions aimed at controlling infection transmission. Over the past decade, the emergence of antimicrobial resistance (AMR) has underscored the significance of clinical microbiology within healthcare systems globally. AMR constitutes a serious health threat, elevating morbidity and mortality risks, particularly within vulnerable populations. A comprehensive review estimated that approximately 4. 95 million deaths in 2019 could be attributed to bacterial AMR, emphasising the urgent need for improved infection control measures and treatment protocols (Dar et al., 2016). Clinical microbiologists play a critical role in monitoring resistance patterns and recommending the most effective antibiotics based on laboratory findings. This information forms the basis for the development of policies at local, national, and international levels aimed at controlling AMR, demonstrating that clinical microbiology is essential not only during direct patient care but also in broader public health initiatives. Furthermore, clinical microbiology significantly contributes to healthcare research and development. Advances in microbiological techniques and instrumentation continually deepen our understanding of pathogens and their interactions with human hosts. This knowledge underpins the development of novel vaccines, diagnostic tools, and therapies. For example, research into resistance mechanisms facilitates the creation of more potent treatments and the introduction of new antibiotic classes. Additionally, in resource- limited settings, efforts to expand laboratory capacity and information systems address healthcare disparities by strengthening disease surveillance and outbreak response capabilities (Dar et al., 2016). Consequently, the integration of clinical microbiology fosters immediate improvements in patient care and establishes a foundation for long- term innovation and public health progress.

Key Areas of Focus Within Clinical Microbiology

Clinical microbiology is a vital part of the wider healthcare sector, focusing on the interaction between microorganisms and human disease. It involves the detection and identification of pathogenic agents such as bacteria, viruses, fungi, and parasites. Understanding microbial pathogenesis mechanisms is essential for accurate diagnosis and appropriate treatment. The ability to distinguish between different pathogens, especially with the rise of new antibiotic resistance, is crucial for clinical decision-making. Research in clinical microbiology also supports the development of new antimicrobials and vaccines, bolstering public health efforts against infectious diseases. Addressing infectious disease challenges with emphasis on these areas enables practitioners to respond to the changing microbial threat profile (Shah, 2025). Title: The Role of Clinical Microbiology in Understanding Pathogens and Preventing Infectious Diseases. An additional vital aspect of clinical microbiology involves understanding modes of infection transmission. Infection control is only effective when healthcare providers are aware of how infectious agents are transmitted, whether directly, via air, or through vectors. Clinical microbiologists also contribute to managing infection prevention and control (IPC) in healthcare settings, which includes monitoring infection rates, patterns of antimicrobial resistance, and implementing policies to reduce transmission risks. Moreover, the growing focus on personalised medicine requires understanding host-microbe interactions to enable targeted therapies based on individual microbial flora. This integrated approach improves treatment outcomes and supports comprehensive public health strategies (Daniel et al., 2025). Education and collaboration are also essential in advancing clinical microbiology. Continuous training of healthcare professionals in microbiological principles helps promote best practice in clinical environments. This encompasses interpreting laboratory results and understanding their implications for patient management. Collaboration among clinicians, public health officials, epidemiologists, and microbiologists is vital in controlling outbreaks and strengthening community health initiatives. For example, joint efforts to improve surveillance systems facilitate earlier outbreak detection and more effective responses to infectious disease crises. Incorporating simulation-based training enhances learning retention and boosts confidence in managing complex cases. Through these multidisciplinary training programmes and collaborations, the practice of clinical microbiology can continue to develop and adapt to the demands of modern medicine (Shah, 2025).

1.1. Historical Development of Clinical Microbiology

The field of clinical microbiology has undergone significant development from its early days to its current status as a vital branch of medicine. Its history can be traced back to pre-scientific times when infectious diseases were attributed to supernatural forces or miasmatic theories. The advent of the germ theory of disease in the late 19th century marked a turning point, as scientists Louis Pasteur and Robert Koch demonstrated the link between microorganisms and specific diseases. This breakthrough transformed the understanding of pathogens and underscored the importance of strict microbiological methods in diagnosing and controlling infections. The historical context shows how advancements in microbiology worked hand in hand with public health initiatives and epidemiological investigations, ultimately shaping modern clinical practice and infection control.

By the end of the 20th century, major technological and methodological innovations had radically transformed clinical microbiology. Culturing techniques allowed for the isolation and identification of causative agents, improving diagnostic accuracy. Additionally, the introduction of antimicrobial therapies dramatically changed infection control strategies and contributed to a decline in infectious disease mortality rates. The discovery of antibiotics in the mid-20th century established them as the cornerstone of bacterial infection treatment, though their overuse has now led to the rise of antibiotic-resistant bacteria, which calls for ongoing surveillance and research. Advances such as polymerase chain reaction (PCR) and serological assays further enabled rapid, specific pathogen detection, reflecting the continuous evolution of microbiological methods and their ongoing importance to public health. The historical development of clinical microbiology provides a foundation for understanding contemporary challenges. Bioterrorism incidents, notably the 2001 anthrax letter attacks, highlighted the critical need for robust microbial surveillance and research capacities as society faced the malicious use of biological agents. Such events, alongside emerging diseases and global health threats, emphasise the importance of integrating microbiological research into public health strategies to meet future challenges. As documented in existing literature, the history of pathogens and their significance influences the formulation of effective measures to combat infectious diseases and improve clinical practice. By learning from historical progress, contemporary clinical microbiology continues to evolve and innovate, ensuring it remains at the forefront of medical science and public health (Nickel, 2005; Rose, 2006).

1.1.1. Pioneers in Microbiology and Their Contributions

The development of microbiology has been significantly influenced by pioneering scientists whose discoveries established the foundation of our understanding of pathogens and diseases. Louis Pasteur is especially prominent in this field, known for his pioneering research on the germ theory of disease, which explained infectious diseases in terms of microorganisms. His experiments refuted spontaneous generation and demonstrated that microorganisms are responsible for fermentation and decay. This work not only revolutionised microbiology but also highlighted the importance of sterilisation techniques in clinical practice.

Pasteur's findings led to advancements such as vaccines, including those he developed for anthrax and rabies. As a result, Pasteur's work links fundamental science with practical applications in disease prevention and treatment. Another major figure, Robert Koch, contributed greatly to microbiology and its clinical use. He is famous for formulating Koch's postulates, which connect specific pathogens to particular diseases. His research on tuberculosis and anthrax provided essential insights into isolating and identifying pathogens, improving diagnostic accuracy for clinicians. Koch's techniques for cultivating bacteria in pure cultures improved microbiological examinations' reliability, supporting better diagnosis and management of infectious diseases. His research laid the foundations for modern microbiological procedures and significantly shaped public health policies. By identifying disease-causing agents, Koch's work was instrumental in establishing standards for disease prevention and global clinical microbiology practice (Figure 1.2).

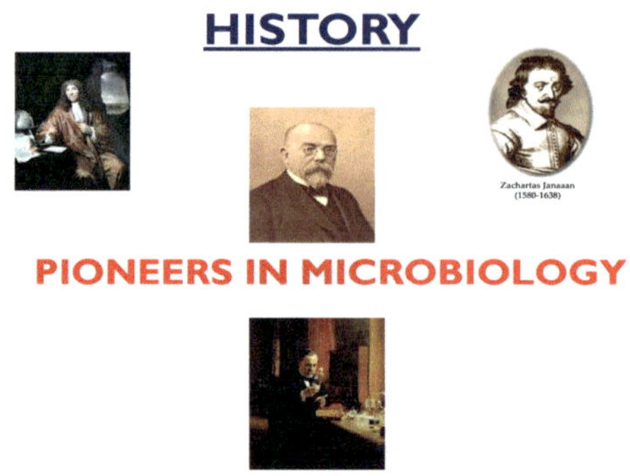

Figure 1.2. The history of pioneers in microbiology.

Source: https://external-content.duckduckgo.com/iu/?u=http%3A%2F%2Fslidetodoc.com%2Fpresentation_image_h%2F25e0cdaf2cee9c370af8d820904c0bd3%2Fimage-2.jpg&f=1&nofb=1&ipt=54d42aaa68d0bc536af1aafb2f3ddd83e1f381ae799251bb1f372337871287c7.

In contemporary settings, the work of early microbiologists continues to influence current research and clinical practices, most notably in combatting antibiotic resistance. Visionaries like Pasteur and Koch established a paradigm for microbial pathogenesis that remains fundamental as new challenges arise. For example, recent studies analyse resistance patterns of common pathogens, such as those discussed in the SWOTARE 2016 series, providing vital epidemiological data on antibiotic resistance in Wisconsin. These findings are crucial for shaping empirical treatment guidelines and enhancing antimicrobial stewardship in clinical environments. As antimicrobial resistance becomes more prominent, it is clear that the research of early microbiologists remains relevant, highlighting the need for ongoing research and adaptation in clinical microbiology to meet evolving healthcare demands.

1.1.2. Evolution of Microbiological Techniques

The progression of microbiological techniques has significantly revolutionised clinical microbiology, addressing both diagnostic and research requirements. From the inception of culture methods that established the foundation for microbial identification to the integration of molecular techniques, the discipline has experienced continuous methodological development. Traditional culture techniques, although fundamentally vital, often involved prolonged incubation periods and were labour-intensive when identifying fastidious organisms. The subsequent emergence of molecular biology methods, including polymerase chain reaction (PCR) and next-generation sequencing (NGS), has transformed the capacity for rapid and accurate diagnosis. These technologies, characterised by enhanced sensitivity and specificity, enable the detection of pathogens even at minimal levels, thereby facilitating treatment protocols and infection control measures within healthcare settings. Recently, machine learning (ML) has become an influential force in clinical microbiology, particularly in optimising laboratory procedures and data analysis. The increasing costs associated with the convergence of laboratory automation and computational science have rendered advanced analytics more accessible. As previously indicated, the application of ML has advanced toward quality assurance of laboratory results and automated diagnostics (Bruyne et al., 2020) (Figure 1.3).

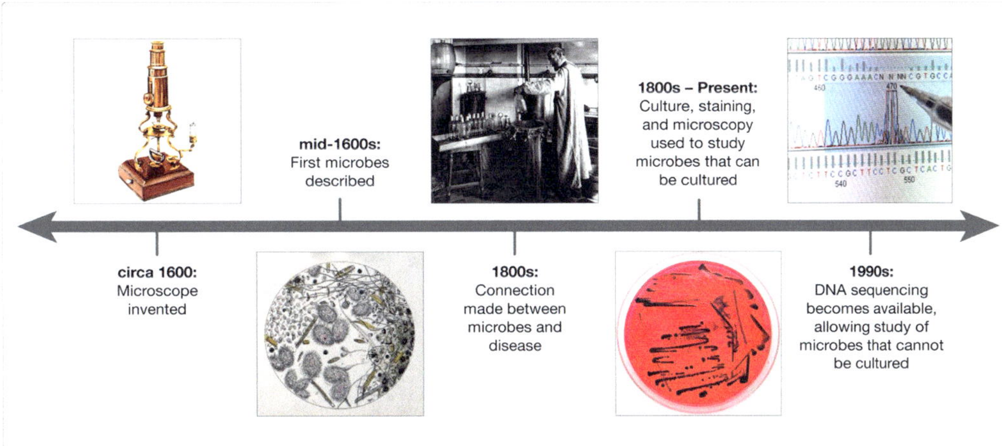

Figure 1.3. Microbiology technology timeline.

Source: https://external-content.duckduckgo.com/iu/?u=https%3A%2F%2Fi.pinimg.com%2Foriginals%2F1d%2Fc6%2F31%2F1dc6319ddd2f10a627d0530bc384109f.jpg&f=1&nofb=1&ipt=3e651c4855dec3d3089de9e1c700a6559ac3f4ae62cb3dd643393d53aeefb9e8.

A pertinent illustration within the field of microbiology involves the detection and identification of microbiologically significant pathogens, as well as the anticipation of antimicrobial resistance. The application of machine learning algorithms enables clinicians to analyse extensive datasets efficiently, thereby augmenting their capacity to interpret complex biochemical information and enhance patient outcomes. This technological progression underscores the imperative of continuously updating microbiological methodologies to maintain clinical microbiology at the vanguard of patient care. Furthermore, the growing emphasis on microbiome research has facilitated the development of innovative microbial strategies to investigate microbial communities in diverse contexts beyond the human host. The term' microbiome, ' inclusive of both microbial species and their collective genetic material, remains without a universally accepted definition but is nonetheless central to understanding health and disease dynamics (Berg et al., 2020). Recent initiatives aim to standardise research methodologies, as existing inconsistencies impede comparability. Advancements in sequencing technologies and bioinformatics have empowered researchers to explore the complexity of microbiome composition, stability, and functionality more thoroughly, thereby enhancing comprehension of microbe-host interactions. These developments not only shape the future of personalised medicine but also offer promising avenues for addressing emergent health challenges, heralding a bright future for microbial research and its clinical applications.

1.1.3. Milestones in the Understanding of Infectious Diseases

The understanding of infectious diseases has fundamentally evolved over several centuries, emphasising rigorous scientific investigation and technological advancements. The initial significant milestones date to the late 19th century with the development of the germ theory of disease, predominantly through the efforts of scientists such as Louis Pasteur and Robert Koch. This theory revolutionised microbiology by identifying specific microorganisms as the causative agents of disease, thereby shifting the paradigm from miasma- based contagion theories to a more empirical approach.

Their groundbreaking insights catalysed the development of effective treatment and prevention strategies, thereby shaping public health initiatives worldwide. This transition underscores the crucial role of scientific inquiry in conquering infectious agents and paves the way for ongoing progress in clinical microbiology and disease control. As researchers further investigated microbial pathogens, the latter half of the 20th century witnessed a notable increase in the discovery of antibiotics. Early antibiotics such as penicillin became formidable tools in combating bacterial infections, significantly reducing mortality from formerly lethal diseases. However, this promising era was subsequently overshadowed by mounting concerns regarding antibiotic resistance. As the PEW Charitable Trust Report (2016) elucidates, although initial progress was achieved, the absence of new antibacterial drug approvals since the 1980s and the emergence of resistant organisms constitute the greatest threats to global health. This paradox necessitates a heightened focus on innovative research techniques, stewardship strategies, and international collaboration- each offering promising prospects yet also presenting new challenges that demand adaptive responses within clinical microbiology. Concurrently, some infectious diseases, including human African trypanosomiasis (HAT), have experienced debilitating epidemics and unprecedented progress toward control and elimination. The consistent decline in reported cases since the early 2000s exemplifies the positive impact of global cooperation, including enhanced screening and treatment modalities. There has also been an emphasis on vector control measures to reduce transmission risks, adopting a comprehensive approach to disease management. Nonetheless, as Davis et al. (2020) note, the potential for resurgence remains a concern, emphasising the importance of sustained investment in public health infrastructure and research. Most importantly, all of these developments serve as a reminder that, despite substantial advancements in understanding infectious diseases, continued vigilance and adaptable strategies are imperative to effectively manage the complexities and uncertainties still inherent in this field.

1.2. Types of Microorganisms in Clinical Microbiology

In the field of clinical microbiology, microorganisms are predominantly classified into several major groups, including bacteria, viruses, fungi, and parasites. Each of these groups encompasses numerous species capable of inducing infections and diseases in humans. Bacteria are unicellular organisms characterised by their rapid proliferation and diverse metabolic capabilities. They may be categorised as pathogenic or non- pathogenic, contingent upon their potential to cause disease. Pathogenic bacteria, such as species of *Streptococcus* and *Staphylococcus*, are responsible for a broad spectrum of illnesses ranging from benign skin infections to severe, life- threatening conditions. The detection and identification of these bacteria are crucial, as they directly influence diagnostic and therapeutic strategies in clinical settings. Viruses differ fundamentally from bacteria in that they are acellular entities requiring a host cell for replication. They are generally classified according to their structural attributes, genetic material, and transmission routes. Notable clinically relevant viruses include the influenza virus and Human Immunodeficiency Virus (HIV), both posing significant global health challenges. The high mutation rates and rapid evolution of viruses render their study challenging, complicating vaccine development and antiviral interventions. A comprehensive understanding of viral replication and pathogenic mechanisms is essential for the advancement of preventive and therapeutic measures, thereby necessitating continuous research and surveillance. Fungi and parasites also constitute vital categories within clinical microbiology. Fungi, such as yeasts and moulds, are opportunistic pathogens that predominantly affect immunocompromised individuals; for example, *Candida* species are associated with severe infections among hospitalised patients. The threat posed by fungal infections is exacerbated by the emergence of antifungal resistance, underscoring the need for ongoing monitoring and the development of improved therapeutic options. Parasites, including protozoa and helminths, are responsible for a variety of diseases, ranging from malaria caused by *Plasmodium* species to schistosomiasis caused by trematodes of the genus *Schistosoma*. Implementing effective control measures against these infections is of paramount importance. This importance is further emphasised by research into contamination risks within healthcare environments, which demonstrates how microorganisms can transfer upon contact with patients and hospital settings (Laatsch-Lybeck et al., 1995; White et al., 2012).

1.2.1. Bacteria: Classification and Characteristics

The classification of bacteria entails a systematic methodology employed to comprehend the extensive diversity of microorganisms. Bacteria are primarily categorised according to their morphological characteristics, genetic makeup, and biochemical properties. This taxonomy is conventionally depicted through a hierarchical framework encompassing domains, phyla, classes, orders, families, genera, and species. The three principal domains—Bacteria,

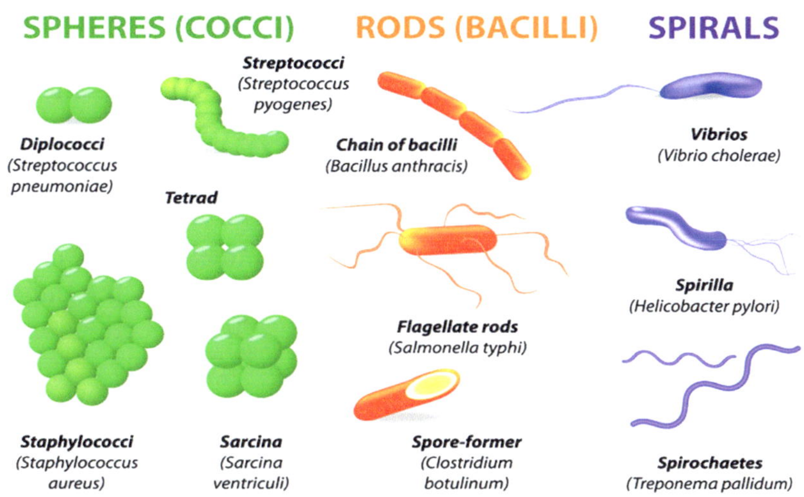

Figure 1.4. The classification of bacteria.

Source: https://external-content.duckduckgo.com/iu/?u=https%3A%2F%2Fmicrobenotes.com%2Fwp-content%2Fuploads%2F2019%2F02%2FClassification-of-Bacteria-on-the-Basis-of-Shape.jpg&f=1&nofb=1&ipt=f0a87f47798ee119bd6914ef283afc414a7046223b8d1433d6ffc10db0e51d67.

Archaea, and Eukarya—underline the evolutionary divergence of microorganisms, with particular emphasis on the fundamental differences between prokaryotic and eukaryotic cells. Consequently, the scientific investigation of bacterial taxonomy transcends mere theoretical inquiry; it constitutes the fundamental basis of microbiology, facilitating the identification and comprehension of specific bacterial roles in health and disease by researchers and healthcare professionals. In clinical microbiology, a thorough understanding of bacterial traits is vital for the diagnosis of infections and the formulation of effective treatment protocols. Attributes such as Gram staining, metabolic activity, and motility significantly impact pathogenicity and antimicrobial resistance. For instance, categorising bacteria as Gram-positive or Gram-negative, based on their cell wall architecture, is essential for determining suitable antimicrobial therapies. Gram-positive bacteria generally possess a thick peptidoglycan layer, while Gram-negative bacteria exhibit a more intricate structure featuring an outer membrane. This distinction assists clinicians in predicting the behaviour of bacterial pathogens and in implementing appropriate infection control measures, thereby underscoring the significance of bacterial classification and awareness of their characteristics in clinical practice (Figure 1.4).

Advancements in molecular biology techniques have further improved bacterial characterisation and classification. Techniques such as 16S rRNA sequencing have become invaluable tools for precisely identifying bacterial species and their functional roles in various environments, including the human microbiota. For example, high-throughput sequencing methods used in recent studies have provided crucial insights into the composition of bacterial vaginal microbiomes in pregnant women, highlighting the important role of Lactobacillus species in health and infection prevention.

This achievement demonstrates the limitations of traditional culture methods and underscores the need to incorporate more advanced techniques to address these gaps. Additionally, issues related to bacteria such as *Mycobacterium avium* subsp. Paratuberculosis emphasises the ongoing necessity for developing sensitive diagnostic tests capable of accurately detecting and characterising pathogens vital to agriculture and public health, illustrating the close connection between classification and clinical applications in microbiology (Englund, 2002; Kaakoush et al., 2016).

1.2.2. Viruses: Structure and Pathogenicity

In clinical microbiology, viruses present a unique challenge due to their distinctive structural features and replication modes. Unlike bacterial or fungal pathogens, viruses are acellular and depend on the host's cellular machinery to replicate. They consist of genetic material, either DNA or RNA, encased in a protein layer called a capsid, and, in most cases, enveloped by a lipid membrane. This envelope, derived from the host cell membrane, contains viral glycoproteins that are crucial for initial infection steps such as attachment and entry into target cells (Figure 1.5). Understanding the complexity of viral structures is vital for designing vaccines and treatments, as specific viral components serve as targets for intervention (e.g., blocking the fusion of the viral envelope with the host cell) (Dar et al., 2016).

Viral pathogenicity results from interactions with host cells and the subsequent immune response. Viral infections can cause a range of diseases, from mild respiratory illnesses to life-threatening systemic conditions, depending on the virus and the host. For instance, some viruses, including influenza, are highly mutable and can evade host immunity, making vaccination challenging. Conversely, other viruses can remain latent in host cells, leading to chronic infections that may recur and cause long-term disease. As seen during the COVID-19 pandemic, understanding viral pathogenesis is essential for informing public health strategies and developing effective therapies to reduce morbidity and mortality caused by viral infections (Huan et al., 2020).

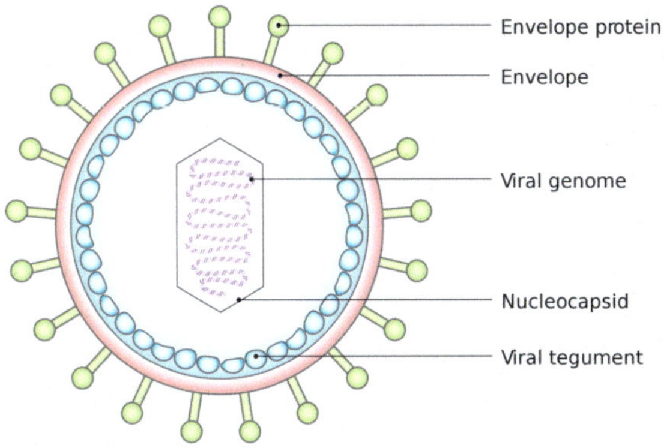

Figure 1.5. Virus structure.

Source: https://external-content.duckduckgo.com/iu/?u=https%3A%2F%2Fopen.oregonstate.education%2Fapp%2Fuploads%2Fsites%2F54%2F2019%2F08%2F2000px-Viral_Tegument.svg_-1-1024x666.png&f=1&nofb=1&ipt=84a21142131b0aec804b67e8e44450d8c805b5f74e265f65ef10636e66df149a.

Investigations into the pathogenesis of specific viral pathogens reveal the interconnected nature of viral structure and disease outcome. For instance, the presence of antiviral peptides, such as antimicrobial peptides (AMPs), offers potential in modulating viral infections by targeting viral envelopes or replication processes. These AMPs, part of the innate immune response, display broad-spectrum activity against various classes of pathogens, including viruses. Recent research has focused on how effective these peptides are against emerging viruses, indicating their new role in the treatment of drug-resistant infections (Siddiqui et al., 2020). Understanding these mechanisms not only offers therapeutic promise but also highlights the strategic focus of recent research on viral morphology and host-pathogen interactions as key aspects of clinical microbiology (Dar et al., 2016; Huan et al., 2020).

1.2.3. Fungi and Parasites: Roles in Human Disease

Parasite, fungus, and human disease interactions are a crucial area of research in clinical microbiology, shedding light on the complexities of infectious diseases. Yeasts are well known to cause a wide spectrum of infections in immunocompromised individuals. These infections range from superficial to systemic and can lead to severe morbidity and mortality. Unlike fungi, protozoa, helminths, and arthropods have evolved complex life cycles and can evade host immunity. This ability facilitates diseases such as malaria and giardiasis, which pose significant health challenges worldwide. Understanding how these fungi and parasites function is essential for developing effective diagnostic tools and drugs to combat human diseases caused by these pathogens.

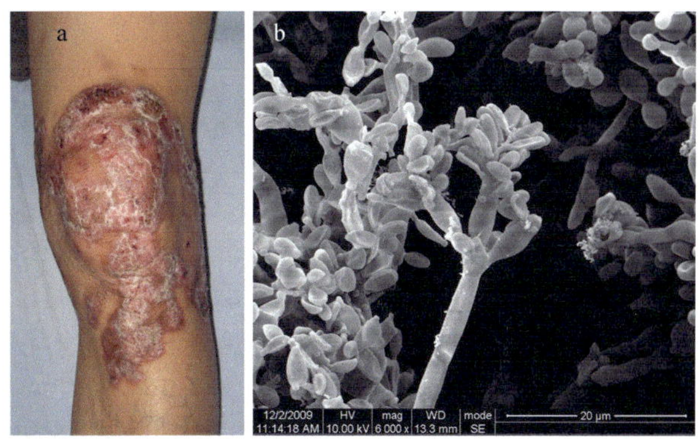

Figure 1.6. Fungal diseases.

Source: https://www.physio-pedia.com/Fungal_Diseases.

The impact of antimicrobial resistance in worsening infections caused by fungi and parasites cannot be overstated. As more antibiotic-resistant bacteria emerge, attention has been diverted away from developing drugs for antiparasitic and antifungal treatments, leading to a resurgence of fungal and parasitic diseases with increased incidence and severity. Multidrug-resistant strains of fungi, like *Candida auris*, are particularly hazardous because they can thrive in hospital environments and develop resistance to standard treatments. To make matters worse, the global spread of resistant parasites has been intensified by the overprescription and misuse of drugs in agriculture. This silent pandemic adds to the disease burden caused by fungi and parasites, impeding public health initiatives and weakening healthcare systems (Salam et al., 2023) (Figure 1.6).

Considering these challenges, research into new therapeutic solutions has become more essential than ever. Antimicrobial peptides (AMPs) are emerging as a promising tool in the fight against resistant fungal and parasitic pathogens. These peptides are naturally produced and exhibit broad-spectrum antimicrobial activity, targeting various pathogens such as bacteria, fungi, and parasites through multiple mechanisms. Their ability to bypass traditional resistance pathways makes them highly appealing for medical use. Consequently, significant research is focused on understanding their mechanisms of action, optimising variant designs, and exploring their applications in medicine and agriculture (Huan et al., 2020). By developing innovative strategies to combat these infectious organisms, clinical microbiology can address critical issues related to parasites and fungi in human disease, ultimately improving global health outcomes.

1.3. Laboratory Techniques in Clinical Microbiology

Clinical microbiology heavily depends on accurate laboratory procedures for pathogen identification and testing. Culture methods remain a fundamental aspect of microbiological diagnosis, allowing bacteria to be cultivated from patient samples. For example, species identification, such as *Brachyspira,* relies on traditional culture techniques combined with biochemical reactions, which have proven effective in recognising these pathogens. While culture methods provide valuable information about the viability and characteristics of microorganisms, they can sometimes be incomplete due to the specific requirements of certain organisms. Additionally, genetic variation among bacterial species complicates diagnosis. Therefore, a combined methodology approach is essential to improve diagnostic accuracy, with studies indicating that integrating culture and DNA-based techniques is the most effective strategy for detecting *Brachyspira* species (Råsbäck, 2007).

Molecular methods have transformed clinical microbiological diagnostics, especially through the use of polymerase chain reaction (PCR) technology. The development of real-time PCR-based assays has significantly accelerated the diagnosis of infectious diseases, providing timely information critical for patient management. Various research efforts focus on optimising automated platforms that streamline the PCR process and increase diagnostic throughput. These tools have been vital during infectious disease outbreaks, such as influenza, where swift identification can influence containment measures. Notably, while molecular techniques deliver rapid and precise data, they also demand effective control of costs and resources, as highlighted in recent reviews. Ultimately, integrating rapid diagnostic devices into routine laboratory practices can help address the growing demand for cost-effective and accurate microbiological analysis (Ince & McNally, 2009). Moreover, traditional immunoassay methods are regaining importance as supplements to modern molecular strategies. Although highly sensitive, PCR can sometimes be resource-intensive; in contrast, immunoassays offer a more economical alternative. Biosensor-immunoassays leverage the specificity and sensitivity of classical serological methods, enhancing their applicability in clinical settings. These devices enable a broader range of antigen detection and provide rapid results with minimal infrastructure requirements.

Combining these traditional methods with molecular diagnostics provides a thorough understanding of microbial infections. This integrated approach will be vital in the future of clinical microbiology, balancing effectiveness with cost, and allowing laboratories to meet diverse clinical needs (Ince & McNally, 2009).

1.3.1. Culture Methods for Isolating Pathogens

Culture methods for isolating pathogens in clinical microbiology are essential techniques used to identify and study infectious agents. These methods involve cultivating microorganisms in specially controlled laboratory conditions to improve their detection and analysis. A key technique that is widely used and highly important is the employment of selective and differential media. Selective media inhibit the growth of non-target organisms while allowing the target pathogens to grow; for example, MacConkey agar is used to isolate Gram-negative bacteria, such as *Enterobacteriaceae*. Differential media enable identification based on observable characteristics of colonies, including colour changes in lactose fermenters like *Escherichia coli*. When applied carefully, these techniques provide clinical microbiologists with valuable information about pathogen diversity and their antimicrobial susceptibility patterns. Culture techniques are extensively utilized in many clinical settings, especially for diagnosing bloodstream infections (BSIs). In a cross-sectional study conducted at a tertiary care hospital, blood cultures were used to isolate bacterial pathogens in patients suspected of having BSIs, thereby demonstrating the importance of such methods in clinical practice (Satapathy et al., 2024) (Figure 1.7).*Escherichia coli*

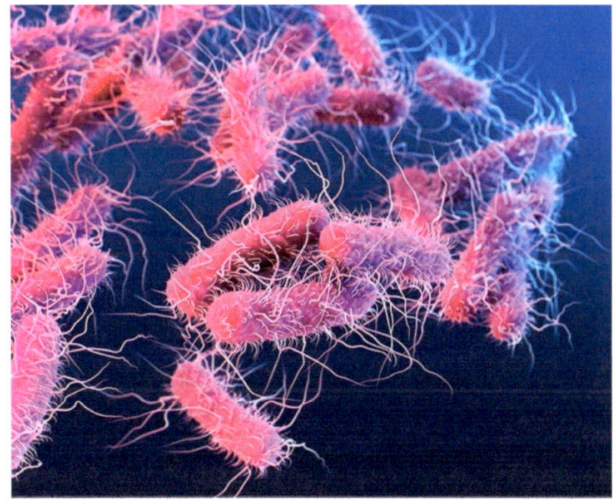

Figure 1.7. Enterobacteriaceae.

Source: https://external-content.duckduckgo.com/iu/?u=https%3A%2F%2Ftecscience.tec.mx%2Fen%2Fwp-content%2Fuploads%2Fsites%2F9%2F2024%2F03%2Fantimicrobial-resistance.jpg&f=1&nofb=1&ipt=f1c7c9d0a9aafdaccdd3fc721059a21632171db4231f46f4e88352d3285444ca.

Blood cultures are analysed using BACTEC systems and then cultured on MacConkey agar and blood agar. By carefully observing colonial morphology, along with Gram staining and biochemical screening, clinicians can effectively identify pathogens. The method identified *Klebsiella pneumoniae* as the most common pathogen, highlighting how essential sound cultural techniques are for obtaining reliable results. These findings improve diagnostic accuracy and guide future clinical practice, especially in modifying antimicrobial therapy. Additionally, culturing technology continues to develop through enhancements in microbial detection systems. Techniques like the agar well diffusion method, used in studies with plant extracts for antimicrobial assessment, demonstrate the value of integrating new methods into standard procedures. For instance, screening *Jatropha tanjorensis* leaf extracts against clinical pathogens showed good culture practices, revealing large zones of inhibition against resistant antibiotic strains (Komolafe et al., 2024). This exemplifies the dual benefit of culture techniques: to isolate pathogens and test their sensitivity to novel antimicrobial compounds. As interdisciplinary research between microbiologists and other fields grows, optimisation of culture methods becomes crucial to tackling public health issues such as antibiotic resistance and advancing clinical microbiology.

1.3.2. Molecular Techniques: PCR and Sequencing

In clinical microbiology, molecular techniques such as Polymerase Chain Reaction (PCR) and sequencing have revolutionised the detection and identification of pathogens. PCR amplifies target DNA sequences, enabling rapid and sensitive identification of microbial pathogens present in clinical samples. This method is especially important where standard culture techniques fall short due to the fastidious nature of certain organisms or their inadequate growth in laboratory conditions. PCR also facilitates the detection of low-abundance pathogens, which can be crucial for disease control and may have significant health implications, such as preterm delivery caused by microbial infection in pregnant women. The role of high-throughput sequencing complements PCR by providing vast amounts of genetic data, revealing the diversity of microbial communities and identifying taxa beyond the scope of the traditional culture approach (Kaakoush et al., 2016) (Figure 1.8).

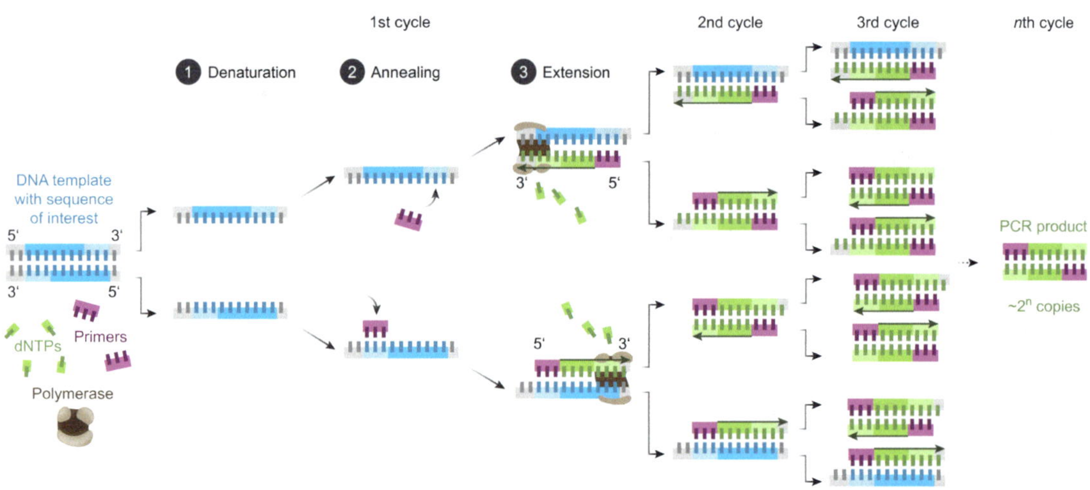

Figure 1.8. Polymerase chain reaction (PCR).

Source: By Enzoklop - Own work, CC BY-SA 4.0, https://commons.wikimedia.org/w/index.php?curid=96042657

The use of sequencing technologies has greatly expanded our understanding of microbial diversity and its potential implications for human health. With methods such as 16S rRNA sequencing and metagenomics, it is possible to describe the microbiome in detail, identifying both common and rare species within a microbial community. This capability has significant clinical implications, particularly in treating conditions where traditional diagnostics are inadequate. For example, the composition of vaginal microbiome during pregnancy significantly influences maternal and neonatal health, as research indicates that dysbiosis is associated with adverse outcomes like preterm birth. Molecular methods enable clinicians and scientists to better monitor and manage these microbial communities, allowing for targeted interventions to reduce risk during pregnancy (Kaakoush et al., 2016). Increasingly, molecular tools are essential for developing diagnostic strategies against pathogens that threaten livestock health, such as *Brachyspira* species, which are linked to serious gastrointestinal infections in pigs. The reliance on PCR and sequencing provides precise identification and epidemiological monitoring of these pathogens, facilitating early intervention and treatment in animal populations. Research has shown that conventional culture and biochemical testing alone lack sufficient diagnostic specificity; therefore, combining molecular diagnosis with traditional methods greatly enhances disease management. For example, a new strain, *B. suanatina*, was identified using a combination of culture, biochemical testing, and molecular analysis, illustrating the importance of integrating different diagnostic measures. Ultimately, merging traditional approaches with modern molecular techniques creates a robust foundation for comprehensive diagnostic systems, improving animal productivity and health.

1.3.3. Antimicrobial Susceptibility Testing

Antimicrobial susceptibility testing (AST) is a crucial procedure in clinical microbiology that determines the effectiveness of specific antimicrobial agents against causative microorganisms. By assessing bacterial susceptibility to antibiotics, clinicians can make more accurate treatment decisions. This process is vital in tackling the growing issue of antimicrobial resistance (AMR), now recognised as a global public health threat. Evidence indicates that AMR significantly contributes to morbidity and mortality, with around 4.95 million bacterial AMR-related deaths reported worldwide in recent years (Dar et al., 2016). Understanding susceptibility and resistance patterns allows clinicians to personalise treatment regimens, ultimately enhancing patient outcomes and preventing treatment failure. The methods used in antimicrobial susceptibility testing are diverse, ranging from phenotypic tests such as disk diffusion and broth dilution techniques to more advanced molecular methods. For instance, in the disk diffusion method, antibiotic-impregnated disks are placed on an agar plate inoculated with the test organism, and the zone of inhibition around each disk is measured to determine susceptibility (Figure 1.9).

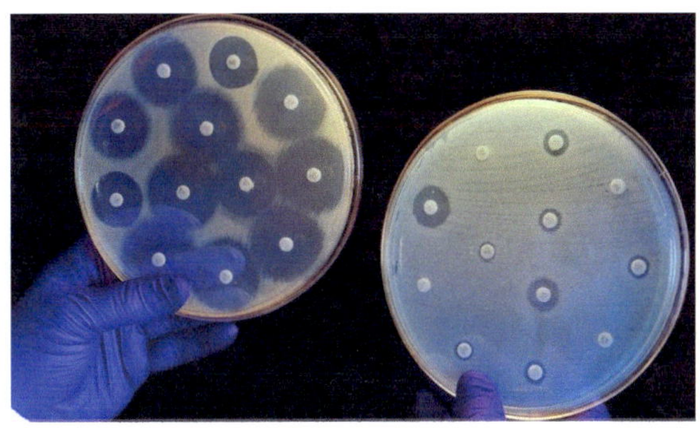

Figure 1.9. Antimicrobial susceptibility testing.

Source: https://blog.biomall.in/wp-content/uploads/2019/08/0619_bacteria_antibiotico_1280a-e1565765010256.jpg.

Conversely, molecular techniques can yield faster results and more detailed resistance profiles. These advancements are critical, especially given the need for rapid and accurate diagnosis of infections caused by multidrug-resistant organisms like *Pseudomonas aeruginosa* and *Acinetobacter baumannii*, which are highly resistant and prevalent in hospitals (Mekonnen et al., 2021). Such pathogens play a major role in nosocomial infections, underscoring the importance of reliable AST protocols in clinical settings.

Additionally, the significance of AST results is vital in guiding appropriate treatment decisions. The emergence of resistant strains highlights the need for continuous surveillance and research aimed at monitoring resistance patterns and developing new antimicrobial agents. Notably, the burden of AMR is most severe in low-resource settings, where access to effective antibiotics may be limited. Addressing these challenges requires collaborative efforts, including enhanced laboratory facilities and better data systems to support evidence-based interventions (Dar et al., 2016). In this way, antimicrobial susceptibility testing functions not only as a diagnostic tool but also as a key component of antimicrobial stewardship, which seeks to preserve the effectiveness of existing antibiotics and promote the development of new drugs.

1.4. Role of Clinical Microbiologists

The role of clinical microbiologists is central to identifying and combating infectious diseases, making them key players in today's healthcare networks. Clinical microbiologists are responsible for the identification, characterisation, and analysis of microbial pathogens that cause disease in humans. Using advanced microbiological techniques, such as culture methods and molecular diagnostics, clinical microbiologists can efficiently diagnose infections, which is critical for successful treatment. Rapid identification of pathogens not only enables personalised patient care but also supports epidemiological investigations of disease outbreaks. Additionally, advancements in genomic technologies have enabled the sequencing of microbial genomes, providing valuable insights into resistance and virulence factors, both of which are crucial for developing effective therapeutic strategies and enhancing public health management. Beyond diagnosis, clinical microbiologists play an essential role in infection control within healthcare settings. They collaborate with healthcare staff to develop procedures that minimise the risk of nosocomial infections, thereby safeguarding both patients and staff.

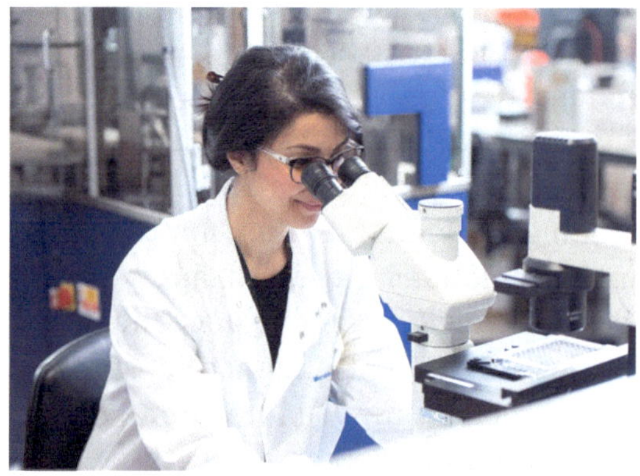

Figure 1.10. Role of clinical microbiologists.

Source: https://www.rcpath.org/static/7b939abe-e076-453a-9c11fa57c48fa291/1113x742_highestperformance__4a7c7e45a350/Sarah170523The-Royal-London-Hospital-0005-1.jpg.

By monitoring infection rates and advising on antibiotic stewardship programmes, they ensure antimicrobials are used responsibly — a vital aspect in addressing the rising challenge of antibiotic resistance. Moreover, by training healthcare professionals in laboratory procedures and safe practices, they help improve standards of care and foster a culture of safety within clinical environments. This comprehensive practice highlights the crucial role of clinical microbiologists in infection prevention and control, which is essential for public health. Their educational and research activities also strengthen their role, keeping clinical microbiologists at the forefront of microbiological innovation. Events like the Young Microbiologists Symposium encourage interaction and exchange of innovative ideas among emerging researchers (Caly et al., 2012) (Figure 1.10).

Through their reporting of results, clinical microbiologists educate the wider scientific community, guiding future research as well as diagnostic and therapeutic progress. Emphasis on continuous professional development ensures that clinical microbiologists stay familiar with evolving methods and new pathogens, improving their ability to respond to changing health concerns. Ultimately, their dedication to research and learning not only boosts individual competence but also enhances healthcare quality, reflecting the vital role of clinical microbiologists in the fight against infectious diseases in today's world.

1.4.1. Responsibilities in Diagnostic Laboratories

In diagnostic laboratories, healthcare providers play a diverse and crucial role in safeguarding patient safety and ensuring the accuracy of laboratory test results. These laboratories operate within the scope of clinical microbiology, engaging in activities such as collecting, processing, and analysing biological specimens. Laboratory technicians must strictly adhere to quality control practices and regulatory requirements, especially when implementing the European Union Regulation (EU) 2017/746, which introduces specific demands for *in vitro* diagnostic medical devices. This regulation requires robust evidence of analytical performance, including accuracy and reliability, thereby fostering a culture of compliance and continuous improvement (Shuroug et al., 2023). Fulfilling these responsibilities not only enhances the quality of care but also supports the overall performance of diagnostic services provided to healthcare systems. Equally important is the ongoing education and training of laboratory staff and stakeholders to foster a comprehensive understanding of emerging technologies and diagnostic strategies. The adoption of advanced diagnostic technologies, such as artificial intelligence, holds significant potential for enhancing diagnostic accuracy, but it also raises important ethical and technical challenges (Shuroug et al., 2023). Laboratories must navigate these challenges to successfully integrate such innovations, necessitating professionals to be well-versed in both the technical aspects and relevant regulatory frameworks.

Furthermore, working with educational institutions and other healthcare providers is vital for the ongoing progress of laboratory medicine, especially in personalised medicine. Such interactions combine expertise, thereby enhancing diagnostic capabilities in line with the evolving needs of patient care. Furthermore, diagnostic laboratories must be equipped to meet the diverse needs of their patient populations, especially during public health crises. Since diagnostic facilities play a vital role in monitoring diseases and outbreaks, they must be capable of responding swiftly and effectively to emerging pathogens. Outbreak preparedness involves not only rapid diagnostic testing but also aligning practices with global guidelines to minimise risks (Dombrink et al., 2022). In this context, laboratories serve as a bridge between clinical microbiology and public health, providing vital data to guide treatment and public health interventions. Therefore, a clear understanding of the roles within diagnostic laboratories is essential, not only for improving patient outcomes but also for strengthening the overall health system's response to infectious diseases (Figure 1.11).

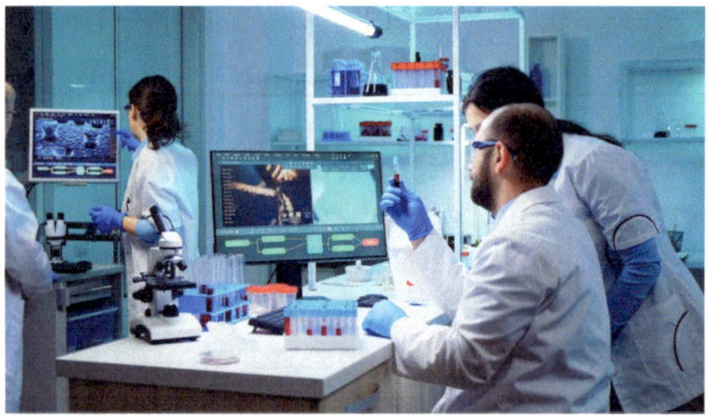

Figure 1.11. The responsibilities of healthcare professionals.

Source: https://external-content.duckduckgo.com/iu/?u=https%3A%2F%2Fjadashbiomedical.com%2Fwp-content%2Fuploads%2F2022%2F10%2Fmicrobiologist-doctor-taking-blood-sample-tube-from-rack-with-machines-analysis-lab-background-1024x576.jpg&f=1&nofb=1&ipt=3755c20141939c718f2c70eb87f35234db98f789d327e0cdef147d7516e31c22.

1.4.2. Collaboration with Healthcare Teams

Effective teamwork with health teams is essential in preventing and controlling clinical site infections. In clinical microbiology, collaboration among healthcare professionals, including doctors, pharmacists, and infection preventionists, plays a crucial role in managing multidrug-resistant microorganisms (MDROs) and ensuring the proper use of antimicrobial agents. The intricate details of infection prevention and antimicrobial stewardship (AS) require cohesive effort, as emphasised in the literature highlighting how these fields are interconnected. Strategic partnerships among various healthcare teams not only optimise the efficiency of infection prevention programmes but also support the primary goal of patient safety by reducing infection-related risks. Collaboration is therefore not only advantageous; it is a fundamental element necessary for the success of many healthcare initiatives in protecting patient health (Ashley et al., 2018) (Figure 1.12).

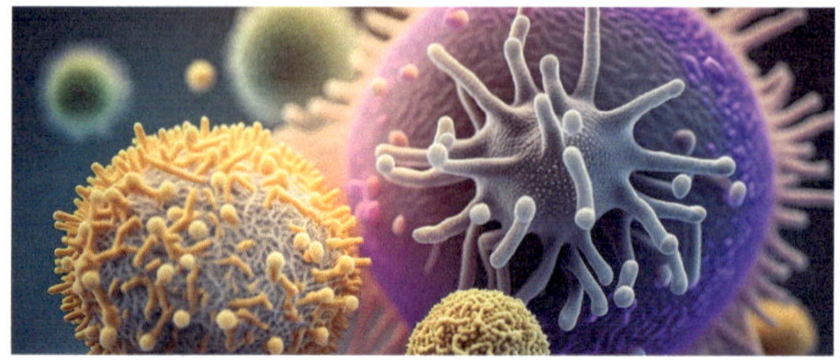

Figure 1.12. Multi-drug-resistant organisms (MDROs).

Source: https://external-content.duckduckgo.com/iu/?u=https%3A%2F%2Fwww.wchc.nhs.uk%2Fwp-content%2Fuploads%2F2023%2F03%2FMDROs.jpg&f=1&nofb=1&ipt=a8010ed48b0ee9c7ffa43840af9b9c49a06510d9095d54b3abb0c29cf4ebffb4.

Furthermore, interprofessional education programmes represent a significant step towards improved healthcare outcomes. For example, when an antimicrobial stewardship curriculum is introduced and highlights the importance of collaboration between pharmacy and medical students through joint learning experiences, it reflects the value of interprofessional practice. This curriculum features interactive, branched-logic clinical case presentations that require students to engage with each other, thereby defining the roles and responsibilities of each profession within the context of antimicrobial use. Results from such programmes demonstrate a notable increase in students' understanding of collaborative approaches after completing these learning modules. By enabling effective communication and teamwork across disciplines, these students are better prepared to address the complex demands of infection control and antimicrobial resistance in their professional lives (Chin-Hong et al., 2017). Ultimately, the benefits of effective healthcare team collaboration extend to their overall healthcare delivery. A coordinated approach among healthcare workers creates a conducive environment for the exchange of vital information, leading to improved clinical decision-making. The ongoing development of team-based strategies ensures the efficient transfer of skills across specialities, all aimed at supporting collective goals of infection control and prevention. The importance of this collaborative framework cannot be overstated, as it not only supports current infection management but also prepares for future healthcare challenges. The synergy fostered by such collaboration offers a remarkable leap forward in clinical microbiology, bringing together efforts to resolve complex health issues and ensuring that safety standards for effective antibiotic treatment are maintained for future generations (Ashley et al., 2018).

1.4.3. Contributions to Public Health and Epidemiology

The epidemiological and public health roles of clinical microbiology are crucial, with understanding antimicrobial resistance (AMR) being especially vital because it poses a significant threat to global health. In 2019, AMR was estimated to be responsible for around 4.95 million deaths worldwide, including 1.27 million directly caused by resistant infections. This sharp increase in mortality highlights the necessity for strong microbiological science and clinical practice to monitor and limit the spread of resistant bacteria. Surprisingly, pathogens such as *Escherichia coli* and *Staphylococcus aureus* are associated with high rates of illness and death, underscoring the importance of the public health sector to prioritise surveillance and control efforts. Effective public health strategies depend on extensive microbiological data, emphasising the importance of integrating clinical microbiology with epidemiology to combat rising resistance and improve wellbeing across various groups (Dar et al., 2016). Additionally, countries like Denmark provide valuable examples of understanding the interaction between clinical microbiology and epidemiology. Denmark's national healthcare database collects high-quality information on public health, enabling epidemiological research by linking healthcare delivery with data collection. This allows detailed analysis of infectious disease trends within the population and helps identify patterns of microbial infections. Conducting longitudinal research using these data sources enhances our comprehension of the public health impact of microbial pathogens and guides effective intervention strategies. The affordability and practicality of matching individual-level data underscore the epidemiological need for precise disease monitoring and highlight the essential role of clinical microbiology in shaping effective public health policies (Schmidt et al., 2019). Overall, integrating public health and clinical microbiology not only deepens our understanding of infectious diseases but also provides epidemiologists with essential tools to address global health challenges. By assessing the burden of disease caused by resistant pathogens and employing robust data systems, public health officials can implement precise prevention and control measures. Information from microbiological investigations is vital for policy development that enhances the effectiveness of public health interventions, ultimately leading to a healthier population. As antimicrobial resistance continues to emerge, the importance of clinical microbiology in epidemiological research grows increasingly, reinforcing the need for ongoing collaboration between microbiologists and public health officials to protect human health (Dar et al., 2016; Schmidt et al., 2019).*Escherichia coliStaphylococcus aureus*

1.5. Infectious Diseases and Their Management

Infectious diseases represent a broad field of interest within clinical microbiology, characterised by the complexity of etiological agents and the challenges they pose in management. Antimicrobial resistance (AMR) ranks among the most significant threats to infection control globally and increasingly strains healthcare systems. Recent research estimates that approximately 4. 95 million deaths in 2019 were attributable to bacterial AMR, underscoring the urgent need for a paradigm shift towards the implementation of comprehensive strategies to address this critical issue. The principal pathogens responsible for AMR- related mortality are those causing commonplace infections, such as *Escherichia coli* and *Staphylococcus aureus*. These findings emphasise the importance of surveillance and early detection of resistant strains, as well as the necessity of planning targeted prevention and control measures to mitigate the burden of infectious diseases without further jeopardising public health (Dar et al., 2016).

The management of infectious diseases requires a multifaceted approach that encompasses antimicrobial therapy, infection control interventions, and the development of novel treatments. Notably, bacteriophage therapy has demonstrated efficacy, especially in treating complex infections such as diabetic foot ulcers. Unlike traditional antibiotics, which frequently eradicate the patient's microbiota and result in additional complications and extended recovery periods, bacteriophage therapy can specifically target pathogenic organisms without harming beneficial microbiota, thereby preserving overall intestinal health. Clinical trials suggest that this approach may be as effective, or even more so, than conventional antibiotics in particular cases, rendering it a promising alternative for clinical application and prompting further research into innovative therapeutic strategies (MacKenzie et al., 2007). Healthcare professionals and researchers must actively foster interdisciplinary collaboration to effectively combat the threat of infectious diseases and AMR. This entails cooperation among public health officials, infectious disease clinicians, epidemiologists, and microbiologists to enhance data collection and laboratory infrastructure, particularly in resource-limited settings. A comprehensive understanding of disease burden and causative pathogens is essential for informing evidence-based policies and interventions. Considering the constant evolution of infectious diseases, ongoing education and research remain imperative. By establishing an improved system for infectious disease control, the medical community will be better positioned to confront current challenges and anticipate future threats, ultimately improving patient outcomes and global health (Dar et al., 2016; Jean- François et al., 2020).*Escherichia coliStaphylococcus aureus*

1.5.1. Common Bacterial Infections and Treatments

*Escherichia coliStaphylococcus aureusEscherichia coli*Bacterial infections continue to pose a significant public health challenge, impacting multiple diseases and bodily systems. Among the most common bacterial infections are those caused by *Escherichia coli* and *Staphylococcus aureus*, resulting in urinary tract infections (UTIS) and skin infections, respectively. The genetic diversity of these bacteria, coupled with their ability to develop resistance to frequently used antibiotics, complicates treatment strategies.

For example, ESBL-producing *E. coli* UTIS are becoming increasingly prevalent, prompting clinicians to explore alternative therapeutic options beyond conventional antibiotics. Understanding bacterial virulence factors and resistance mechanisms is imperative for the development of effective treatment protocols, thereby improving patient outcomes and curbing the spread of resistant strains within the community. In addition to traditional antibiotics, innovative approaches are under investigation to combat bacterial infections, especially those involving resistance. Notably, a study assessing the anti-biofilm activity of Manuka honey against ESBL (extended-spectrum beta-lactamase)-producing bacteria such as *Escherichia coli* and *Klebsiella pneumoniae* is of particular interest. Biofilms are instrumental in chronic infections by shielding bacteria from immune responses and antibiotics, thus making infections more challenging to eradicate (Figure 1.13). The findings of this research indicate that Manuka honey may serve as a valuable adjunct to standard treatment regimens, decreasing biofilm biomass and potentially improving infection resolution. This investigation into novel therapeutic agents is especially pertinent in response to the urgent necessity for alternative strategies to address the escalating prevalence of antibiotic-resistant bacteria, which presents a significant threat to contemporary medicine.

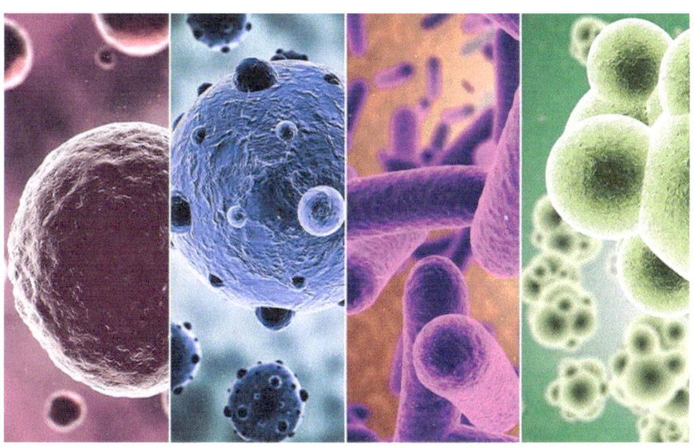

Figure 1.13. Bacterial infections.

Source: https://www.uhhospitals.org/-/media/images/blog/2022/12/cell-collage-464462144-blog-mainarticleimage.jpg?h=450&w=720&la=en&hash=F9147D3E9FDB202A54F81AE99B29C188.

Understanding the dynamics of changing bacterial pathogens and their relationship with human health is of great importance, as this knowledge will guide clinical practices. *Helicobacter pylori* serves as a prime example of this dynamic, given its role in causing peptic ulcers and gastric cancer, while also maintaining a complex interaction with its human host. The bacterium can oscillate along a spectrum from mutualism to pathogenicity, influenced by host, environmental, and genetic factors, necessitating a similarly sophisticated approach to treatment. As scientific research continues to unveil the cellular mechanisms underlying bacterial activity and host interactions, future therapeutic strategies must incorporate these insights into their design. Addressing the challenges posed by common bacterial infections will require a concerted effort in both clinical practice and public health initiatives, promoting a proactive rather than reactive approach to controlling bacterial diseases.

1.5.2. Viral Infections: Prevention and Control

Effective prevention and control of viral infections are crucial for safeguarding public health. One of the primary strategies employed is immunisation through vaccination, which elicits protective immunity against specific viral pathogens. For example, the administration of live attenuated or inactivated vaccines has demonstrated a considerable impact in reducing morbidity and mortality associated with viral diseases. Data from veterinary research indicate that vaccination against infectious bovine rhinotracheitis, viral diarrhoea, parainfluenza 3, and respiratory syncytial infection can decrease the incidence of these viral diseases to approximately 15%, thereby significantly reducing the occurrence of outbreaks. The combined application of vaccination and surveillance measures can effectively diminish the dissemination and severity of viral infections in both human and animal populations, emphasising the vital importance of prophylactic interventions in the management of viral diseases (Kornieikov et al., 2019) (Figure 1.14).

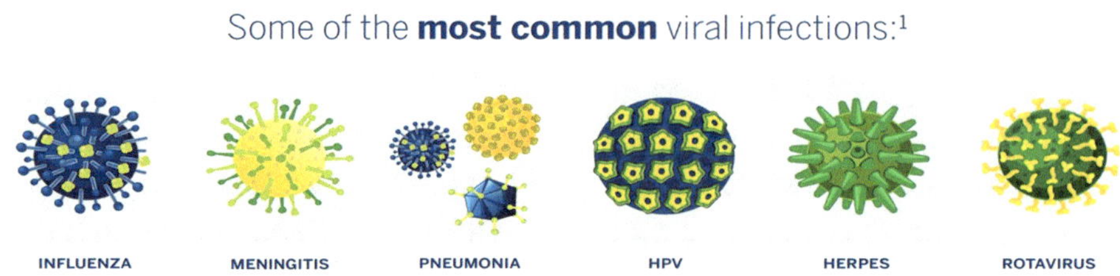

Figure 1.14. The most common viral infections.

Source: https://s7g10.scene7.com/is/image/biomerieux/Viral%20sepsis%20-%20Image%2002?qlt=85&wid=480&ts=1646918695659&dpr=on,2.625.

In addition to vaccination, public health education plays an essential role in the prevention of viral infections. Public education focusing on modes of transmission, signs and symptoms, and the importance of cleanliness can empower individuals to undertake preventive measures against infections. Initiatives such as hand hygiene, respiratory etiquette, and awareness campaigns regarding vaccination can induce significant behavioural changes and reduce the incidence of viral diseases. Specifically, concerning the human immunodeficiency virus (HIV), targeted educational interventions among high-risk populations have demonstrated effectiveness in controlling outbreaks. The transmission of HIV subtypes, notably subtype F1, among specific demographic groups in Belgium, underscores the necessity for tailored educational approaches to prevent transmission (Vinken et al., 2019). Consequently, comprehensive public health strategies are vital components of the broader framework for the prevention of viral infections.

Lastly, the implementation of comprehensive surveillance systems is instrumental not only in supporting preventive strategies but also in facilitating prompt responses to viral outbreaks. By monitoring infection trends and identifying new viral strains, health authorities are equipped to intervene promptly and allocate resources effectively. The data collected can further inform vaccine development and treatment protocols, thereby enhancing the efficacy of preventative and therapeutic measures. In the context of the Belgian HIV-1 epidemic, it was observed that improvements in surveillance have enabled a better understanding of transmission dynamics, which in turn has contributed to controlling the spread of infection. This adaptable public health approach—comprising vaccination, education, and surveillance—demonstrates a multifaceted strategy for the prevention and management of viral infections, and upholds clinical microbiology as a central component of public health initiatives (Vinken et al., 2019).

1.5.3. Emerging Infectious Diseases and Challenges

The incidence of infectious diseases presents a critical challenge to public health systems globally, necessitating a sophisticated comprehension of clinical microbiology. As globalisation heightens human interaction and facilitates the facile movement of people, animals, and goods across regions, microorganisms can disseminate more rapidly than ever before. Factors such as urbanization, global warming, and habitat encroachment further exacerbate this issue by disturbing ecosystems and fostering closer contact between humans and zoonotic reservoirs. Additionally, the development of antimicrobial resistance renders simple infections resistant to treatment swiftly, which is anticipated to lead to increased morbidity and mortality. Timely monitoring and responsive public health interventions are essential to mitigate the consequences of these novel diseases and to establish a comprehensive system that reflects the multifaceted transmission pathways of pathogens among various industries and geographical locations (Dar et al., 2015). Undoubtedly, one of the most significant challenges in managing emerging infectious diseases lies in the rapid identification and characterisation of novel pathogens. Advances in genomic technologies, such as Next-Generation Sequencing (NGS), have transformed pathogen discovery by enabling microbiologists to detect novel viral agents cost-effectively within clinical laboratories. This innovation plays a pivotal role in outbreak preparedness and response, as early detection facilitates rapid epidemiological assessments and the deployment of pertinent public health countermeasures. Furthermore, the incorporation of molecular approaches can augment screening capabilities for potential infectious agents in vaccines and other biological products. Despite these technological progressions, notable challenges persist, including data management and the bioinformatics analysis necessary for interpreting large datasets generated by these approaches.

hese scientific challenges must be addressed by clinicians to accurately identify evolving pathogens and develop relevant treatment protocols. An interdisciplinary approach is essential in managing the issues posed by emerging infectious diseases. Embracing the One Health philosophy, which recognises the interconnectedness of human, animal, and environmental health, is crucial in formulating effective public health policies. Such an approach promotes intersectoral coordination, enabling comprehensive policy review and targeted interventions that are tailored to local contexts and specific needs. Ensuring the proper use of antimicrobials, establishing robust surveillance mechanisms, and implementing effective infection control and prevention measures are vital in reducing the incidence and transmission of infectious diseases. It is imperative to prioritise these strategies in low- and middle-income countries, where the burden of infectious diseases is typically highest. A concerted global effort, grounded in sound evidence and policy-focused research, is necessary to sustain global health security and enhance preparedness and response capabilities for future outbreaks (Dar et al., 2015).

1.6. Antimicrobial Resistance

The global AMR phenomenon presents a significant public health challenge that warrants urgent attention within the domain of clinical microbiology. As pathogens evolve and develop mechanisms to evade the effects of widely used drugs such as antibiotics, treatment protocols become increasingly ineffective. This issue is of particular concern, as it complicates the management of common infections and contributes to elevated morbidity and mortality rates among affected populations. The resistance observed in pathogens such as multidrug-resistant *Escherichia coli* and *Klebsiella pneumoniae* highlights the necessity for clinicians to adopt increasingly sophisticated strategies for diagnosis and treatment, thereby underscoring the link between clinical practice and microbial resistance. Research reveals a concerning trend of antibiotic resistance across various regions worldwide, with especially notable increases in low- to middle-income countries. Recent studies indicate that hospitals in Tanzania and Zambia report a rising prevalence of methicillin-resistant *Staphylococcus aureus* (MRSA) and extended-spectrum beta-lactamase (ESBL) producers. These findings emphasise the need for enhanced clinical microbiology services capable of providing systematic surveillance and data collection to inform national health guidelines.

Furthermore, the literature review demonstrates a clear association between rising AMR rates and suboptimal antibiotic stewardship. This underscores underlying challenges faced by healthcare systems, including the necessity for updated guidelines to combat resistance and improve patient outcomes (Mshana et al., 2013). The complex nature of AMR necessitates a One Health approach, recognising the interconnectedness of animal health, human health, and the environment. The application of antibiotics in veterinary medicine, whether therapeutically or as feed additives, exacerbates the resistance issue. Clinical microbiology experience indicates that resistance patterns can transcend species and impact both human and animal health sectors. Effective strategies for controlling AMR must include robust surveillance systems, adherence to best practices in antibiotic usage, and intersectoral collaboration involving healthcare professionals, veterinarians, and policymakers. The integration of these sectors offers substantial potential to advance the management and mitigation of antimicrobial resistance (Barnard, 2019) (Figure 1.15).*Escherichia coliStaphylococcus aureus*Barnard, 2019

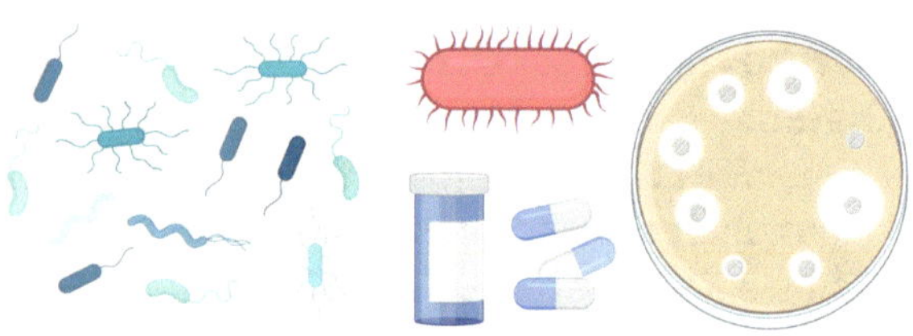

Figure 1.15. Antimicrobial resistance (AMR).

Source: https://microbenotes.com/wp-content/uploads/2022/10/Antimicrobial-resistance-AMR-and-Antibacterial-Resistance-ABR.jpg.

1.6.1. Causes and Implications of Resistance

The phenomenon of antimicrobial resistance represents one of the most significant challenges in clinical microbiology, attributable to various factors associated with human behaviour, agriculture, and healthcare systems. Misuse and excess prescription of antibiotics in both humans and animals are primary contributors. As indicated in a previous review of literature from certain African nations, there has been a concerning rise in multidrug-resistant pathogens such as *Escherichia coli* and *Klebsiella pneumoniae*, which are frequently involved in nosocomial infections. This increase in resistance complicates treatment protocols, extends hospital stays, escalates medical expenses, and exerts additional pressure on public health resources. The involvement of veterinary clinics in antibiotic usage introduces further complexity to this issue, necessitating a One Health approach that integrates human, animal, and environmental health to address the shared threat of antimicrobial resistance collectively (Mshana et al., 2013). On a broader scale, beyond patient-level therapy, antimicrobial resistance impacts public health initiatives and clinical outcomes. As resistance intensifies, the efficacy of standard treatments diminishes, leading to higher morbidity and mortality rates from infections once deemed manageable. For example, the rising prevalence of methicillin-resistant *Staphylococcus aureus* (MRSA) underscores the need for enhanced clinical microbiology services, particularly in resource-limited settings. Improved microbiological diagnostics can facilitate more effective surveillance, thereby informing local treatment guidelines and shaping national policies to mitigate antimicrobial resistance. Consequently, recommendations emphasise the crucial necessity of improving practices in antibiotic prescription and production, alongside implementing systemic responses to emerging resistance patterns (Mshana et al., 2013). Furthermore, research into alternative antimicrobial therapies and biocidal agents presents promising avenues for reducing resistance issues. Emerging evidence on ozone's capacity to inactivate foodborne pathogens underscores the importance of innovative microbiological methodologies. Studies on pathogens such as *Campylobacter jejuni* and *Salmonella enteritidis* highlight the significance of a multidisciplinary strategy for effectively combating bacterial resistance. Combining novel treatment approaches with traditional antibiotics can strengthen clinical microbiology's capacity to confront this challenge. Additionally, such research can contribute to the development of enhanced food safety protocols, ultimately reducing the transmission of resistant pathogens. Translating these scientific advances into clinical practice may serve as a foundational element in the ongoing efforts to combat the widespread issue of antimicrobial resistance, reinforcing the importance of continued research and development in this critical field.*Escherichia coliStaphylococcus aureus*

1.6.2. Strategies to Combat Antimicrobial Resistance

The increasing prevalence of antimicrobial resistance (AMR) presents a significant public health challenge that necessitates the rigorous implementation of appropriate control strategies. Central to managing AMR is the judicious use of antibiotics. Limiting unnecessary prescriptions, especially in outpatient settings, is crucial to minimise bacterial adaptation and resistance development. Education for both patients and healthcare professionals can significantly influence prescribing behaviours, promoting more responsible use of antibiotics. Adherence to established guidelines regarding the duration and selection of therapy ensures the effectiveness of antibiotics while preventing resistance. Through stewardship interventions that oversee and regulate antibiotic prescribing, healthcare institutions can foster an environment of awareness regarding AMR, thereby reducing the rates of acquired resistance within clinical settings (Pachisia et al., 2025). Complemented by stewardship initiatives, the exploration of novel therapeutic approaches remains essential to diminish AMR. This includes the development of new adjuvant compounds and antibiotic classes capable of augmenting the activity of existing drugs. The investigation of combination therapies — that is, utilising multiple antibiotics or agents with synergistic effects — has become a focal point of research aimed at counteracting bacterial defence mechanisms, such as those exhibited by *Klebsiella pneumoniae*. For example, recent regimens such as Ceftriaxone/Sulbactam/EDTA-based therapy have demonstrated efficacy against carbapenem-resistant organisms, owing to their capacity to target multiple bacterial survival pathways (Reddy et al., 2024).

Furthermore, the screening and validation of innovative treatment modalities, such as bacteriophage therapy and antimicrobial peptides, present promising avenues for research. Successful implementation of these modalities could revolutionise the management of resistant infections. Additionally, infection prevention and control are critical components in the fight against AMR. Healthcare hygiene practices, including proper hand hygiene and the use of personal protective equipment, substantially reduce infection rates and consequently diminish the need for antibiotics. Surveillance systems for antibiotic-resistant infections enable healthcare facilities to respond proactively by monitoring emerging resistance trends, thereby informing treatment protocols and policy development. Patient education regarding infection prevention strategies – such as vaccination and wound care – also plays a vital role in reducing infection susceptibility and dependence on antimicrobials. By adopting a comprehensive approach that encompasses prudent antibiotic prescribing, innovative therapy research, and stringent infection control measures, healthcare professionals can make significant advances in combating the pervasive threat of antimicrobial resistance, ultimately preserving the efficacy of current antibiotics and safeguarding public health.

1.6.3. Role of Clinical Microbiology in Monitoring Resistance

The role of clinical microbiology as a sentinel for antimicrobial resistance is increasingly recognised as vital to patient safety and public health. As pathogens develop resistance to the most commonly used drugs, clinical microbiology laboratories are at the forefront of detecting resistant strains and guiding therapy. Among various activities, surveillance of antimicrobial resistance provides clinicians with the data needed to select suitable empiric treatments for infections. By continuously gathering and reporting resistance pattern information, laboratories not only aid clinicians in making informed decisions but also support wider epidemiological surveillance efforts. Furthermore, early detection of resistance through screening of blood cultures allows healthcare facilities to respond promptly, reducing the impact of resistant infections on patient outcomes (MacKenzie et al., 2007). This ongoing feedback loop ultimately sustains antibiotic stewardship and helps to maintain the efficacy of available antimicrobial agents. Beyond susceptibility testing, clinical microbiology also directly contributes to antibiotic stewardship programmes within healthcare settings. The activities of clinical microbiologists often extend beyond individual patient care to include organisational policies aimed at limiting unnecessary antibiotic use. Using current data on resistance trends, microbiology laboratories enable hospitals to manage their antibiotic prescribing effectively. Research indicates that hospitals participating in formal stewardship and continuous monitoring experience lower antibiotic consumption, thereby preventing the emergence of resistant strains (Dar et al., 2015). This synergy exemplifies how clinical microbiology can support local and global strategies to contain antibiotic resistance, emphasising the need for cautious antimicrobial use and the preservation of existing therapeutics. Lastly, the role of clinical microbiology in tracking resistance forms part of a One Health approach, integrating human, animal, and environmental health sectors. Tackling AMR necessitates coordinated action across these interconnected disciplines, with clinical microbiologists providing essential surveillance data to inform policy-making. By uniting public health officials, veterinarians, and environmental scientists, the information generated by clinical laboratories can be contextualised within a broader understanding of how resistance emerges and spreads across different ecosystems. Such an integrated strategy responds to global calls for increased AMR action, highlighting the importance of research and policy development tailored to local contexts and specific sector needs (Dar et al., 2015). Clinical microbiology is progressively playing a key role in the worldwide fight against antimicrobial resistance through these collective efforts.

SUMMARY

Clinical microbiology increasingly plays a central role in managing modern public health emergencies, such as biological incidents and disease outbreaks. The rapid dissemination of pathogens necessitates proactive measures, exemplified by training programmes designed to equip medical personnel with the skills needed for effective response procedures. Institutional training programmes like those at De Montfort University have demonstrated the importance of combining theory with practical experience in competency development to support public health interventions. These learning methods not only enhance individual preparedness but also foster collaboration in tackling biological threats, thereby reducing potential public health risks and creating safer communities (Pena et al., 2019).

Furthermore, advances in pathogen genomics, especially with next-generation sequencing (NGS), hold significant promise for improving public health responses. Utilising bacterial pathogen genomics enhances outbreak detection, tracing origins, and conducting preventative surveillance of antimicrobial resistance. The ability of NGS to provide high-resolution transmission route inference is vital for implementing more effective control and prevention measures. However, routine application of whole-genome sequencing faces inherent challenges such as data integration and quality assurance. Overcoming these obstacles through interdisciplinary collaborations among epidemiologists, clinicians, and bioinformaticians is essential to establishing successful genomic surveillance systems (Boon et al., 2019).

Lastly, clinical microbiology remains a crucial science-public health interface that requires ongoing research, education, and strategic planning. Developing effective training programmes that blend theoretical knowledge with practical application improves the preparedness of health professionals against biological hazards. As the infectious disease landscape continues to evolve, integrating new technologies and fostering collaboration will be key to guiding prevention and control strategies. Strengthening the links between clinical microbiology and public health infrastructure will ultimately lead to more resilient health systems capable of withstanding infectious disease impacts and safeguarding population health worldwide.

An intrinsic understanding of clinical microbiology involves respecting established practices while embracing innovative approaches that have the potential to enhance patient outcomes. The primary considerations are derived from the analysis of n-of-1 trials, which are crucial for optimising the evaluation of health technologies on an individualised basis. These trials encompass administering treatments in a randomised sequence to a single patient over specified periods, thereby facilitating personalised treatment strategies. The National Institute for Health Research's DIAMOND project highlighted the importance of stakeholder input in this domain, exemplifying collaborative efforts in the development of successful n-of-1 trials. This initiative resulted in the formulation of twenty key points serving as a reference for clinicians and researchers, emphasising concerns such as the number of treatment cycles and the selection of appropriate comparators (Chatters et al., 2024). This methodology exemplifies the potential for advancing understanding and fostering innovation within clinical practice.

Furthermore, ongoing breakthroughs in therapies, particularly for challenging conditions such as migraine, exemplify the evolving landscape of clinical microbiology. Recent advancements have underscored the significance of alternative treatments, especially considering that nearly fifty percent of patients may not respond effectively to standard therapies targeting calcitonin gene-related peptide (CGRP). Emerging therapeutic targets include novel drug classes such as zavegepant and primarily lasmiditan, designed to address various facets of migraine's complex pathophysiology. Clinical trial data indicate that research efforts should focus on identifying new targets, emphasising the synergy between clinical and preclinical studies as essential methods for developing efficacious treatments (Wells-Gatnik et al., 2023). This reflects a broader movement within clinical microbiology, whereby continuous knowledge generation and application are vital for advancing patient care. Lastly, the integration of personalised approaches in clinical microbiology challenges traditional paradigms of treatment design. By prioritising patient-centric models in trials such as n-of-1, clinicians and researchers can tailor interventions to meet individual patient needs. This significant shift is accompanied by an increasing recognition of disease heterogeneity and the vital role of personalised medicine in effective disease management.

Additionally, investigations into novel treatments for disorders such as migraine demonstrate the potential for targeting specific biological pathways to enhance therapeutic efficacy. Overall, these developments underscore the growing importance of refined clinical trials and the necessity for responsive and adaptive healthcare policies within clinical microbiology (Chatters et al., 2024; Wells-Gatnik et al., 2023). This synthesis of knowledge paves the way for widespread improvements in treatment approaches across various medical domains and disciplines.

CLOSER LOOK

THE DEVELOPMENT AND PROGRESSION OF CLINICAL MICROBIOLOGY

Clinical microbiology has traveled a far distance from its early days in the 19th century when pioneers like Louis Pasteur and Robert Koch founded it by establishing the relationship between infectious disease and microorganisms. Their discoveries, such as the germ theory of disease and Koch's postulates, revolutionized medical science and highlighted the need for microbiological diagnoses within the clinical environment (Figure 1.16).

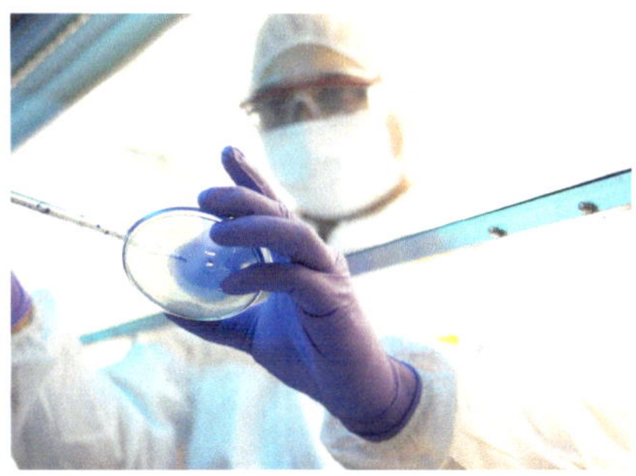

Figure 1.16. A clinical microbiologist conducts laboratory work in a sterile environment, using a petri dish and pipette to analyse microbial samples.

Source: https://career-advice.jobs.ac.uk/wp-content/uploads/Clinical-Microbiology-teaching-fellow-jobs.jpg.optimal.jpg.

Early in the 20th century, clinical microbiology developed as a subspecialty of laboratory medicine. The advent of culture techniques, staining processes (e.g., Gram staining), and biochemical tests allowed bacteria and fungi responsible for infections to be identified. The development of antibiotics like penicillin during the 1940s further emphasized the role of the microbiologist in recommending appropriate antimicrobial treatment through susceptibility testing. The second half of the 20th century also witnessed the addition of serology and immunology to clinical microbiology, which enabled the detection of parasitic and viral infections. Advanced technology saw the development of automated microbial sensitivity and identification tests, offering quicker and more reliable clinical diagnosis. In the last decades, molecular biology has transformed clinical microbiology. Techniques such as PCR (polymerase chain reaction), nucleic acid amplification, and genome sequencing allow for rapid and precise diagnosis of pathogens, even those difficult to grow. These methods also facilitate outbreak tracking, identification of antimicrobial resistance, and epidemiological monitoring. Clinical microbiology plays a key role in the present in patient management, infection prevention, and public health. It supports evidence-based treatment, prevents transmission of healthcare-associated infections, and responds to new infectious threats such as COVID-19 and antimicrobial-resistant bacteria. It evolves in an ongoing fashion through diagnostic development, bioinformatics, and precision medicine and is currently an essential science in modern healthcare.

REFERENCES

1. Dar, O. A., Hasan, R., Schlundt, J., Harbarth, S., Caleo, G., Dar, F. K., Littmann, J., Rweyemamu, M., Buckley, E. J., Shahid, M., Kock, R., Li, H. L., Giha, H., Khan, M., So, A. D., Bindayna, K. M., Kessel, A., Pedersen, H. B., Permanand, G., Zumla, A., ... Heymann, D. L. (2016). Exploring the evidence base for national and regional policy interventions to combat resistance. *Lancet (London, England)*, *387*(10015), 285–295. https://doi.org/10.1016/S0140-6736(15)00520-6(accessed on 16th July 2025).
2. Alowais, S. A., Alghamdi, S. S., Alsuhebany, N., Alqahtani, T., Alshaya, A., Almohareb, S. N., Aldairem, A., et al. (2023). Revolutionizing healthcare: The role of artificial intelligence in clinical practice. BMC Medical Education, 23. https://doi.org/10.1186/s12909-023-04698-z (accessed on 16th July 2025).
3. Goudie, A. C., Olateju, F., Anderson, J. G., Rowan, N., & MacGregor, S. J. (2003). Inactivation of pathogens on food and contact surfaces using ozone as a biocidal agent. Poster session presented at Society for General Microbiology – 152nd Meeting – –, University of Edinburgh. (accessed on 16th July 2025).
4. Ashley, E. S. D., Cosgrove, S. E., Fakih, M. G., Manning, M., et al. (2018). *Antimicrobial stewardship and infection prevention—Leveraging the synergy: A position paper update.* https://core.ac.uk/download/155271805.pdf (accessed on 16th July 2025).
5. Baho, S., Czapnik, P., & Samarasinghe, S. (2019). *Preliminary analysis of the anti-biofilm efficacy of manuka honey on extended spectrum β-lactamase producing* Escherichia coli *TEM-3 and* Klebsiella pneumoniae *SHV18, associated with urinary tract infections.* https://core.ac.uk/download/228189014.pdf (accessed on 16th July 2025).
6. Barnard, N. (2019). *Prevalence of Gram-negative infections in cervico-facial sepsis.* https://core.ac.uk/download/289120735.pdf (accessed on 16th July 2025).
7. Caly, D. L., Coulthurst, S. J., Geoghegan, J. A., Malone, J. G., & Ryan, R. P. (2012). Socializing, networking and development: a report from the second 'Young Microbiologists Symposium on Microbe Signalling, Organization and Pathogenesis'. *Molecular microbiology*, *86*(3), 501–512. https://doi.org/10.1111/mmi.12016(accessed on 16th July 2025).
8. Berg, G., Rybakova, D., Fischer, D., Cernava, T., Champomier Vergès, M. C., Charles, T. C., Chen, X., et al. (2020). Microbiome definition re-visited: Old concepts and new challenges. Microbiome, 8. https://doi.org/10.1186/s40168-020-00875-0 (accessed on 16th July 2025).
9. Boon, N. A. M., Descamps, T., Devleesschauwer, B., Robert, A., et al. (2019). *Status and potential of bacterial genomics for public health practice: A scoping review.* https://core.ac.uk/download/227041617.pdf (accessed on 16th July 2025).
10. MacKenzie, F. M., Gould, I. M., Bruce, J., Mollison, J., Monnet, D. L., Krcmery, V., Cookson, B., & van der Meer, J. W. (2007). The role of microbiology and pharmacy departments in the stewardship of antibiotic prescribing in European hospitals. *The Journal of hospital infection*, *65 Suppl 2*, 73–81. https://doi.org/10.1016/S0195-6701(07)60019-X(accessed on 16th July 2025).
11. Chatters, R., Hawksworth, O., Julious, S., & Cook, A. (2024). The development of a set of key points to aid clinicians and researchers in designing and conducting n-of-1 trials. Trials, 25. https://www.semanticscholar.org/paper/92d637c0cbc381ffbd47fe08e12d39663b872932 (accessed on 16th July 2025).

12. Chin-Hong, P. V., Kim, L., MacDougall, C., Nanamori, M., et al. (2017). *An interprofessional curriculum on antimicrobial stewardship improves knowledge and attitudes toward appropriate antimicrobial use and collaboration.* https://core.ac.uk/download/323074459.pdf (accessed on 16th July 2025).

13. PEW Charitable Trust Report (2016). *A scientific roadmap for antibiotic discovery: A sustained and robust pipeline of new antibacterial drugs and therapies is critical to preserve public health.* https://core.ac.uk/download/75785719.pdf (accessed on 16th July 2025).

14. Daniel, A., Nagandla, K., & Daniel, S. (2025). Application of Gagné's instructional design in clinical simulation: Enhancing learning in obstetric emergency management. Cureus, 17. https://www.semanticscholar.org/paper/425f2b0302283741a4c321b78572b1b880e3c905 (accessed on 16th July 2025).

15. Davis, C., Keeling, M. J., & Rock, K. S. (2020). Human African trypanosomiasis: Current status and eradication efforts. https://core.ac.uk/download/288396366.pdf (accessed on 16th July 2025).

16. De Bruyne, S., Speeckaert, M. M., Van Biesen, W., & Delanghe, J. R. (2020). Recent evolutions of machine learning applications in clinical laboratory medicine. Critical Reviews in Clinical Laboratory Sciences, 58, 131–152. https://doi.org/10.1080/10408363.2020.1828811 (accessed on 16th July 2025).

17. Dombrink, I., Lubbers, B. R., Simulescu, L., Doeswijk, R., Tkachenko, O. Y., Dequeker, E., Fraser, A. G., et al. (2022). Critical implications of IVDR for innovation in diagnostics: Input from the BioMed Alliance Diagnostics Task Force. HemaSphere, 6, e724–e724. https://doi.org/10.1097/hs9.0000000000000724 (accessed on 16th July 2025).

18. Englund, S. (2002). *Molecular biology techniques as a tool for detection and characterization of Mycobacterium avium subsp. paratuberculosis.* https://core.ac.uk/download/11694594.pdf (accessed on 16th July 2025).

19. Gallagher, J. E., K.C., S., Johnson, I., Al-Yaseen, W., Jones, R., McGregor, S., Robertson, M., et al. (2020). A systematic review of contamination (aerosol, splatter and droplet generation) associated with oral surgery and its relevance to COVID-19. BDJ Open, 6. https://doi.org/10.1038/s41405-020-00053-2 (accessed on 16th July 2025).

20. Gillen, A. L., Oliver, D., & Sherwin, F. (2010). *Robert Koch, creation, and the specificity of germs.* https://core.ac.uk/download/225131973.pdf (accessed on 16th July 2025).

21. Huan, Y., Kong, Q., Mou, H., & Yi, H. (2020). Antimicrobial peptides: Classification, design, application and research progress in multiple fields. *Frontiers in Microbiology, 11.* https://doi.org/10.3389/fmicb.2020.582779 (accessed on 16th July 2025).

22. Hueppchen, E., Munson, E., & Zeman, H. (2017). *Surveillance of Wisconsin organisms for trends in antimicrobial resistance and epidemiology (SWOTARE): Epidemiologic correlates for 2016 surveillance isolates.* https://core.ac.uk/download/213087724.pdf (accessed on 16th July 2025).

23. White S, Topping A, Humphreys P, Rout S, Williamson H. The cross-contamination potential of mobile telephones. *Journal of Research in Nursing*. 2012;17(6):582-595. doi:10.1177/1744987112458670

24. Huon, J. F., Montassier, E., Leroy, A. G., Grégoire, M., Vibet, M. A., Caillon, J., Boutoille, D., et

al. (2020). Phages versus antibiotics to treat infected diabetic wounds in a mouse model: A microbiological and microbiotic evaluation. mSystems, 5. https://doi.org/10.1128/msystems.00542-20 (accessed on 16th July 2025).

25. Ince, J., & McNally, A. (2009). *Development of rapid, automated diagnostics for infectious disease: Advances and challenges.* https://core.ac.uk/download/30633630.pdf (accessed on 16th July 2025).

26. Johnson, A. E. W., Bulgarelli, L., Shen, L., Gayles, A., Shammout, A., Horng, S., Pollard, T., et al. (2023). MIMIC-IV, a freely accessible electronic health record dataset. Scientific Data, 10. https://doi.org/10.1038/s41597-022-01899-x (accessed on 16th July 2025).

27. Kaakoush, N., Mendz, G., & Quinlivan, J. (2016). *New techniques to characterize the vaginal microbiome in pregnancy*. https://core.ac.uk/download/84111222.pdf (accessed on 16th July 2025).

28. Laatsch-Lybeck, Linda Jean; Ong, Poh Chye; and Kloth, Luther C., "In vitro Effects of Two Silver Electrodes on Select Wound Pathogens" (1995). Physical Therapy Faculty Research and Publications. 111. https://epublications.marquette.edu/phys_therapy_fac/111 (accessed on 16th July 2025).

29. Komolafe, C. J., Adetoyinbo, I. I., Alao, F., & Ogunsola, J. F. (2024). Phytochemical analyses and antibacterial activities of *Jatropha tanjorensis* J. L. Ellis and Saroja leaves extract against clinical pathogens. *Asian Journal of Applied Chemistry Research.* https://www.semanticscholar.org/paper/b4a46b60b7de0f47d20022576e3013c2a2b5d54b (accessed on 16th July 2025).

30. Kornieikov, O., Prokhoriatova, O. V., Kolchik, O. V., Oleshko, A., Borodai, N. I., & Al Jabari, M. (2019). The efficiency of different approaches to the prevention and control of bovine pneumoenteritis. *Veterinary Medicine: Inter-departmental Subject Scientific Collection.* https://www.semanticscholar.org/paper/e0d7509803da91a7e118eab0fa76909a5fb4d24d (accessed on 16th July 2025).

31. Koskella, B., & Lin, D. (2014). *Friend and foe: Factors influencing the movement of the bacterium* Helicobacter pylori *along the parasitism-mutualism continuum.* https://core.ac.uk/download/323080778.pdf (accessed on 16th July 2025).

32. Maimaiti, Z., Li, Z., Xu, C., Chen, J., & Chai, W. (2023). Global trends and hotspots of phage therapy for bacterial infection: A bibliometric visualized analysis from 2001 to 2021. Frontiers in Microbiology, 13. https://doi.org/10.3389/fmicb.2022.1067803 (accessed on 16th July 2025).

33. Mshana, S. E., Matee, M., & Rweyemamu, M. (2013). Antimicrobial resistance in human and animal pathogens in Zambia, Democratic Republic of Congo, Mozambique and Tanzania: an urgent need of a sustainable surveillance system. *Annals of clinical microbiology and antimicrobials, 12*, 28. https://doi.org/10.1186/1476-0711-12-28(accessed on 16th July 2025).

34. Mekonnen, H. S., Seid, A., Fenta, G. M., & Gebrecherkos, T. (2021). Antimicrobial resistance profiles and associated factors of Acinetobacter and Pseudomonas aeruginosa nosocomial infection among patients admitted at Dessie Comprehensive Specialized Hospital, North-East Ethiopia: A cross-sectional study. PLoS ONE, 16, e0257272–e0257272. https://doi.org/10.1371/journal.pone.0257272 (accessed on 16th July 2025).

35. Murray, C. J. L., Ikuta, K. S., Sharara, F., Swetschinski, L. R., Robles Aguilar, G., Gray, A. P., Han, C., et al. (2022). Global burden of bacterial antimicrobial resistance in 2019: A systematic analysis.

The Lancet, 399, 629–655. https://doi.org/10.1016/s0140-6736(21)02724-0 (accessed on 16th July 2025).

36. N/A. (1974). *Barnes Hospital Bulletin.* https://core.ac.uk/download/70380984.pdf (accessed on 16th July 2025).

37. Nickel, J. (2005). Management of urinary tract infections: Historical perspective and current strategies: Part 2—Modern management. *The Journal of Urology, 173*(1), 27–32. https://www.semanticscholar.org/paper/5debc56010bc5285f33a1ddb34f23e062a6ec774 (accessed on 16th July 2025).

38. Pachisia, A. V., Govil, D., Pal, D., Gupta, A., Todi, S., Singh, Y. P., Jain, S., et al. (2025). A retrospective, multi-center study to evaluate the effectiveness of different antibiotics/combinations being used in patients with bloodstream infection caused by CRE (Klebsiella pneumoniae, Escherichia coli), CRAB & CRPA (Outcome Study). Indian Journal of Critical Care Medicine: Peer-reviewed, Official Publication of Indian Society of Critical Care Medicine, 29, S159–S160. https://www.semanticscholar.org/paper/f7287fb8eb36fa65f4681ab22296ec97ac0f52d2 (accessed on 16th July 2025).

39. Peña, M. A., & Peña-Fernández, A. (2019). *Implementation of environmental recovery training response to biological incidents in a human health degree.* https://core.ac.uk/download/228192477.pdf (accessed on 16th July 2025).

40. Råsbäck, T. (2007). *Laboratory diagnostics of Brachyspira species.* https://core.ac.uk/download/11695182.pdf (accessed on 16th July 2025).

41. Reddy, S. P., Singh, C. D., Kumar, S., & Muthusamy, R. (2024). Prevalence and antibiotic resistance of Klebsiella pneumoniae in diabetic foot ulcer. Cureus, 16. https://www.semanticscholar.org/paper/901c0892e9a996685fbcbf9257a3c8d7388fb9bd (accessed on 16th July 2025).

42. Rose, J. (2006). Small scares. *Nature Biotechnology, 24*, 507. https://www.semanticscholar.org/paper/84607ec97376e59a4449d3d760185fd2011f09e8 (accessed on 16th July 2025).

43. Salam, M. A., Al-Amin, M. Y., Tabassoom Salam, M., Pawar, J. S., Akhter, N., Rabaan, A. A., & Alqumber, M. A. A. (2023). Antimicrobial resistance: A growing serious threat for global public health. Healthcare, 11, 1946–1946. https://doi.org/10.3390/healthcare11131946 (accessed on 16th July 2025).d

44. Satapathy, S., Mandavi, D., Panda, D. K., & Samal, D. (2024). Isolation and identification of bacterial pathogens from blood cultures in a tertiary care hospital and their clinical correlation. *South Eastern European Journal of Public Health.* https://www.semanticscholar.org/paper/83e5bd180872cf1dcc6098875b2e37d8a5aba024 (accessed on 16th July 2025).

45. Schmidt, M., Schmidt, S. A. J., Adelborg, K., Sundbøll, J., Laugesen, K., Ehrenstein, V., & Sørensen, H. T. (2019). The Danish health care system and epidemiological research: From health care contacts to database records. *Clinical Epidemiology, 11*, 563–591. https://doi.org/10.2147/clep.s179083 (accessed on 16th July 2025).

46. Shah, S. (2025). Epidemiological and clinical profiles of infectious endophthalmitis: A comparative study of traumatic and non-traumatic aetiologies in a tertiary eye care center in rural tribal areas of Western India. Journal of Ophthalmology and Advance Research. https://www.semanticscholar.org/paper/863c73870d795d830f5566d8786530b52e5224f6 (accessed on 16th July 2025).

47. Vinken, L., Fransen, K., Cuypers, L., Alexiev, I., Balotta, C., Debaisieux, L., Seguin-Devaux, C., et al. (2019). Earlier initiation of antiretroviral treatment coincides with an initial control of the HIV-1 sub-subtype F1 outbreak among men-having-sex-with-men in Flanders, Belgium. Frontiers in Microbiology, 10. https://www.semanticscholar.org/paper/873d564e16def85ca878659446b2ae664441d3fa (accessed on 16th July 2025).

48. Wells-Gatnik, W., Wences Chirino, T. Y., Onan, F. N., Onan, D., & Martelletti, P. (2023). Emerging experimental drugs in clinical trials for migraine: Observations and key talking points. *Expert Opinion on Investigational Drugs, 32*, 761–771. https://www.semanticscholar.org/paper/0013cb82cef816418fa5eeec5160d6f9431338b1 (accessed on 16th July 2025).

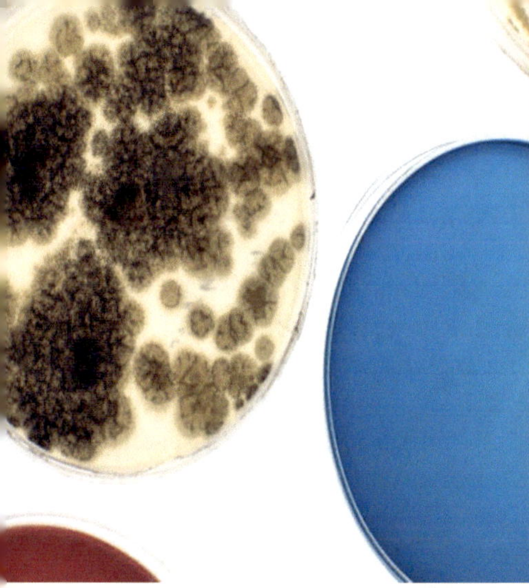

Chapter 2

MICROBIAL TAXONOMY AND CLASSIFICATION

Contents

Introduction

Taxonomy and classification of microbial life have become increasingly important in understanding biodiversity and ecosystem interactions. Microorganisms, despite their small size, represent a vast and diverse range of species that play vital roles in most biogeochemical cycles. The complex interactions between prokaryotes and their environment require robust classification systems to reveal their evolutionary histories. Traditional taxonomic methods based on phenotypic traits often fail to capture the full extent of microbial diversity, leading to misclassifications and gaps in knowledge. Therefore, a more advanced approach to microbial taxonomy has become necessary — one that utilizes molecular tools to provide a clearer and more complete picture of these organisms' complexities. The integration of molecular methods, such as DNA sequencing and genomics, has revolutionised the field of microbial taxonomy. These techniques enable detailed analysis of genetic material, allowing identification of prokaryotes based on genetic similarity and evolutionary lineage. The old models of taxonomy, reliant on visible characteristics, are being replaced by genome-oriented frameworks that offer greater precision in delineating species and higher taxonomic ranks. The development of these molecular techniques underscores the need to update taxonomic guidelines, fostering ongoing scientific progress and enhancing the consistency and accuracy of microbial classification. Alongside this, establishing standardised protocols for genomic data usage is essential to guide researchers and ensure compatibility across studies. As microbial taxonomy advances, the incorporation of new standards and methodologies remains a priority to keep pace with technological progress. The rapid growth of genomic data demands a flexible approach to classification methodologies, addressing recent technological advances effectively. This dynamic context necessitates a re-evaluation of existing recommendations to include modern methods and tackle practical challenges faced by practitioners, such as data accessibility and interpretative frameworks. By establishing minimal standards and recommendations that incorporate these developments, scientists can improve the precision and relevance of microbial classifications. As noted in the literature, the future of this field not only aims to refine taxonomic systems but also seeks to bridge the gap between scientific discovery and practical applications in microbial ecology and other areas (Belhadi et al., 2025; Raúl et al., 2024).

Definition of Microbial Taxonomy

Microbial taxonomy pertains to the systematic identification, classification, and nomenclature of microorganisms, including bacteria, archaea, fungi, algae, and viruses. Its significance lies in facilitating an understanding of microbial diversity and evolutionary relationships.

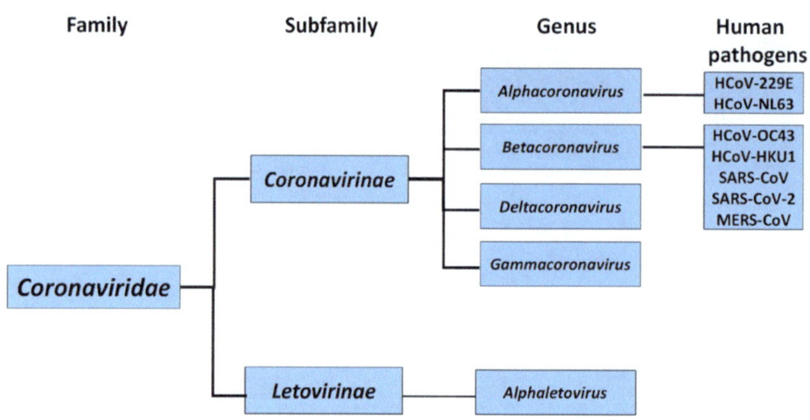

Figure 2.1. Microbial taxonomy.

Source: https://cms-media.bartleby.com/wp-content/uploads/sites/2/2021/06/17151018/Microbial-Taxonomy-1.jpg.

This discipline integrates morphological characteristics, genetic data, and ecological roles to accurately categorise these organisms. As microbial ecology increasingly gains importance across various disciplines, from environmental science to medicine, the necessity for precise taxonomic classification has become paramount. The integration of traditional methods, such as morphology assessment, with advanced molecular techniques, including phylogenetic analysis, serves to refine classification and delineate species boundaries with greater accuracy. Through rigorous classification, researchers are better equipped to comprehend microbial biodiversity and ecological impacts within their respective ecosystems. Current challenges in microbial taxonomy are exemplified by the rise of genomic technologies that provide deeper insights into microbial evolution. The utilisation of molecular methods, including whole-genome sequencing, enables precise identification of microbial lineages and the designation of taxonomic units based on genetic relatedness. Nonetheless, consensus on a standardised genome-based definition of genera remains elusive, with ongoing debates regarding the appropriate criteria for classification. This lack of uniformity may lead to over-splitting at the genus level, complicating scientific communication and potentially destabilising microbial nomenclature. Addressing these issues necessitates the development of a standardised methodological framework, as recent research suggests, which rigorously examines prokaryotic genera using objective criteria. Such an approach is essential to enhance the accuracy and stability of microbial classification and taxonomy (Val-Calvo et al., 2023) (Figure 2.1. 1).

Furthermore, microbial taxonomy has practical implications beyond research; it is essential for applied purposes such as environmental monitoring and public health. For instance, an accurate definition of species enhances the detection of pathogenic microorganisms and facilitates the monitoring of the transmission of antibiotic-resistant microorganisms. Understanding the taxonomy of harmful algal blooms, as demonstrated in *Prorocentrum* species studies, underscores the importance of precise delineation at both the species and interspecies levels within complex ecosystems (Zheng et al., 2024). Increased taxonomic confidence advances ecological management activities, bioinformatics applications, and conservation practices, thereby fostering more effective responses to microbial threats. In conclusion, microbial taxonomy provides a fundamental framework not only for the systematic study of microorganisms but also for the development of effective methods regarding their ecological functions, health implications, and environmental impacts.

Importance of Classification in Microbiology

Microorganism classification constitutes a fundamental activity within microbiology, facilitating the comprehension of microbial diversity and ecological relationships. By systematically categorising microorganisms, researchers are enabled to identify and distinguish between species based on shared characteristics such as genetic, morphological, and biochemical features. Systematic classification not only assists in predicting microbial behaviour but also enhances understanding of their roles within ecosystems and their interactions with other organisms. For instance, differentiating pathogenic from non-pathogenic bacteria is crucial in clinical diagnosis and treatment planning, thereby underscoring the immediate utilitarian importance of microbial taxonomy within health sciences. Ultimately, classification provides a foundation for ongoing advancements in microbiological research and education, fostering the integration of various scientific disciplines to realise the full potential of microorganisms. Cutting-edge methodologies embedded in microbial classification are increasingly vital for improving the accuracy and reliability of taxonomic identification. Among these, metabarcoding employs high-throughput sequencing techniques to analyse the genetic material of environmental samples. Although effective, metabarcoding often encounters variability due to differences in bioinformatics tools and reference databases across laboratories. For example, variability stemming from the choice of variable regions within the 16S rRNA gene can pose challenges to comparative analyses (Babis et al., 2024). The use of robust algorithms and validated protocols can mitigate these issues, yielding more consistent results and a deeper understanding of microbial ecology. Consequently, developing advanced classification methods is essential to address the taxonomic challenges faced in contemporary microbiology research. The integration of artificial intelligence and machine learning into microbial classification holds transformative potential for future research and breakthroughs. Through the analysis of big data, it is possible to train sophisticated neural networks to identify and classify microorganisms with remarkable accuracy. Studies indicate that employing AI in this context can achieve classification accuracies of up to 99%, effectively capturing the complex genetic and morphological diversity inherent in microorganisms (Abhishek et al., 2023). Such precision not only enhances our understanding of microbial functions but also bears significant implications across disciplines, including biotechnology, medicine, and environmental science. As the scientific community continues to develop these advanced classification techniques, the potential for automated taxonomic classification to revolutionise our approach to exploring the microbial world and its intricate relationship with human health and environmental sustainability is profound.

2.1. Historical Background of Microbial Taxonomy

The establishment of microbial taxonomy entails a comprehensive understanding of the complexities involved in classifying microorganisms. Early taxonomists primarily relied on basic morphological traits to categorise organisms, which frequently resulted in ambiguities, particularly in microbial entities where physical features can be exceedingly subtle. This limitation became increasingly apparent as microbiology advanced, notably through the development of microscopy, which revealed a vast diversity of microbial life and challenged existing classification systems. A transition towards a more systematic framework commenced in the mid-20th century, characterised by a renewed emphasis on genetic attributes and biochemical properties in biological classification. This shift marked a significant departure from observational taxonomy towards a more analytical approach, thereby enabling the application of molecular techniques that provided deeper insights into microbial phylogeny and taxonomy. These scientific advancements underscored the necessity for a robust framework capable of accommodating the extensive diversity and intricate interrelations of microbial organisms. The recognition of microorganisms as a distinct and significant class of life emerged in the 20th century, driven by philosophical and methodological developments that enhanced the understanding of biodiversity. Scientists began to perceive microbial life not merely as single-celled entities but as vital components within Earth's ecosystems. This reevaluation was supported by evidence of microbial cooperation, communication, and evolutionary dynamics, which highlighted their roles in health and environmental processes. O'Malley notes that recognising microorganisms as comparable to macroorganisms bears profound implications for theories such as evolution, ontology, and taxonomy, necessitating a deeper insight into biodiversity (Brune et al., 2013). The advent of genetic sequencing technologies catalysed a paradigm shift, allowing classification based on genetic composition rather than solely on physical attributes. This gene-based methodology now constitutes the foundation of contemporary microbial taxonomy, leading to more accurate and reliable classification systems. Additionally, the development of biocollections has significantly transformed the historical context of microbial taxonomy. Collections of microbial specimens serve as vital tools for empirical validation and biodiversity exploration (Pavlinov, 2016). The systematic collection and organisation of microbial specimens into biocollections have enhanced the taxonomic framework, providing representative samples that reflect the diversity of microbial life. These collections, functioning as scientific resources and biodiversity repositories, illuminate evolutionary history and ecological relationships among microorganisms. As biological research progresses, preserving microbial diversity has become imperative not only for scientific inquiry but also for conservation initiatives. This paradigm shift underscores the importance of continual research and development in microbial taxonomy, recognising the fragile web of relationships among microbial life forms and their habitats.

2.1.1. Early Classification Systems

The advent of early classification schemes in microbial taxonomy marked the beginning of a more structured understanding of microbial diversity. Initial classifications were primarily based on observable morphological characteristics, which served as the main criteria for differentiating organisms. Taxonomists such as Carl Linnaeus established the foundation of binomial nomenclature, a system that assigned a unique two-part name to each species. This method not only facilitated scientific communication but also provided a hierarchical framework for organising organisms. However, reliance on morphology proved increasingly limiting, as it often failed to account for the extensive biochemical and genetic diversity present within microbial populations. Consequently, the development of initial classification systems evolved as scientists recognised the need to incorporate additional criteria for taxonomic placement, leading to the emergence of more advanced and multidimensional classification systems (Figure 2.2).

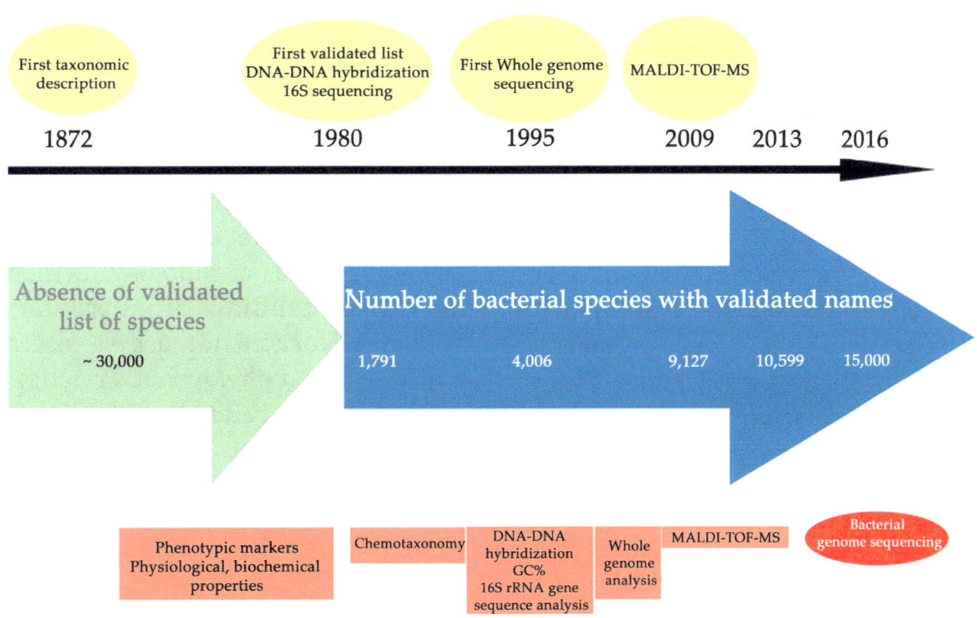

Figure 2.2. Evolution of bacterial taxonomy.

Source: https://www.researchgate.net/figure/Evolution-of-bacterial-taxonomy-The-most-important-changes-in-bacterial-taxonomic-tools_fig2_315832389.

With the increasing research into microorganisms, the development of early classification systems faced several challenges and limitations. The main limitation was the inability of morphological properties to capture the subtlety of microbial life. For example, many bacteria share common morphological features but differ significantly in genetic makeup and metabolic functions. This disparity created a need for alternative classification strategies and encouraged the use of biochemical methods, such as enzymic activity and metabolic profiling, alongside morphological data. Additionally, the advent of molecular techniques in the second half of the twentieth century, like DNA sequencing, began to provide new avenues for classification beyond morphology alone. These advances marked a breakthrough, suggesting that an integrative approach—incorporating morphological, biochemical, and genetic traits—could better reflect microbial diversity. Consequently, early classification systems laid the groundwork for modern developments in microbial taxonomy and established a more systematic approach. The development of phylogenetics in the latter half of the 20th century, which utilized genetic information to elucidate evolutionary relationships, revolutionised the field. Techniques such as ribosomal RNA sequencing shed light on microbial phylogeny, allowing researchers to differentiate relationships that were previously obscured by morphological similarities. Today, contemporary classification methods place greater emphasis on genetic information alongside traditional characteristics, providing a more comprehensive view of microbial life. This paradigm shift reflects the ongoing evolution of classification systems, as scientists recognise the complex interplay of morphology, biochemistry, and genetic makeup in microbial taxonomy. Ultimately, the early classification systems initiated the trajectory towards the current depth of understanding at the heart of microbiology.

2.1.2. Contributions of Key Scientists

Microbial classification has been profoundly influenced by the research of pioneering scientists who laid the foundation for understanding the complexity of microbial life. Among these influential figures is Carl Woese, who transformed the classification of prokaryotes by introducing the three-domain system — Bacteria, Archaea, and Eukarya. Woese's research, particularly through ribosomal RNA sequencing, provided a molecular basis for classification beyond traditional morphological-based methods. His studies focused on the evolutionary and genetic relationships among organisms, which were previously obscured by phenotypic variability. This paradigm shift marked a turning point, facilitating an accurate depiction of microbial diversity and the development of genomics-based taxonomic methods. Woese's contributions highlight the importance of molecular phylogenetics in the classification of microorganisms, thereby enabling future research to build upon a robust evolutionary framework. Roger Stanier is another prominent figure in microbial taxonomy, whose contributions to bacterial physiology and morphology further enhanced the understanding of microbial diversity. Stanier advocated for a systematic approach that integrated phylogenetic relationships with physiological traits, thereby increasing the taxonomic resolution of bacteria. He played a significant role in the creation of an initial comprehensive census of bacterial isolates, which continues to underpin subsequent taxonomic research. His interest in polyphasic taxonomy — a methodology combining morphological, cultural, and genomic data — has influenced modern microbial identification techniques.

Additionally, Stanier's collaborative efforts culminated in the publication of foundational texts such as Berge's Manual of Determinative Bacteriology, which remains vital for bacterial identification and classification, reflecting the enduring impact of his work within the discipline. The collective efforts to advance microbial taxonomy are also exemplified by initiatives led by organisations such as Berge's International Society for Microbial Systematics (BISMiS). This society has played a crucial role in promoting the dissemination of information among microbiologists and in advocating for the systematic study of prokaryotes. As highlighted in recent scholarly literature, the evolution of prokaryotic systematics has transitioned from morphological to genomics-based approaches, inspired by authoritative references such as Berge's Manual of Systematics of Archaea and Bacteria (BMSAB) (Jiao et al., 2024). The collaborative environment fostered by BISMiS provides an innovative platform for researchers to address emerging challenges in taxonomy. Moreover, the society's commitment to integrating post-genomic data into classification schemes underscores the necessity of revising traditional taxonomic protocols in response to technological innovations, thereby transforming microbial systematics into an effective discipline in the era of genomics and bioinformatics.

2.1.3. Evolution of Taxonomic Methods

The evolution of taxonomic methods in microbial taxonomy signifies a substantial departure from traditional morphological classification towards molecular-based techniques. Historically, taxonomists primarily relied on phenotypic characteristics, such as morphology and biochemical traits, for microorganism classification. However, this approach proved insufficient as scientists recognised the extensive diversity of microbial life, which often exhibited significant genetic variation despite sharing similar phenotypic traits. This disparity underscored the necessity for a more robust classification system capable of accurately representing microbial relationships and diversity. Consequently, the development of tools such as DNA sequencing marked a paradigm shift, enabling scientists to classify organisms using genetic information- an approach that provides a more reliable predictor of evolutionary relatedness. The advent of genomic methodologies has heralded a revolutionary era in microbial taxonomy, offering an alternative means of species identification. Recent proposals have suggested a genomic definition of species, wherein strains within the same species share more than 95% Average Amino Acid Identity (AAI) and Average Nucleotide Identity (ANI) (Thompson et al., 2013). The utilisation of genomic data for species delineation allows researchers to categorise taxonomic groups in accordance with phylogenetic relationships, replacing traditional morphological attributes that do not necessarily correlate with genetic diversity. This genomic approach not only enhances the precision of microbial classification but also fosters a more cohesive understanding of microbial ecology- an aspect of increasing importance as our knowledge of microbial diversity and scope expands.

Furthermore, taxonomic methodologies have been profoundly influenced by advancements in metagenomic technology, which facilitates the analysis of microbial diversity in environmental DNA pools. Traditional PCR techniques tend to underestimate microbial diversity due to amplification biases and sequencing limitations (Sharpton et al., 2011). Conversely, metagenomic approaches, such as those enabled by PhylOTU, allow researchers to define operational taxonomic units (OTUs) without the biases inherent in PCR-based methods. Recent studies have demonstrated that metagenomic libraries not only detect a broader taxonomic range but also often identify previously overlooked taxa, thereby enriching our understanding of microbial life. The synergy of genomic and metagenomic approaches signifies a groundbreaking era in microbial taxonomy, promoting more accurate and comprehensive classifications aligned with evolutionary history.

2.2. Fundamental Concepts in Taxonomy

Taxonomy is the foundation of biological classification, with a systematic approach to naming, defining, and classifying organisms. Microbiologists have also historically emphasised morphology and genetic features in taxonomic methods. However, fundamental principles in taxonomy also involve the phylogenetic relationships of organisms, which are crucial for fully appreciating the vast microbial diversity. The introduction of molecular techniques has transformed microbial taxonomy, allowing scientists to examine genetic material and phylogenetic connections in ways previously unimaginable. This has led to a reevaluation of traditional classification systems and highlighted the need for a more nuanced understanding of microbial diversity, acknowledging the complexity of genetic transfer and adaptation within microbial communities, and addressing the limitations of earlier biological categorisation systems in accurately reflecting ecological interactions. In recent years, incorporating new microbial phenomena into taxonomic discourse has greatly enriched our understanding of taxonomy itself. For example, advances in knowledge about microorganisms' cooperative activities — such as biofilm formation and quorum sensing — challenge the view of microorganisms as primarily single-celled entities. These cooperative behaviours demonstrate that microbial life exists within complex social networks, suggesting a form of taxonomy that extends beyond traditional classifications. Recognising these developments, it becomes clearer that microbial taxonomy is not a static system but one that is dynamic and influenced by modern microbiological research. This broader perspective fosters a taxonomy rooted in ecological realities and evolutionary principles, urging researchers to reconsider long-standing assumptions in the field. Furthermore, the philosophical significance of microbial classification has prompted questions about the nature of biological categories and the conceptual frameworks used to classify them. Ethnobiological complexity highlights debates in this area and supports a multidimensional framework capable of capturing the intricacies of classification in both traditional and microbial contexts. While such frameworks promise greater understanding, they also pose challenges regarding the relevance of natural kinds within microbial taxonomy. Specifically, the difficulty lies in reconciling empirical observations with higher-level classifications that may offer limited explanations for the variability and fluidity observed among microbial entities. Consequently, as these discussions deepen, they underline the necessity for ongoing dialogue concerning the philosophical foundations of taxonomy and the adaptive strategies essential for effectively classifying the vast diversity of microbial life present in different ecosystems (Brune et al., 2013; Ludwig, 2018).

2.2.1. Taxonomic Hierarchy

Taxonomic ranking constitutes the fundamental principle of microbial taxonomy, as it offers an organised framework within which biological organisms are systematically classified and grouped. This structured hierarchy consists of a series of ranks, including domain, kingdom, phylum, class, order, family, genus, and species, each representing different levels of relatedness and taxonomic importance. For microorganisms, particularly bacteria and archaea, the implementation of this taxonomic hierarchy is of considerable significance, as it facilitates systematic naming based on shared phenotypic characteristics and genetic relationships. Recent advancements in genomic analysis have, in recent years, enabled scientists to refine the taxonomic hierarchy, better reflecting the diversity and interrelationships of both eukaryotic and prokaryotic organisms. Approaches such as Average Nucleotide Identity (ANI) analysis allow researchers to delineate species boundaries with high precision, thereby advancing our understanding of microbial ecology and evolution. Within the taxonomic framework, the species and genus levels assume particular importance in microorganism classification, as they offer critical insights into the characteristic features of specific microorganisms (Figure 2.3).

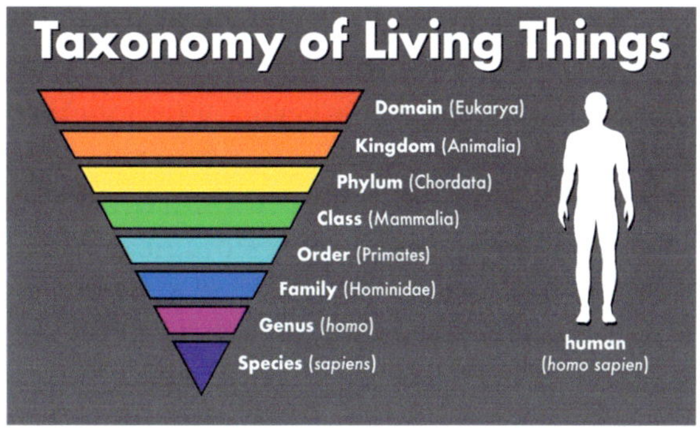

Figure 2.3. Taxonomic hierarchy.

Source: https://assets.ltkcontent.com/images/6106/human-classification_7abbbb2796.jpg.

For instance, the genus Dickeya includes some pathogenic bacteria that are well-documented to cause significant agricultural damage through soft rot diseases. Recent genomic studies on *Dickeya dadantii* have revealed its environmental adaptability and virulence factors, emphasising its relevance in plant pathology. The identification of numerous virulence genes, as well as antibiotic resistance traits in isolates such as CCRMP144 and CCRMP250, demonstrates the importance of genomic techniques in clarifying the taxonomic status of the organism. These methods not only aid accurate identification but also enable the development of targeted management practices to reduce crop loss caused by these pathogens, highlighting the practical significance of taxonomy in agriculture. Land use changes influence microbial diversity, reflecting the dynamic relationship between taxonomic hierarchies and environmental change. Research indicates that converting natural ecosystems into agricultural land significantly alters microbial communities, leading to taxonomic and functional homogenisation. For example, a study analysing 1185 soil samples found that land conversion affected 20% of phylotypes, with notable variations in the abundance of microbial groups such as *Chloroflexi* and *Gemmatimonadota*. While the overall functional structure remains relatively stable, key functional genes involved in nutrient cycling decline in agricultural ecosystems, indicating ecological imbalance. These findings reveal the profound impacts of human activity and underscore the necessity of conserving microbial biodiversity at taxonomic levels, which is crucial for ecosystem resilience and function (Peng et al., 2024; Pereira et al., 2024).

2.2.2. Nomenclature Rules

Nomenclature rules are highly important in classifying microorganisms, ensuring consistency and accuracy in naming within the ever-evolving field of microbiology. Nomenclature is an official system that enables researchers to discuss species and their taxonomy clearly. With the growing diversity of microbes, especially with the advent of genome sequencing, strict nomenclature guidelines are now seen as essential. Traditional classification methods, mainly based on phenotypic traits, often fell short in adequately capturing the complexity of microbial life. Consequently, recent efforts aim to modernise nomenclature by incorporating genomic data, so names reflect evolutionary relationships and genetic similarities among microorganisms, thus improving scientific discussions on microbial classification (Raúl et al., 2024). A significant milestone in nomenclature is the development of the Genome Taxonomy Database (GTDB). This addresses the increasing submission of genomic sequences from both cultured and uncultured microbes. GTDB offers an integrated system for annotating these genomes through automated processes that compare average nucleotide identity and measure relative evolutionary divergence. A unique aspect of GTDB is its reliance on the List of Prokaryotic names withstanding in Nomenclature (LPSN), which acts as a critical reference for valid naming rules. By establishing these standards, GTDB not only aids in discovering and classifying new organisms but also encourages further study and international collaboration among microbiologists, strengthening its role in microbial taxonomy and nomenclature (Chuvochina et al., 2023). Despite advancements in genomic techniques and classification systems, challenges remain, especially concerning uncultured taxa. The Code of Nomenclature of Prokaryotes Described from Sequence Data, known as SeqCode, was created to overcome these limitations. It provides a systematic approach for naming uncultured microbes. Traditional codes, like the International Code of Nomenclature of Prokaryotes (ICNP), are limited because they do not cover organisms that cannot be cultured in isolation. SeqCode establishes nomenclatural types based on genomic sequences, allowing names to be linked with organisms that have not yet been cultivated. This dual approach not only addresses existing gaps in the nomenclature system but also promotes the integration of molecular data into taxonomy, creating a more comprehensive system for microbial nomenclature (Chuvochina et al., 2023).

2.2.3. Types of Classification Systems

Microorganism classification is a complex endeavour involving multiple independent systems that reflect the diversity and intricacy of microbial life. Traditional taxonomic methods predominantly depend on morphological, physiological, and ecological attributes to categorize organisms into hierarchical ranks such as domain, kingdom, phylum, class, order, family, genus, and species. However, with advancements in microbial genetics, classification frameworks have progressively incorporated genomic data. Molecular techniques, including 16S rRNA gene sequencing, have augmented microbial taxonomy by allowing researchers to identify organisms based on genetic similarity, rather than solely on phenotypic traits. This evolution acknowledges the limitations inherent in traditional methods and fosters a more precise depiction of microbial relationships and taxonomy. Genomic classification schemes are increasingly emerging as a primary tool in microbial taxonomy, signifying significant methodological progress in the discipline. There is a notable trend among researchers to define species based on genomic information. Current studies demonstrate that strains classified within the same microbial species exhibit over 95% Average Amino Acid Identity (AAI) and Average Nucleotide Identity (ANI) (Thompson et al., 2013) (Figure 2.4).

This approach highlights the significance of genomic data in characterising microbial species and allows for a better understanding of microbial relationships within a genus. Additionally, the use of draft genomes in describing new taxa has become standard practice, helping researchers create an integrated genomic profile of new microorganisms. This genome-focused strategy not only improves existing classification systems but also offers a solid foundation for discovering novel species within complex microbial communities. Furthermore, applying classification systems in practice involves integrating various data sources, which is crucial for conservation and biodiversity programmes.

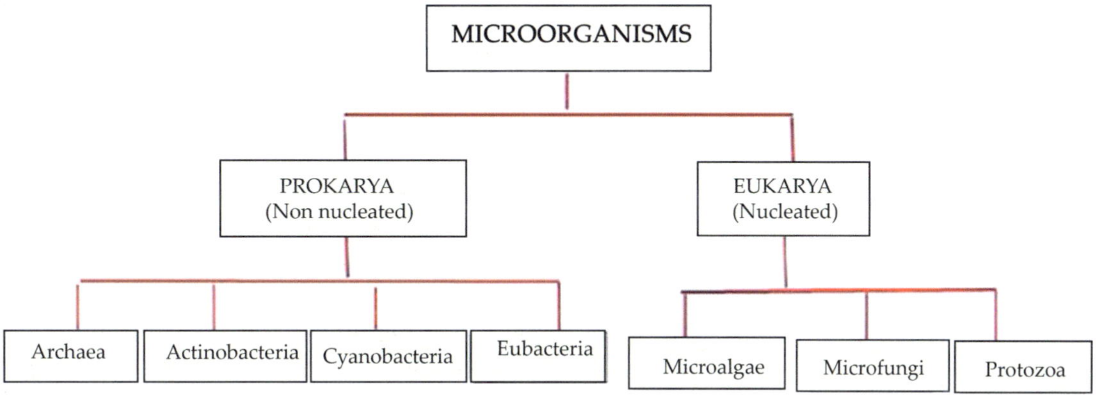

Figure 2.4. The broad classification of microorganisms.

Source: https://www.researchgate.net/publication/337870971/figure/fig1/AS:834614427914240@1575998994227/The-broad-classification-of-microorganisms.png.

As ecosystems face increasing pressure from human activities, robust classification systems are essential for making informed decisions in biodiversity conservation. The cycle of biodiversity data encompasses planning, collection, certification, description, preservation, discovery, integration, and analysis—forming the basis for generating reliable indicators for conservation purposes (Gadelha et al., 2018). With biodiversity informatics, researchers can compile vast amounts of raw data from field surveys, automated sensors, and molecular studies to refine microbial classification systems. This consolidation not only deepens understanding of microbial diversity but also facilitates accurate communication of this knowledge to policymakers, underscoring the importance of classification systems in addressing global biodiversity challenges.

2.3. Modern Techniques in Microbial Classification

The microbiological classification landscape has undergone rapid evolution owing to advancements in contemporary methodologies that leverage technological innovations. Traditional techniques, which predominantly rely on morphological and biochemical traits, face limitations in classifying the extensive diversity of microorganisms. Molecular approaches, such as DNA sequencing, have revolutionised the identification and classification of microbial communities in comparison to conventional methods. The progression of high-throughput sequencing technologies permits more precise and efficient analysis of complex microbial assemblages. For example, the employment of next-generation sequencing (NGS) enables researchers to generate extensive collections of sequence data, thereby tracking the genetic variability within microbial communities across diverse environments. This paradigm shift has broadened the scope of microbial taxonomy, especially in extreme environments such as hypersaline and soda lakes, where unique bacterial features can be elucidated through genomic studies (Dhundale et al., 2021). Metagenomics represents another pivotal advancement in microbial taxonomy, offering insights into the uncultivated components of microbial life. By examining genetic material directly obtained from environmental samples, researchers can circumvent the limitations associated with laboratory cultivation of microorganisms. Notably, metagenomics challenges traditional taxonomy classification due to the vast number of short sequence fragments generated by next-generation sequencing technologies, thereby necessitating effective classification tools capable of managing large data sets. Reliable and accessible methods such as EnSVM (Ensemble Support Vector Machine) have emerged as robust solutions, providing systematic approaches to fragment identification. EnSVM and its enhanced variant, EnSVMB, exhibit high sensitivity and specificity, facilitating efficient classification of microbial taxonomy even in complex datasets (Jiang et al., 2017).

The integration of advanced molecular techniques with computational processes has elevated microbial identification to unprecedented levels of accuracy and specificity. The synergy of metagenomic analysis and sophisticated classification algorithms enhances our capacity to explore and interpret microbial diversity across various ecological contexts, from extreme environments to more common habitats. Moreover, as our understanding of microbial communities deepens, these innovations hold critical importance for ecological monitoring, biotechnological applications, and public health. The transition toward a data-driven era in microbial taxonomy not only expands our scientific knowledge but also highlights the importance of interdisciplinary approaches in addressing global challenges related to microbial diversity and its implications. Ultimately, cutting-edge techniques in microbial classification exemplify the union of technology and biology, paving the way for further advances in microbial ecology and taxonomic frameworks.

2.3.1. Molecular Methods (e.g., DNA Sequencing)

The advancement of molecular methodologies, particularly DNA sequencing, has significantly enhanced microbial classification and taxonomy. Traditional approaches primarily depended on phenotypic characteristics, which often provided limited insights into microbial diversity. Molecular techniques offer a more comprehensive and precise understanding of microbial relationships and evolutionary trajectories. The transition from conventional classification frameworks to genome-based systems highlights the growing importance of DNA sequencing, which has become the primary tool for delineating not only bacterial species but also higher taxonomic groups. The constraints of phenotypic traits in capturing the complexity of microbial diversity are now addressed through techniques that enable comprehensive genomic analysis, thereby facilitating the development of a more robust taxonomy that accurately reflects the evolutionary history and diversity of prokaryotic microorganisms within a modern scientific context (Raúl et al., 2024) (Figure 2.5).

Furthermore, the use of molecular methods in microbiological classification has presented both challenges and opportunities for data comparison across laboratories. Metabarcoding has created difficulties for scientists, as DNA sequencing is used to analyse environmental samples, but variations in bioinformatics tools and methods make these analyses complex. For example, the accuracy of taxonomic identification often depends on the choice of variable sites in the 16S rRNA gene. Using algorithms like DADA2, researchers can optimise data processing, as demonstrated in a study involving activated sludge samples. In addition to highlighting the importance of selecting the right variable regions, the study also evaluated different databases for their ability to accurately classify operational taxonomic units (OTUs). The findings emphasise the need for standardisation in molecular techniques to resolve inconsistencies and improve reproducibility in microbial taxonomy research (Babis et al., 2024).

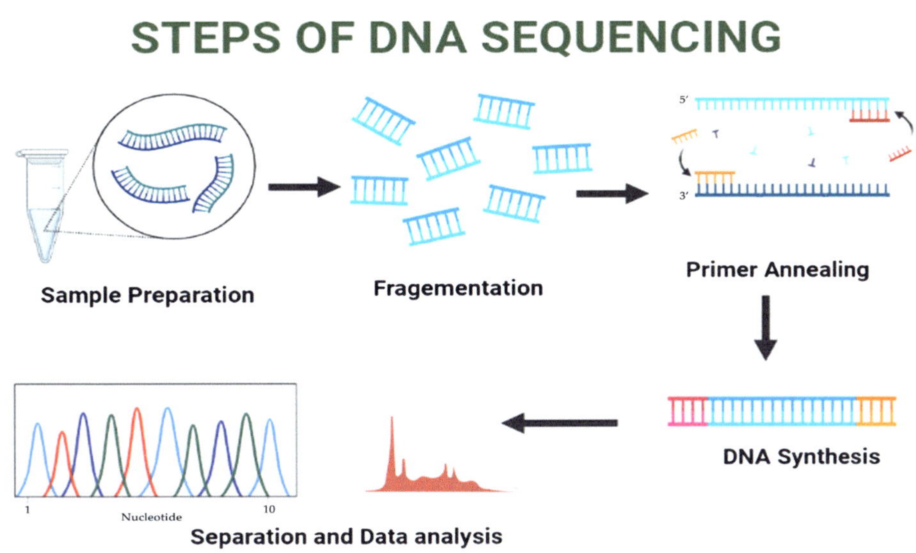

Figure 2.5. Steps of DNA sequencing.

Source: https://sciencevivid.com/dna-sequencing/.

Ultimately, these molecular methods also have applications in ecological and evolutionary studies, expanding the understanding of microbial diversity. As DNA sequencing technologies continue to advance, researchers gain unprecedented access to genomic data that can inform classification systems and reveal not only taxonomic information but also functional capacities within microbial communities. By classifying and describing microbes at a genetic level, it becomes possible to track biodiversity and ecosystem health more effectively. Such developments are vital for addressing environmental and biotechnological challenges. Therefore, efforts to refine and standardise molecular techniques in microbial taxonomy hold great promise for transforming the field, leading to a more comprehensive and systematic study of microbial classification across various ecological contexts (Raúl et al., 2024).

2.3.2. Phenotypic Methods (e.g., Biochemical Tests)

Phenotypic methods, especially biochemical assays, have long been the primary approach for species identification and classification of microorganisms. These assays rely on the metabolic and physiological traits of microorganisms to classify them based on observable characteristics. Common biochemical tests such as catalase tests, fermentation assays, and enzyme activity studies offer extensive information about the ecology and behaviour of microorganisms. By analysing the metabolic pathways and by-products of a microorganism, researchers can draw logical conclusions regarding evolutionary relationships and taxonomic levels between species. Although phenotypic methods are often used because they are straightforward and inexpensive, they may not always fully capture the diversity and complexity of microbial life. In recent years, advanced single-cell analytical techniques, such as Single-cell Raman Spectroscopy (SCRS), have been developed as supplements to traditional phenotypic methods. SCRS delivers high-resolution, non-invasive single-cell characterisation, allowing researchers to observe phenotypic variability associated with growth phase and metabolism. This innovative approach enables the collection of large datasets from multiple microbial strains, supporting not only taxonomic classification but also providing insights into their potential functions within ecological settings. As noted in previous research, SCRS models can improve classification accuracy to 96.1% in taxonomic identification and show promise in bridging the gap between laboratory results and real environmental samples (Figure 2.6).

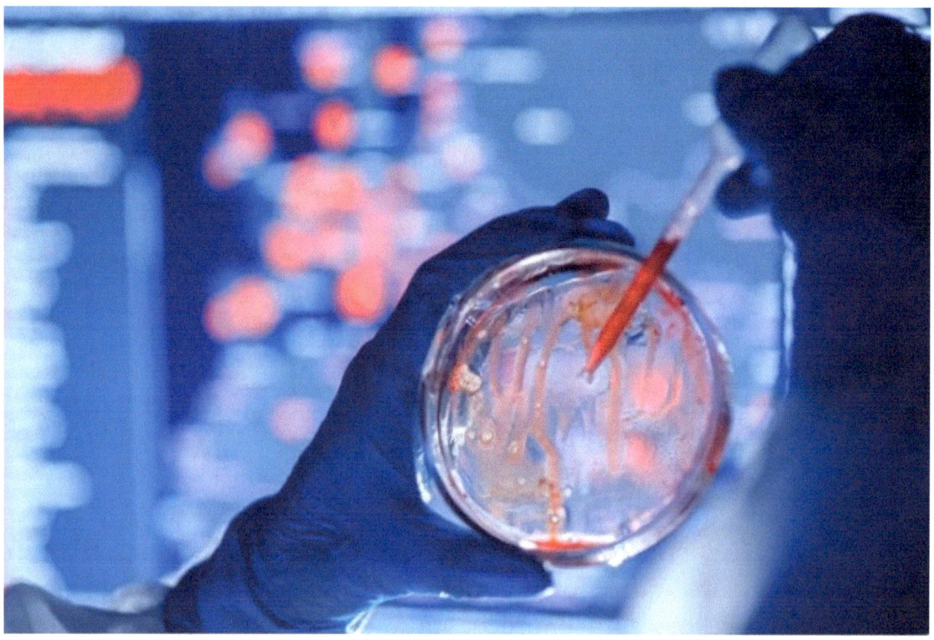

Figure 2.6. Biochemical tests.

Source: https://www.news-medical.net/image-handler/picture/2021/1/shutterstock_1672798186.jpg.

These developments reflect the fluid nature of microbial taxonomy, suggesting that phenotypic methods are being complemented by molecular and technologically advanced techniques to provide a more comprehensive account of microbial diversity. While paradigm shifts at the level of molecular methods are transforming how microbial classification is viewed, phenotypic methods remain a part of taxonomic systems. Biochemical tests continue to be useful, especially where rapid identification is required or when molecular methods are impractical. Additionally, combining genotypic and phenotypic data offers a robust approach to characterising microbial taxonomy, as seen in revised classification criteria involving DNA sequencing and traditional phenotypic traits. These integrative methods can promote more consistent practices in microbial taxonomy, enabling scientists to better represent the diversity within microbial biodiversity and ecological processes. This interaction between different classification techniques not only deepens our understanding of microbial evolution but also facilitates new biotechnological applications based on precise microbial identification and classification.

2.3.3. Bioinformatics in Taxonomy

The integration of bioinformatics into microbial taxonomy marks a transformative development in how scientists categorise and understand microbial diversity. Using advanced computational tools, bioinformatics helps manage large amounts of genomic and metagenomic data, enabling efficient identification and classification of microbial species. The use of software packages and algorithms allows researchers to reassess sequences from numerous samples and discover phylogenetic patterns that were previously difficult to detect with traditional methods. Additionally, bioinformatics techniques provide deeper insights into microbial communities by clarifying metabolic processes used by different taxa, thus offering valuable information about their functional roles in various habitats. Mock communities have also become essential for testing and refining bioinformatics methods in microbial taxonomy. Resources like Mockrobiota, which compile datasets of known taxa, provide ways to validate the accuracy and reproducibility of computational methods (Shiffer et al., 2016). Applying these standardised mock communities enables researchers to optimise their bioinformatics pipelines for peak performance and comparability across studies. This tool promotes open access and encourages collaboration within the scientific community, ultimately streamlining taxonomic procedures. The combined analysis and interpretation of complex datasets will not only enhance microbial classification but also create new opportunities for research across multiple disciplines. The metaproteomics approach highlights the potential for expanding microbial classification through bioinformatics by integrating taxonomy with functional capacity. This method uses mass spectrometry to characterise microbial proteins, helping to reveal taxonomic diversity and functional roles of microbial communities in various fields such as medical and environmental sciences (Heyer et al., 2019). Improved workflows in metaproteomics have increased the efficiency and speed of data analysis, leading to more protein identifications and better annotations. These advances underline the essential role of bioinformatics, not only in discovering microorganisms but also in understanding their biochemical and ecological functions. The emergence of metaproteomics is set to further boost microbial taxonomy and classification, fostering a greater understanding of microbial life and its importance in both ecological and applied contexts.

2.4. Major Domains of Life

The Earth's life is broadly classified into three main domains: Bacteria, Archaea, and Eukarya. This classification has significant implications for the taxonomy of microorganisms because understanding these domains provides the foundation for establishing and categorising microorganisms. Bacteria, which are highly genetically diverse, are characterised by their prokaryotic cell structure, absence of a nucleus, and usually one large circular chromosome. Their ecological adaptability allows them to thrive in a wide range of environments, from highly stressful conditions to symbiotic relationships. This is important for clarifying numerous biogeochemical processes, highlighting the role bacteria play in different environments. Recognising the factors that differentiate bacteria from other domains helps scientists improve their classification methods and develop targeted studies on microbial interactions and functions within ecological niches. In contrast to Bacteria, Archaea are similarly diverse but distinct groups of prokaryotic organisms with different biophysical and biochemical properties. Typically inhabiting extreme environments, such as hot springs and salt lakes, Archaea have unique adaptations that set them apart from their bacterial relatives. Genomic research has uncovered that Archaea possess distinctive membrane lipids and a specialized RNA polymerase that more closely resembles that of Eukarya, indicating their evolutionary importance. Consequently, the genomic taxonomy of Archaea is being increasingly refined, with recent proposals suggesting the application of the genomic species concept based on shared genetic features, as discussed in recent literature (Thompson et al., 2013) (Figure 2.7).

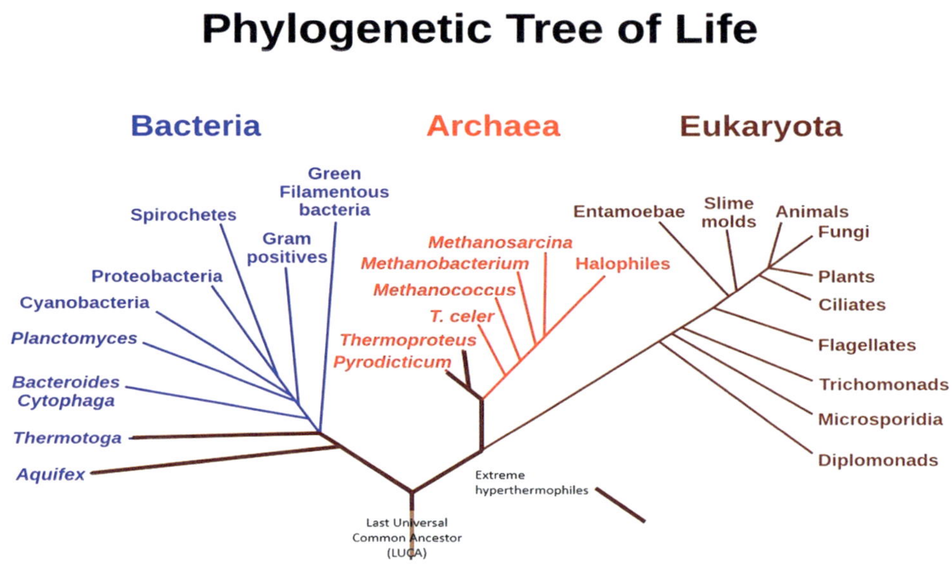

Figure 2.7. Major domains of life.

Source: https://www.thoughtco.com/thmb/41HGMKbMXDiMEhSKnzNvA8LslDc=/1500x0/filters:no_upscale():max_bytes(150000):strip_icc()/three_domain_system-57c48baa3df78cc16eb59931.jpg.

This definition aims to incorporate genomic information into an existing classification framework, thus offering a more comprehensive view of microbial diversity in the Archaea domain. The most developed of the three domains is Eukarya, which includes a broad range of organisms such as fungi, plants, and animals. Microbial eukaryotes like protozoa and algae in this domain play significant roles in ecological functions and possess diverse metabolic abilities. Classifying eukaryotic microorganisms requires a detailed study of their evolutionary history, especially through genomic analyses that reveal substantial genetic divergence. It has been observed that extensive genomic variation among these microorganisms is associated with lineage-specific genes, which emerge quickly, and segmentally variable genes (SVGs), which reflect environmental adaptation (Kasif et al., 2004). Such genetic insights are vital to microbial taxonomy, as these species demonstrate the adaptive nature of eukaryotic microorganisms and their capacity for adaptation, underscoring the importance of including genomic data to trace complex evolutionary patterns across different eukaryotic lineages.

2.4.1. Bacteria

The diversity of bacteria is extensive, reflecting the vast array of species characterised by complex metabolic activities, environmental resilience, and ecological roles. Phenotypic characteristics and genetic composition serve as the foundational basis for classification within microbial systematics.

While morphological and biochemical testing previously dominated the classification process, technological advancements have revolutionised our understanding of bacterial phylogeny. New definitions of species emphasise the importance of genomic comparisons, wherein organisms belonging to the same microbial species typically exhibit over 95% Average Amino Acid Identity (AAI) and Average Nucleotide Identity (ANI) (Thompson et al., 2013). This genomic approach permits more precise classification, enabling the determination of species based on genetic profiles rather than superficial phenotypic traits. Consequently, the integration of genomic resources refocuses bacterial taxonomy towards a deeper understanding of microbial diversity. Current research underscores the critical use of specific genetic markers to elucidate relationships among bacterial taxa. For example, within the phylum *Bacteroidetes*, the gyrB gene serves as one of the key phylogenetic markers, allowing for finer discrimination among closely related groups, such as those within the genus *Flavobacterium*. This gene encodes an essential component of DNA gyrase, and sequences derived from it have demonstrated higher discriminatory power than traditional 16S rRNA gene sequences.

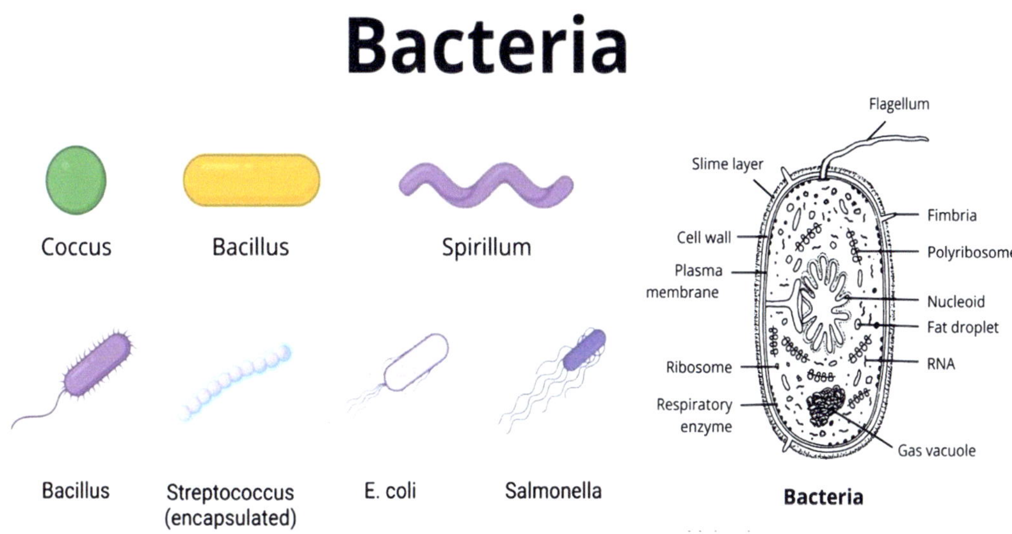

Figure 2.8. Bacteria.

Source: https://biologylearner.com/wp-content/uploads/2024/02/Bacteria-1024x536.jpg.

The utilisation of gyrB offers a more refined comprehension of microbial phylogenetics, elucidating the intricate relationships among various *Flavobacterium* species. The incorporation of such molecular markers within bacterial classification systems enables researchers to delineate bacterial species and their phylogenetic relationships more effectively, which is fundamentally significant for taxonomy and applied microbiology. Furthermore, the ramifications of more precise bacterial classification extend beyond academic interest; they have immediate implications for science, particularly in the fields of medicine, ecology, and biotechnology. Accurate taxonomy is crucial for understanding the activities of specific bacteria in disease and health, ecosystem processes, and industrial applications. For example, the identification of pathogenic strains depends on precise classification to inform treatment strategies and public health policies. Similarly, a more comprehensive understanding of bacterial diversity can be leveraged to advance bioremediation and the development of innovative biotechnological processes. As microbial taxonomy continues to evolve, the integration of genomic data not only redefines our understanding of bacterial diversity but also generates new research avenues and applications that can significantly benefit society as a whole.

2.4.2. Archaea

The taxonomy of Archaea has undergone significant development, reflecting advances in the understanding of microbial diversity. As a distinct domain separate from Bacteria and Eukaryota, Archaea encompasses a variety of extremophiles and methanogens that inhabit specialized ecological niches. The traditional taxonomic framework for Archaea predominantly relied on morphological and biochemical characteristics; however, with the advent of molecular tools such as 16S rRNA gene sequencing, researchers have gained profound insights into their phylogenetic relationships. This molecular approach has uncovered surprising diversity within the Archaea, necessitating new classifications aligned with these discoveries. For example, the identification of several genera, including *Methanoculleus*, illustrates the limitations of conventional methods. These developments underscore the complexities inherent in microbial taxonomy, especially when considering the numerous environmental adaptations of Archaea (see Figure 2.9).

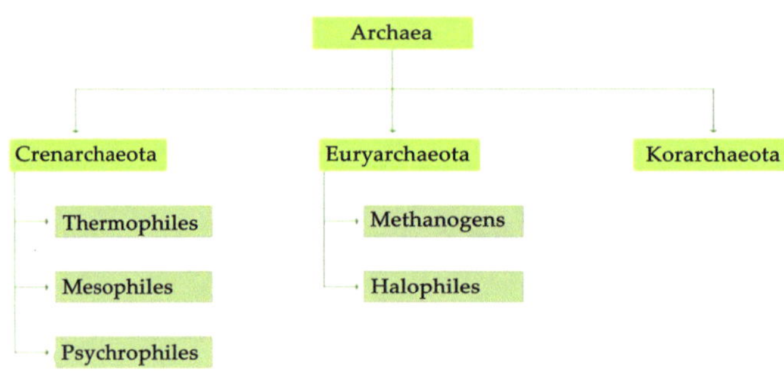

Figure 2.9. Types of archaea.

Source: https://www.sciencetopia.net/wp-content/uploads/2021/01/chart.jpg.

Furthermore, the utilization of high-throughput sequencing technologies has furnished essential tools for the comparative analysis of archaeal populations across diverse ecosystems. For instance, 16S rRNA amplicon sequencing has been employed to investigate the microbiome associated with anaerobic digestion and to reveal biases introduced by primer selection and PCR amplification. The findings demonstrated pronounced biases against particular taxa, such as *Euryarchaeota*, underscoring how standard protocols may temporarily exclude specific genera, exemplified by *Methanoculleus*, in PCR-based methodologies. Consequently, the adoption of multiple techniques, including shotgun DNA sequencing, affords a more comprehensive understanding of archaeal communities within various environments. This multifaceted perspective not only augments our comprehension of microbial diversity but also challenges prevailing paradigms in microbial taxonomy, prompting a re-evaluation of the methods employed in classifying these vital microorganisms. In light of this context, the application of metagenomic approaches emerges as a promising pathway for advancing microbial taxonomy. Through the utilization of computational tools such as PhylOTU, researchers are able to transcend the limitations imposed by conventional Operational Taxonomic Unit (OTU) clustering methods, which often fail to encompass the full spectrum of microbial communities. This is particularly pertinent to Archaea, given that metagenomic analyses have unveiled a broader diversity of operational taxonomic units that were previously overlooked due to biases inherent in PCR-based methodologies. By adopting these innovative approaches, the field of microbial taxonomy can be significantly advanced. The identification of novel taxa across previously uncharacterized phyla broadens our understanding of archaeal diversity and emphasises the importance of implementing agile, integrative taxonomic strategies. Looking ahead, these methodologies will be essential for accurately characterising the vast diversity of Archaea and elucidating their ecological functions across different environments (Sharpton et al., 2011; Campanaro et al., 2018).

2.4.3. Eukarya

Eukarya, one of the three fundamental domains of life, is a diverse group of organisms central to understanding the taxonomy and classification of microorganisms. The eukaryotic cell, characterised by membrane-bound organelles and a true nucleus, can be distinguished from prokaryotes, which lack these features. This distinction results in a more complex organisation, allowing eukaryotic organisms to have specialized functions and interactions with their environments. Eukarya includes various groups such as animals, plants, fungi, and numerous protists, all of which possess unique cellular forms and metabolic activities. The evolutionary relationships among these organisms have been of great interest, especially regarding their roles in the environment and biogeochemical cycles. Therefore, assessing these relationships helps answer broader questions about evolution and how life forms adapt to environmental changes. The taxonomy of eukaryotic organisms incorporates both morphological and molecular approaches, enabling a comprehensive understanding of their diversity. Molecular techniques, like DNA sequencing, have transformed microbial taxonomy by providing insights into the genetic basis of evolutionary relationships. These approaches preserve traditional morphological classifications but also clarify phylogenetic connections among various eukaryotic groups. For instance, ribosomal RNA sequence analysis has revealed significant kinship among diverse organisms in Eukarya and has allowed scientists to construct accurate phylogenetic trees. Additionally, recent functional studies of translational systems across eukaryotic and other kingdoms reveal shared characteristics that can guide evolutionary research. These interdisciplinary methods exemplify the interconnected nature of eukaryotic organisms and their ecological significance across diverse environments (Briones & Amils, 1998) (Figure 2.10).

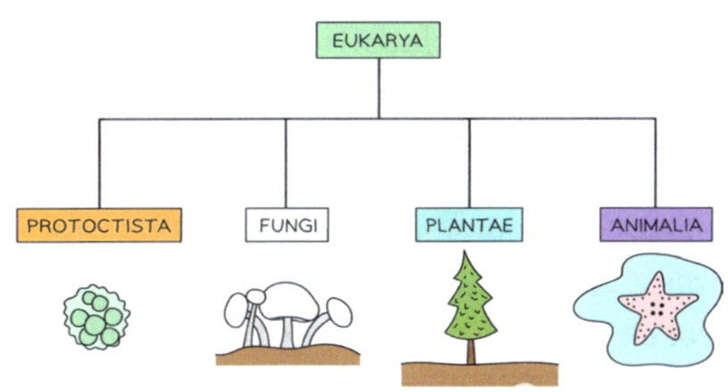

Figure 2.10. Classification of Eukarya.

Source: https://cdn.savemyexams.com/cdn-cgi/image/w=1920,f=auto/uploads/2021/03/The-Kingdoms-of-Eukarya.png.

In particular, the interaction of eukaryotic microorganisms with their environment exemplifies their role in biogeochemical cycling and their influence on global climate variables. An instance is the investigation of wet tundra ecosystems, which reveals the complexities of microbial populations within permafrost and highlights the niches occupied by eukaryotic microorganisms in methane production and carbon cycling. The findings indicating that microbial communities consist of all three domains of life, with a substantial representation of eukaryotes, underscore the pervasive impact of eukaryotes on ecosystem processes. Moreover, an understanding of substrate limitation, as influenced by organic matter quality, enhances models that predict trace gas fluxes from such systems, thereby holding significance for climate change negotiations. While eukaryotic microorganisms develop resistance to extreme environments, it remains essential to measure their resilience and interactions with other organisms to fully comprehend their taxonomy and classification (Wagner et al., 2005).

2.5. Classification of Bacteria

The bacterium has experienced a significant revision in its classification, driven by advancements in scientific knowledge and technological innovations. Initially, bacterial taxonomy was primarily founded on phenotypic characteristics, including morphology, staining reactions, and metabolic functions. However, this approach proved insufficient for capturing the full diversity of bacterial life. The introduction of molecular techniques, such as nucleic acid sequencing, marked a pivotal step towards adopting more comprehensive classification systems known as polyphasic taxonomy. This methodology combines traditional phenotypic descriptions with genetic data to produce a more precise and complete understanding of bacterial relationships. The advent of genome sequencing has enabled scientists to elucidate evolutionary connections among bacterial species, thereby refining classification accuracy. Consequently, reference works like Bergey's Manual of Systematics of Archaea and Bacteria have become essential resources for microbiologists involved in bacterial taxonomy, significantly facilitating communication and research within the field (Jiao et al., 2024). More recently, the paradigm of bacterial classification has further evolved into the genomic era, wherein genomic data not only contributes to classification but also potentially streamlines the process of delineating taxa. The rapid increase in species descriptions, coupled with ongoing reclassifications, presents substantial challenges for taxonomists striving to maintain a consistent hierarchical system. It is anticipated that genomic methodologies will promote a more stable taxonomy that offers enhanced accuracy and reliability. An illustrative example is the taxonomy of rhizobia, a vital component in nitrogen fixation in legumes, which exemplifies how genomic insights can revolutionize bacterial taxonomy. This scenario highlights how technological and methodological advancements influence our approach to discovering and classifying bacterial species, underscoring the imperative for a systematic and orderly classification framework capable of accommodating the dynamic nature of microbial diversity (Helene et al., 2022). As microbial taxonomy continues to develop, several themes emerge that require concerted attention from researchers and taxonomists. Collaborative efforts, such as those promoted by Bergey's International Society for Microbial Systematics, are essential in addressing issues posed by evolving classification requirements. Key areas include the development of comprehensive databases, standardized nomenclature, and taxonomic schemes that incorporate ecological and functional traits. Such collaborative endeavors enhance the legitimacy of classifications and underscore the importance of adaptable methodologies in a rapidly progressing scientific landscape. Furthermore, ongoing dissemination of knowledge and skills among microbiologists will foster solutions to emerging challenges, thereby maintaining the relevance and robustness of bacterial classification. As this discipline advances, the integration of genomic information with traditional classification systems will increasingly shape our understanding of bacterial diversity and its ecological significance within natural and agricultural ecosystems (Jiao et al., 2024).

2.5.1. Gram-positive versus Gram-negative Bacteria

The classification of bacteria into Gram-positive and Gram-negative is a fundamental aspect of microbial taxonomy, primarily based on differences in their cell wall structures and staining characteristics. The thick peptidoglycan layer in Gram-positive bacteria retains the crystal violet stain during Gram staining, causing them to appear purple. This structural feature not only influences the shape of the bacterium but also enhances its resistance to certain environmental stresses, including antimicrobial agents. Conversely, Gram-negative bacteria have a thinner peptidoglycan layer, supplemented by an outer membrane rich in lipopolysaccharides. This composition results in a pink appearance after staining, indicating a reduced ability to retain the crystal violet dye. Variations in cell wall structure significantly impact the physical properties, pathogenicity, and treatment approaches for bacterial infections. These structural differences also influence their response to antimicrobial drugs, making treatment more complex. For instance, the outer membrane of Gram-negative bacteria acts as an additional barrier, generally rendering them more resistant to specific antibiotics compared to Gram-positive bacteria. This distinction is clinically relevant because Gram-negative bacteria tend to cause more invasive infections, necessitating tailored therapeutic strategies. The antimicrobial resistance observed in many Gram-negative species has driven research into new drugs and treatment protocols, highlighting the evolving nature of microbial taxonomy. Studies, such as the investigation of actinomycetes like *Streptomyces sp.* TN17 for their antimicrobial properties, demonstrate potent inhibition of both Gram-positive and Gram-negative bacteria, providing promising avenues for discovering new antibiotics to combat these often resilient pathogens (Smaoui et al., 2011) (Figure 2.11).

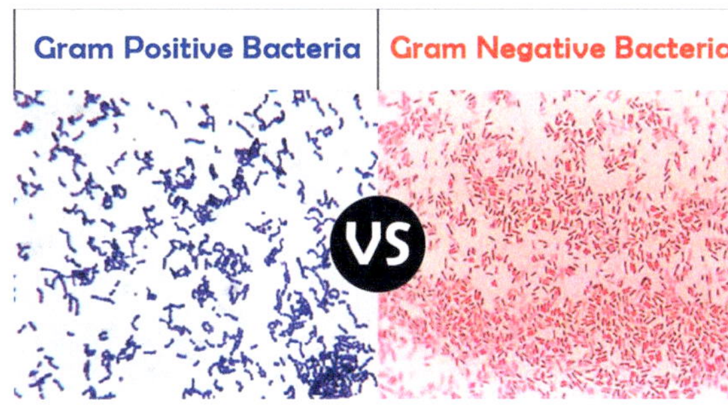

Figure 2.11. Gram-positive versus Gram-negative bacteria.

Source: https://microbenotes.com/wp-content/uploads/2018/07/Differences-Between-Gram-Positive-and-Gram-Negative-Bacteria.jpg.

Furthermore, the taxonomic classification of such bacterial groups is supplemented by molecular research, mainly through the analysis of 16S rRNA gene sequences. This type of genetic analysis provides data on the phylogenetic relationships between different bacterial species, emphasising not only their morphological features but also their evolutionary lineages. For example, a recent paper described a new actinomycete strain, Sg 10, active against Gram-positive bacteria and genetically linked to the *Streptosporangium* genus (Zitouni et al., 2006). This is just one way in which the growing impact of molecular taxonomy helps solve traditional classification issues, making it possible to identify species with useful antibacterial activities. Generally, understanding the differences between Gram-positive and Gram-negative bacteria is crucial for advancing microbial taxonomy and medical interventions.

2.5.2. Classification Based on Shape and Arrangement

Shape and arrangement classification are essential in microbial taxonomy for distinguishing and identifying microbial species. Microbial morphology, size, shape, and spatial pattern provide crucial information for taxonomists. Bacteria, for example, can be classified into three broad shapes: cocci (spherical), bacilli (rod-shaped), and spirilla (spiral). Each morphological form reflects various biological features and evolutionary adaptations, making species identification feasible and enabling ecological interpretation. This classification system is not merely convenient; it establishes a framework for understanding microbial diversity and supports future research on microbial functions and interactions within ecosystems. Furthermore, the architecture of microbial cells adds another level of complexity to their classification. Microorganisms are arranged in various configurations, such as individually, in pairs, chains, or clusters. For example, cocci can form single cells (monococci), pairs (diplococci), or chains (streptococci). Such arrangements can influence the physiological characteristics of the microorganisms, including biofilm formation or resistance to environmental stresses (Figure 2.12).

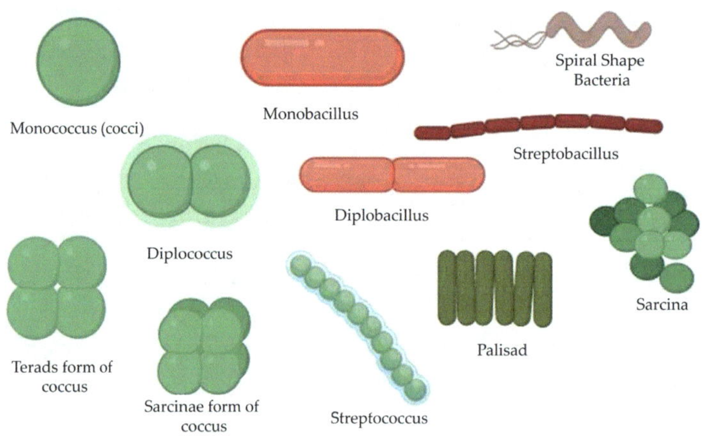

Figure 2.12. Bacteria sizes, shapes, and arrangement.

Source: https://biologynotesonline.com/wp-content/uploads/2024/03/shape-and-arrangement-of-bacteria-1.webp.

One should value such arrangements, especially in clinical microbiology, as the identification of pathogenic bacteria often relies on their morphological characteristics and arrangements. This subtle classification also highlights the close connection between microbial morphology and their ecological niches. In some cases, the use of specialized microscopic techniques has now uncovered unique structures beyond traditional classification methods that only consider shape and arrangement. For example, observed phenotypes in certain stalked bacteria or filamentous microorganisms show that morphology can be dynamic, depending on environmental or developmental signals. There have been reports of multicellular organisation similar to that in multicellular organisms, which raises questions about the evolution and ecology of these microorganisms. As research progresses, particularly with technological advancements, our understanding of classifying microorganisms by shape and arrangement is likely to develop further. Ongoing research into new morphological features, such as those seen in the Devonian stromatoporoid specimen with its distinctive distribution of spicules, underscores the importance of this borderland of classification in expanding our overall knowledge of microbial diversity and taxonomy (Da Silva et al., 2014; Okoh et al., 2014).

2.5.3. Importance of Metabolic Pathways in Classification

Microbial taxonomic classification has traditionally relied on morphological, biochemical, and genetic data. However, the role of metabolic pathways has emerged as a crucial component in achieving accurate microbial taxonomy and classification. Metabolic pathways clarify how microorganisms generate energy, synthesise essential compounds, and respond to their environment. For example, certain metabolic capabilities may distinguish populations that are morphologically similar yet differ significantly in ecological roles or infectivity. Focusing on these pathways enables researchers to differentiate microorganisms with greater precision, revealing evolutionary relationships and functional capacities often overlooked by other methods.

The metabolism of microorganisms - including fermentation, respiration, and biosynthesis - substantially influences their classification. For instance, some bacteria possess metabolic functions that allow them to degrade complex substrates, such as β-glucan, providing insights into their ecological niches within digestive communities. This specificity indicates that gut microbial communities vary according to metabolic capacity, which in turn affects host health outcomes, particularly in humans (Yan, 2025). Additionally, understanding the metabolic interactions within gut microbial communities can facilitate classification beyond genetic data, emphasising functional biological characteristics. Furthermore, microbial metabolic pathways are integral to understanding optimal symbiotic relationships and adaptation mechanisms in diverse environments. For instance, the metabolism of insect pests demonstrates the interaction between microbial activity and host digestive processes, which is vital for nutrient absorption and detoxification (Mondal et al., 2023). Variations in microbial metabolism underpin adaptive strategies in insect populations, influencing their ecological niches, pest status, and resistance mechanisms. By integrating metabolic pathway analysis with traditional classification techniques, researchers can achieve a comprehensive, three-dimensional understanding of microbial taxonomy, ultimately advancing biotechnological applications and microbial community management in agricultural and clinical contexts.

2.6. Role of Microbial Taxonomy in Research and Medicine

The significance of microbial taxonomy in medicine and research is progressively increasing, as it underpins our comprehension of the interactions among various microorganisms and their hosts. Accurate classification of these organisms facilitates the identification of pathogenic species, thereby enabling researchers and clinicians to diagnose and treat diseases with greater efficacy. For instance, the development of targeted antimicrobial therapies relies on an effective taxonomic system that differentiates bacterial strains and their associated virulence factors. Such classification simplifies the monitoring of resistance patterns to antibiotics, providing essential information for public health policy formulation. Furthermore, the advent of advanced genomic techniques has revolutionised microbial taxonomy, allowing researchers to establish more precise classification frameworks and deepen our understanding of microbial functions and diversity, ultimately improving clinical outcomes and therapeutic strategies. Beyond disease diagnosis and treatment, microbial taxonomy plays a pivotal role in understanding host-microbiome interactions. These intricate interactions substantially influence numerous biological processes, including immunity, metabolism, and behaviour. Studies indicate that individual microbiome composition traces back to developmental stages influenced by maternal factors; notably, a substantial proportion of an infant's bacterial microbiome originates directly from maternal gut microbiota (Handley et al., 2019). By characterising and defining these microbial communities, researchers can explore correlations between microbiome structure alterations and health outcomes, thus identifying potential therapeutic avenues.

Additionally, ontological models, such as the Ontology of Host- Microbiome Interactions (OHMI), provide systematic frameworks for describing this complexity, thereby enhancing data integration and reproducibility in HMI studies (Alekseyenko et al., 2019). Such systematic approaches are essential for advancing knowledge concerning microbiomes and their medical applications. Moreover, microbial taxonomy extends beyond personalised medicine, where treatment is tailored according to an individual's microbial profile. Variability among microbial communities across individuals informs treatment strategies aiming to optimise therapeutic efficacy beyond traditional methodologies. The emerging discipline of metagenomics — analysing genetic material directly from environmental samples — exemplifies how microbial taxonomy can uncover previously undocumented species and elucidate their roles in health and disease. This knowledge bears implications for the design of targeted therapies and preventive strategies for conditions influenced by microbiome variation. As our understanding of the microbiome's role in human health progresses, it becomes apparent that precise microbial taxonomy is crucial for guiding future research and clinical management.

2.6.1. Implications for Antibiotic Resistance

The applications of microbial taxonomy profoundly influence the domain of antibiotic resistance, where microbial diversity significantly affects treatment outcomes. Traditional reliance on higher-level taxonomic classifications often fails to capture the complexities inherent at a more granular level of microbial functionality. By pinpointing individual strains and analysing their respective resistomes — the collection of antibiotic resistance genes present within a community — researchers can improve their understanding of the role that specific bacterial populations play in the dissemination of resistance. This insight holds particular importance within hospital environments, where the process of antibiotic selection can serve as a critical determinant in patient management and public health. Consequently, enhancing taxonomic frameworks through genomics-centric and functional knowledge will yield valuable insights into the mechanisms underlying antibiotic resistance and will more effectively inform therapeutic strategies (Sabaria, 2024). The progression of metagenomic sequencing techniques represents a fundamental advancement in elucidating the complexities of antibiotic resistance in relation to microbial taxonomy. High-resolution data facilitate the identification of bacterial guilds-communities comprised of co-occurring taxa that interact within particular environments. Analyses conducted at the guild level have provided evidence of distinct patterns in resistance gene expression and distribution, correlated with health status and disease conditions. For example, the identification of specific guilds with high resistance gene content can be utilized to predict the likely efficacy of antibiotic treatments based on the microbial community composition within a patient's microbiome. As these methodologies gain prominence, they shift focus away from broad-spectrum antibiotics toward more targeted interventions that consider an individual's microbial profile, thereby reducing the selective pressure for the development of resistance (Tang et al., 2024) (Figure 2. 13).

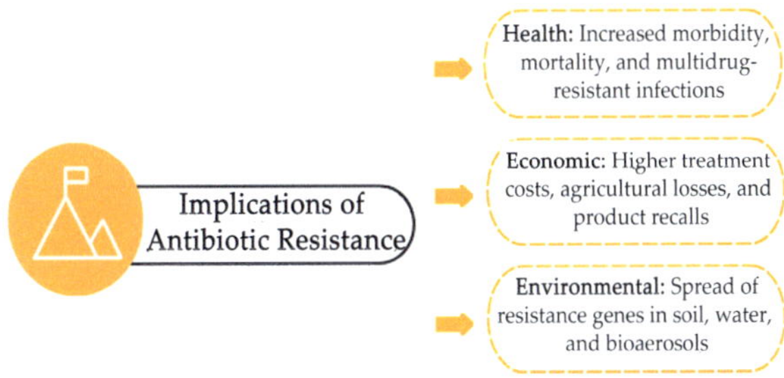

Figure 2.13. The problem of antibiotic resistance.

Source: https://www.mdpi.com/2076-0817/13/12/1123.

Ultimately, the implications of antibiotic resistance derived from microbial taxonomy and classification necessitate a paradigm shift in infectious disease management. As further research unveils the intricate interactions within microbial communities, it becomes increasingly apparent that oversimplified models are inadequate for elucidating the system's dynamic nature. A refined typology incorporating functional genomics enhances scientific comprehension and bears significant applications for public health policy. By concentrating on ecological interactions among microorganisms, we can strategically optimise interventions to prevent the emergence and dissemination of antibiotic-resistant strains. Consequently, the adoption of advanced microbial taxonomy and classification systems represents a crucial advancement in comprehensively and effectively addressing the urgent challenge of antibiotic resistance (Tang et al., 2024).

2.6.2. Importance in Environmental Microbiology

The role of microbial communities in environmental microbiology underpins the understanding of ecological systems and their health. Microorganisms, including bacteria, fungi, and viruses, inhabit nearly every habitat on Earth, fulfilling vital roles in processes such as nutrient cycling, bioremediation, and biodegradation. These processes are not only essential for maintaining ecological equilibrium but also for safeguarding human health and sustainability. For example, microbial communities decompose organic matter, recycling nutrients and promoting plant growth. The biodiversity within microbial taxonomies reflects the functional capabilities of these organisms; consequently, it is possible to propose an integrated approach to environmental management. By categorising and studying microbial taxa, scientists can better predict how alterations in environmental conditions—such as pollution or climate change—impact microbial functions and, consequently, broader ecological interactions. This underscores the importance of microbial classification in both foundational research and applied environmental science. Recent advancements in metagenomic methodologies have considerably expanded our understanding of environmental microbiology, particularly in complex ecosystems. Technologies like metagenomic next-generation sequencing (NGS) enable researchers to deconstruct intricate microbial communities and identify previously uncharacterized taxa and their ecological roles. This approach has been pivotal in identifying numerous pathogens and elucidating their interactions within ecosystems. For instance, data derived from metagenomic NGS-based studies have transformed our comprehension of microbiota across various environments, shedding light on their roles in ecosystem health and resilience. The increasingly systematic categorisation of microbial life facilitated by such discoveries enhances the monitoring and management of microbial ecosystems, which is vital for environmental sustainability. These developments highlight the integrative nature of microbial taxonomy and its practical application in addressing urgent ecological challenges and informing conservation initiatives.

Furthermore, beyond ecological functions, microbial taxonomy bears significant implications for human health and the understanding of disease. Research has demonstrated that microbiota present in environments such as soil and water bodies influence the dynamics of human-associated microbiomes. As the interplay between human health and environmental microorganisms becomes clearer, it emphasises the necessity of integrating environmental microbiology with microbial taxonomy. For example, the gut-brain axis is now widely recognised as a crucial pathway through which environmental microorganisms may affect neurological health, emphasising the connection between individual well-being and environmental conditions. Consequently, the classification of microorganisms not only supports ecological regulation but also plays a critical role in the development of therapeutic interventions for health issues, as alterations in microbial populations may be implicated in disease pathogenesis. This intersection of environmental microbiology and human health exemplifies the broader significance of microbial taxonomy classification in resolving ecological and health-related challenges, highlighting its unparalleled relevance in contemporary research and application (John et al., 2019; Michael et al., 2019).

2.6.3. Applications in Biotechnology

Applications of biotechnology are intricately linked to the principles of microbial taxonomy and classification, particularly in industrial and environmental contexts. A comprehensive understanding of microbial diversity, achieved through taxonomic classification, not only broadens our knowledge of microbial communities but also facilitates the optimisation of biotechnological processes. For example, methods such as metabarcoding have become fundamental in categorising the extensive array of microorganisms present in environmental samples and bioprocesses. Nonetheless, challenges persist, as bioinformatics approaches vary across laboratories, potentially hindering accurate result comparisons. Studies employing techniques such as DADA 2 illustrate how optimising the preprocessing of raw sequence data can improve taxonomic identification efficiency and, consequently, enhance the management of microbial resources for biotechnological applications (Babis et al., 2024). The potential to standardise these processes marks a significant advancement toward achieving maximal efficiency and effectiveness in biotechnological utilisation. Beyond taxonomic classification, the industrial application of microbial enzymes constitutes a vital sector within biotechnology, driven by microbial taxonomy knowledge. Enzymes derived from diverse microbial sources, including bacteria, fungi, and cyanobacteria, are extensively used across various industries, spanning pharmaceuticals, agriculture, and food production. These enzymes are integral to processes requiring specific catalytic properties, often obtained from extremophilic microorganisms capable of surviving in adverse conditions. Typically, submerged fermentation and solid-state fermentation techniques are employed for enzyme production. Accurate classification and separation of microorganisms enable the identification of strains suitable for specific industrial processes, thereby facilitating the use of enzymes tailored to particular industrial needs. This understanding enhances the capacity to leverage biological processes in technology, underscoring the significance of microbial taxonomy in fostering innovation within biotechnological sectors (Slimane & Nabti, 2024). By integrating genetic and taxonomic information with biotechnological applications, the effective utilisation of microbial resources is promoted, thereby advancing sustainable development. As biotechnological methods continue to evolve, the importance of microbial taxonomy in the discovery, classification, and exploitation of microbial entities will only intensify. Furthermore, advances in genomics and bioinformatics hold promise for improved monitoring of microbial populations and insights into their functional potential. Enhanced taxonomic resolution enables researchers to identify novel microbial strains with unique enzymatic or metabolic capabilities, which can be exploited for green technologies such as biofuels and bioremediation protocols. Consequently, the interplay between microbial taxonomy, classification, and biotechnological applications not only fosters scientific inquiry but also inspires innovative solutions to current challenges in medicine, industry, and environmental sustainability.

SUMMARY

The discovery of microbial taxonomy and classification bears considerable significance in enhancing our understanding of the complexity inherent in microbial populations. Looking ahead, it is apparent that emerging technologies, such as the gSpreadComp workflow, will augment our knowledge of microbial dynamics and their implications for public health. This approach exemplifies the efficacy of integrating comparative genomics with conventional taxonomic frameworks to generate insightful analyses of antibiotic resistance and virulence factors. By eliminating the necessity for hypothesis formulation through the application of sophisticated data processing techniques, the gSpreadComp process renders targeted microbial research more accessible, underscoring the demand for such methodologies in an increasingly dynamic scientific landscape (Kasmanas et al., 2025). In conclusion, the adoption of these advanced methods will better equip researchers to address urgent issues in microbial ecology and public health. Moreover, the importance of standardisation in microbial classification practices cannot be overstated. Research efforts related to metabarcoding, especially within environmental microbiology, emphasise issues arising from methodological diversity and the heterogeneity of databases, which consequently hinder effective cross-study comparisons. The employment of efficient algorithms such as DADA 2 for analysing 16S rRNA sequences to optimise the process allows researchers to achieve greater accuracy and reproducibility in taxonomic assignments. The findings that different 16S rRNA gene regions produce variable biodiversity estimates and taxonomic outcomes highlight the critical need for careful selection of markers and databases in microbial investigations (Babis et al., 2024). Such standardisation would not only advance scientific knowledge but also promote collaboration and comparability across laboratory studies, ultimately fostering progress within the broader scientific community engaged in microbial taxonomy and classification. Overall, research in microbial taxonomy and classification constitutes a vital component of microbiological inquiry, with significant applicability to public health and environmental management. As evidenced by workflows such as the gSpreadComp workflow and advancements in metabarcoding techniques, the integration of genomic data with rigorous taxonomic methodologies can provide valuable insights into microbial behaviour and interactions. The incorporation of this knowledge is essential for developing effective strategies to combat antibiotic resistance and to manage the influence of microbial diversity within ecosystems. As approaches and data exchange protocols continue to evolve, the future of microbial taxonomy will undoubtedly enhance our capacity to address complex biological challenges, thereby affording us a clearer understanding of the microbial world (Babis et al., 2024; Kasmanas et al., 2025).

The study of microbial taxonomy and classification is central to understanding the vast heterogeneity that characterises microbial life. Such fundamental advances in genomic profiling have highlighted the potential to identify discrete molecular subgroups within microbial populations, often associated with specific clinical phenotypes and disease courses. This molecular taxonomy not only enhances scientific understanding but also provides a basis for a mechanistic approach to microbial classification. Therefore, it is a basic tool for therapeutic research and clinical decision-making, emphasising the need to integrate genomic information into traditional systems of classification. By developing such a taxonomy, scientists can detect microbial properties and characteristics, leading to more effective control of microbial-related diseases and the development of targeted therapeutic approaches. In fact, studies on soil microbial communities illustrate the importance of taxonomic ranking in ecological management. For example, metagenomic studies have demonstrated the diverse roles of soil microorganisms across various ecosystems, as they perform vital functions such as nutrient cycling and organic matter decomposition. This is well exemplified by the widespread analysis of sandy soil samples within the Tubaiq conservation area, where high-throughput 16S rRNA sequencing revealed a rich diversity of microbes. With thousands of operational taxonomic units (OTUs) distributed across numerous phyla, families, and genera, the results highlight the intricate community structures that exist naturally. These findings are valuable for implementing agricultural practices and environmental policies, as they reveal the functional capacities and ecological significance of different microbial populations in diverse soil ecosystems. This research also enhances understanding of the broader implications of microorganism classification in environmental contexts. Microbial community structure identification not only aids ecological research but also improves comprehension of how such communities develop to adapt to various environments. The dominance of particular phyla, such as *Pseudomonadota*, and the abundance of *Actinomycetes*, exemplify how identification provides evidence of ecological interactions within these groups. Furthermore, functional characterisation of capacities such as amino acid transport and metabolism offers deeper insights into the ecological roles of these microorganisms in soil systems. Such information is essential for developing effective conservation and restoration methods, underscoring the importance of microbial taxonomy and classification in research and practical applications within ecosystem management.

CLOSER LOOK

INTERNATIONAL CODE OF NOMENCLATURE OF PROKARYOTES (ICNP)

The International Code of Nomenclature of Prokaryotes (ICNP) is the global nomenclature standard for naming prokaryotic microorganisms, i.e., bacteria and archaea. Formerly known as the *International Code of Nomenclature of Bacteria*, ICNP ensures consistency, clarity, and universality in prokaryotic nomenclature, enabling researchers globally to communicate effectively about microbial species. The ICNP is governed by the International Committee on Systematics of Prokaryotes (ICSP), which takes into account revisions and amendments to the Code. It establishes rules for naming novel taxa (species, genera, families, etc.), publication of valid names, and nomenclatural controversies. Names must be in Latin grammatical constructions and typically descriptive, honorific, or geographic.

To be validly published, a new prokaryotic name must meet several criteria:

- It must be published in the *International Journal of Systematic and Evolutionary Microbiology (IJSEM)*.
- A type strain of the organism must be deposited in at least two recognized culture collections in different countries.
- A detailed description must accompany the name, including morphological, physiological, and genetic characteristics (Figure 2.14).

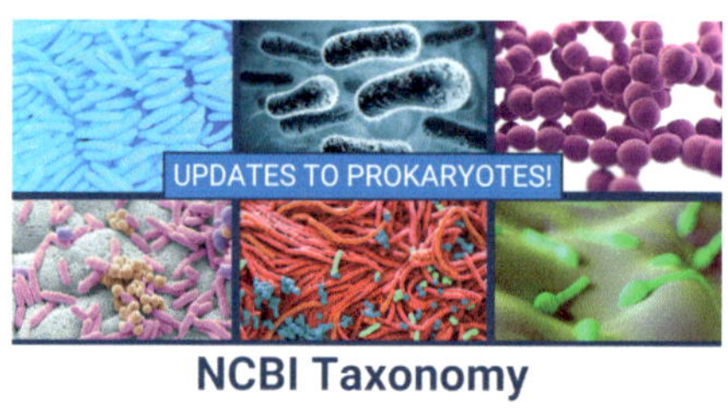

Figure 2.14. Visual representation of diverse prokaryotic microorganisms, highlighting recent updates to prokaryotic classification in the NCBI Taxonomy database.

Source: https://ncbiinsights.ncbi.nlm.nih.gov/wp-content/uploads/2024/10/Proks_NCBI-Taxonomy-2-e1727879532293.png.

The ICNP also gives instructions on dealing with synonyms, homonyms, and corrections of names to maintain taxonomic stability. Regular revision incorporates developments in molecular taxonomy, including genome-based classification, which is progressively impacting prokaryotic systematics. One of the fundamental principles under ICNP is the publication precedence principle, i.e., the first validly published name prevails. Exceptions are, however, allowed in a bid to preserve long-established and widespread names for stability's sake. The ICNP is significant in microbial taxonomy and science because it provides a standardized approach to naming and classifying prokaryotes. As microbial diversity continues to increase through metagenomic and culture-independent approaches, the ICNP continues to develop to facilitate taxonomic integrity and scientific purity throughout the sciences.

REFERENCES

1. S. Abhishek, A. T, P. Prakash and R. B. Bentov, "Microbial Taxonomy: An Artful Exploration of Microbes with Neural Networks," *2023 International Conference on Intelligent Computing, Communication & Convergence (ICI3C)*, Bhubaneswar, India, 2023, pp. 365-370, doi: 10.1109/ICI3C60830.2023.00076.(accessed on 16th July 2025).
2. Al-Awthan, Y. S., Mir, R., Alatawi, F. A., Alatawi, A. S., Almutairi, F. M., Khafaga, T., Shohdi, W. M., et al. (2024). Metagenome analysis identified novel microbial diversity of sandy soils surrounded by natural lakes and artificial water points in King Salman Bin Abdulaziz Royal Natural Reserve, Saudi Arabia. *Life, 14.* https://www.semanticscholar.org/paper/a85854c10a28f15d1f29105e8587a784f2599ae3 (accessed on 16th July 2025).
3. Alekseyenko, A. V., Beiting, D. P., Curtis, J. L., He, et al. (2019). *OHMI: The Ontology of Host-Microbiome Interactions.* https://core.ac.uk/download/286357479.pdf (accessed on 16th July 2025).
4. Almenderj, H., & Ismail, E. S. (2025). Classification and taxonomy of undeniable signatures: From early designs to post-quantum approaches. *European Journal of Pure and Applied Mathematics.* https://www.semanticscholar.org/paper/b4774854a8e6826c63f17a1519285e9f7ee2f6b7 (accessed on 16th July 2025).
5. Campanaro, S., Treu, L., Kougias, P.G. *et al.* Taxonomy of anaerobic digestion microbiome reveals biases associated with the applied high throughput sequencing strategies. *Sci Rep* **8**, 1926 (2018). https://doi.org/10.1038/s41598-018-20414-0(accessed on 16th July 2025).
6. Babis, W., Jastrzębski, J., & Ciesielski, S. (2024). Fine-tuning of DADA2 parameters for multiregional metabarcoding analysis of 16S rRNA genes from activated sludge and comparison of taxonomy classification power and taxonomy databases. *International Journal of Molecular Sciences, 25.* https://www.semanticscholar.org/paper/6f2408ee8156fac6a4e8a48cbd499d0f6570aed7 (accessed on 16th July 2025).
7. Heyer, R., Schallert, K., Büdel, A., Zoun, R., Dorl, S., Behne, A., Kohrs, F., Püttker, S., Siewert, C., Muth, T., Saake, G., Reichl, U., & Benndorf, D. (2019). A Robust and Universal Metaproteomics Workflow for Research Studies and Routine Diagnostics Within 24 h Using Phenol Extraction, FASP Digest, and the MetaProteomeAnalyzer. *Frontiers in microbiology*, *10*, 1883. https://doi.org/10.3389/fmicb.2019.01883(accessed on 16th July 2025).
8. Belhadi, A., Yazidi, A., Lind, P. G., & Djenouri, Y. (2025). EEG data classification: Review and taxonomy. *ACM Transactions on Computing for Healthcare.* https://www.semanticscholar.org/paper/c2dfb68a3a595ad69c6b6054dd794d646c147cda (accessed on 16th July 2025).
9. Bernard, E., Hasserjian, R. P., Greenberg, P. L., Arango Ossa, J. A., Creignou, M., Tuechler, H., Gutiérrez-Abril, J., et al. (2024). Molecular taxonomy of myelodysplastic syndromes and its clinical implications. *Blood, 144*, 1617–1632. https://www.semanticscholar.org/paper/0df05c9f6881a1d4128a8fda62a5e2bfd27744f9 (accessed on 16th July 2025).
10. Briones, C., & Amils, R. (1998). The evolution of function: a new method to assess the phylogenetic value of ribosomal sensitivity to antibiotics. *International microbiology : the official journal of the Spanish Society for Microbiology*, *1*(4), 301–306.(accessed on 16th July 2025).

11. Brune, A., Douglas, A. E., O'Donnell, A. G., Simpson, A. G. B., Underwood, A. J., Griffin, A. S., Bull, A. T., et al. (2013). *Size Doesn't Matter: Towards a More Inclusive Philosophy of Biology.* https://core.ac.uk/download/17297615.pdf (accessed on 16th July 2025).
12. Thompson, C. C., Chimetto, L., Edwards, R. A., Swings, J., Stackebrandt, E., & Thompson, F. L. (2013). Microbial genomic taxonomy. *BMC genomics*, *14*, 913. https://doi.org/10.1186/1471-2164-14-913(accessed on 16th July 2025).
13. Chuvochina, M., Rinke, C., Mussig, A. J., Chaumeil, P. A., Parks, D. H., & Hugenholtz, P. (2023). Genome Taxonomy Database and SeqCode: Microbial taxonomy and nomenclature in the age of big sequence data. *Biodiversity Information Science and Standards.* https://www.semanticscholar.org/paper/cf10f7fffea4a7c8bbd27f2f300ce1460d3d5b3e (accessed on 16th July 2025).
14. Cryan, J. F., O'Riordan, K. J., Cowan, C. S. M., Sandhu, K. V., Bastiaanssen, T. F. S., Boehme, M., Codagnone, M. G., et al. (2019). The microbiota-gut-brain axis. *Physiological Reviews, 99*, 1877–2013. https://doi.org/10.1152/physrev.00018.2018 (accessed on 16th July 2025).
15. Dhundale, V., Hemke, V. M., Desai, D., Joshi, S., Shete, P., & Kaur, G. (2021). Polyphasic approach to understand bacterial community landscape in soda lake environment. *Applied Ecology and Environmental Sciences.* https://www.semanticscholar.org/paper/386db582d67059635 46d9411584386333 0651168 (accessed on 16th July 2025).
16. Sharpton, T. J., Riesenfeld, S. J., Kembel, S. W., Ladau, J., O'Dwyer, J. P., Green, J. L., Eisen, J. A., & Pollard, K. S. (2011). PhylOTU: a high-throughput procedure quantifies microbial community diversity and resolves novel taxa from metagenomic data. *PLoS computational biology*, *7*(1), e1001061. https://doi.org/10.1371/journal.pcbi.1001061(accessed on 16th July 2025).
17. Slim Smaoui, Florence Mathieu, Lilia Fourati Ben Fguira, Georges Merlina, Lofti Mellouli. Taxonomy and antimicrobial activities of a new Streptomyces sp. TN17 isolated in the soil from an oasis in Tunis. Archives of Biological Science, 2011, 63 (4), pp.1047-1056. ff10.2298/ABS1104047Sff. ffhal-04310374(accessed on 16th July 2025).
18. Wagner, D. , Gattinger, A. , Lipski, A. and Schloter, M. (2005): Methane fluxes, microbial activities and community structures in a wet tundra of the Lena Delta , 22. International Polartagung, Jena, September 18-24 . (accessed on 16th July 2025).
19. Handley, S. A., Holtz, L. R., Lim, E. S., Maqsood, et al. (2019). *Discordant transmission of bacteria and viruses from mothers to babies at birth.* https://core.ac.uk/download/286537341.pdf (accessed on 16th July 2025).
20. Okoh C., Roy R., Mehnen J., Redding L. and Harrison A.. Development of an Ontology for Aerospace Engine Components Degradation in Service. DOI: 10.5220/0005090201080119 In Proceedings of the International Conference on Knowledge Engineering and Ontology Development (KEOD-2014), pages 108-119(accessed on 16th July 2025).
21. Helene, L. C. F., Klepa, M. S., & Hungria, M. (2022). New insights into the taxonomy of bacteria in the genomic era and a case study with rhizobia. *International Journal of Microbiology, 2022.* https://www.semanticscholar.org/paper/b977fc6437b3087398316e31d034f47bf4f0011b (accessed on 16th July 2025).
22. Jiang, Y., Wang, J., Xia, D., & Yu, G. (2017). EnSVMB: Metagenomics fragments classification using ensemble SVM and BLAST. *Scientific Reports, 7.* https://www.semanticscholar.org/paper/92349549f2154f157d54d3b07380eb5b242e0f0a (accessed on 16th July 2025).

23. Jiao, J. Y., Abdugheni, R., Zhang, D. F., Ahmed, I., Ali, M., Chuvochina, M., Dedysh, S., et al. (2024). Advancements in prokaryotic systematics and the role of Bergey's International Society for Microbial Systematics in addressing challenges in the meta-data era. *National Science Review, 11.* https://www.semanticscholar.org/paper/360ad886a86802e2db261e7a6579ffb09d9fed3c (accessed on 16th July 2025).

24. Kasif, S., Roberts, R. J., & Zheng, Y. (2004). *Segmentally Variable Genes: A New Perspective on Adaptation.* https://core.ac.uk/download/3451156.pdf (accessed on 16th July 2025).

25. Kasmanas, J. C., Magnúsdóttir, S., Zhang, J., Smalla, K., Schloter, M., Stadler, P. F., de Carvalho, A. C. P. L. F., et al. (2025). Integrating comparative genomics and risk classification by assessing virulence, antimicrobial resistance, and plasmid spread in microbial communities with gSpreadComp. *GigaScience, 14.* https://www.semanticscholar.org/paper/e331729edda62985458bb0ff6f5853a8aba2265f (accessed on 16th July 2025).

26. Li, G., Wang, Z., Wu, C., Wang, D., Han, I., Lee, J., Kaeli, D. R., et al. (2025). Towards high-accuracy bacterial taxonomy identification using phenotypic single-cell Raman spectroscopy data. *ISME Communications, 5.* https://www.semanticscholar.org/paper/5e76db79110d502ed0e99521de5f3bf5bc178a86 (accessed on 16th July 2025).

27. Ludwig, D. (2018). *Letting go of "natural kind": Toward a multidimensional framework of nonarbitrary classification.* https://core.ac.uk/download/131213147.pdf (accessed on 16th July 2025).

28. Mondal, S., Somani, J., Roy, S., Babu, A., & Pandey, A. (2023). Insect microbial symbionts: Ecology, interactions, and biological significance. *Microorganisms, 11.* https://www.semanticscholar.org/paper/cb179d89d57ee5a4b6f95a250ead6d7e9d342fd3 (accessed on 16th July 2025).

29. Pavlinov, I. (2016). *Biodiversity and Biocollections: Problem of Correspondence.* https://core.ac.uk/download/131209780.pdf (accessed on 16th July 2025).

30. Peng, Z., Qian, X., Liu, Y., Li, X., Gao, H., An, Y., Qi, J., et al. (2024). Land conversion to agriculture induces taxonomic homogenization of soil microbial communities globally. *Nature Communications, 15.* https://www.semanticscholar.org/paper/4c15c7c01f90549c007cca63605e3153622d698d (accessed on 16th July 2025).

31. Pereira, M. S., Rodrigues, D. L., Ariute, J. C., Carneiro, D. V. D., Sodrzeieski, P. A., Gama, M. A. S., de Souza, E. B., et al. (2024). Beyond the basics: Taxonomic classification and pathogenomics in recently discovered *Dickeya dadantii* isolates. *Taxonomy.* https://www.semanticscholar.org/paper/8fda0291b3f7d6fb94861f8fa856ea001a115372 (accessed on 16th July 2025).

32. Riesco, R., & Trujillo, M. E. (2024). Update on the proposed minimal standards for the use of genome data for the taxonomy of prokaryotes. *International Journal of Systematic and Evolutionary Microbiology, 74.* https://www.semanticscholar.org/paper/51a47285d669a32251bb3d8fd097122a206d3328 (accessed on 16th July 2025).

33. Sabaria, S. (2024). Harnessing machine learning for metagenomics: Discovering the invisible microbial world. *Communications on Applied Nonlinear Analysis.* https://www.semanticscholar.org/paper/e20229232884cb33a9de9fc2cc5081d73f040573 (accessed on 16th July 2025).

34. Shiffer, A., Wolfe, B., Maurice, C. F., Caporaso, J. G., Rideout, J. R., Neufeld, J. D., Bokulich, N. A., et al. (2016). *Mockrobiota: A Public Resource for Microbiome Bioinformatics Benchmarking.* https://core.ac.uk/download/323066010.pdf (accessed on 16th July 2025).

35. Slimane, M., & Nabti, E.-h. (2024). Recent status in production, biotechnological applications, commercial aspects, and future prospects of microbial enzymes: A comprehensive review. *International Journal of Agricultural Science and Food Technology.* https://www.semanticscholar.org/paper/386c2023d5010c1e14e12a006f76365f57d70224 (accessed on 16th July 2025).

36. Tang, S., Wu, G., Liu, Y., Xue, B., Zhang, S., Zhang, W., Jia, Y., et al. (2024). Guild-level signature of gut microbiome for diabetic kidney disease. *mBio, 15.* https://www.semanticscholar.org/paper/081042becd75fadacd853d51cbf6738c323cbcbb (accessed on 16th July 2025).

37. Val-Calvo, J., & Vázquez-Boland, J. (2023). Mycobacteriales taxonomy using network analysis-aided, context-uniform phylogenomic approach for non-subjective genus demarcation. *mBio, 14.* https://www.semanticscholar.org/paper/3d8885b60d3beb32cc85cf9e4327f07bca608d2b (accessed on 16th July 2025).

38. Wilson, M. R., Sample, H. A., Zorn, K. C., Arevalo, S., Yu, G., Neuhaus, J., Federman, S., et al. (2019). Clinical metagenomic sequencing for diagnosis of meningitis and encephalitis. *New England Journal of Medicine, 380*, 2327–2340. https://doi.org/10.1056/nejmoa1803396 (accessed on 16th July 2025).

39. Yan, J. (2025). Immune and metabolic pathways of microbial population structure remodeling in biopharmaceuticals for intestinal diseases. *Molecular & Cellular Biomechanics.* https://www.semanticscholar.org/paper/fb5f99b5baa0d84d35bcb9d21326a7f13d1c3229 (accessed on 16th July 2025).

40. Zhang, Q., Ahmed, K., Sharda, N. K., & Wang, H. (2024). A comprehensive survey of animal identification: Exploring data sources, AI advances, classification obstacles and the role of taxonomy. *International Journal of Intelligent Systems.* https://www.semanticscholar.org/paper/989de81caecfe7e8f2a1c4ddc49e9685b3ed9c4b (accessed on 16th July 2025).

41. Zhang, Y., Yang, R., Xu, X., Li, R., Xiao, J., Shen, J., & Han, J. (2024). TELEClass: Taxonomy enrichment and LLM-enhanced hierarchical text classification with minimal supervision. *Proceedings of the ACM on Web Conference 2025.* https://www.semanticscholar.org/paper/6083c840b4f9d5edbae0d60c7d330a76cd965a6a (accessed on 16th July 2025).

42. Zheng, D., Zou, L., Zou, J., Li, Q., & Lu, S. (2024). Refining taxonomic identification of microalgae through molecular and genetic evolution: A case study of *Prorocentrum lima* and *Prorocentrum arenarium*. *Microbiology Spectrum, 12.* https://www.semanticscholar.org/paper/d20583deaf77eace82cea215a5ce4ab175b17b0e (accessed on 16th July 2025).

43. Zitouni, A., Lebrihi, A., Athalye, et al. (2006). *Taxonomy and chemical characterization of antibiotics of Streptosporangium Sg 10 isolated from a Saharan soil.* https://core.ac.uk/download/12039754.pdf (accessed on 16th July 2025).

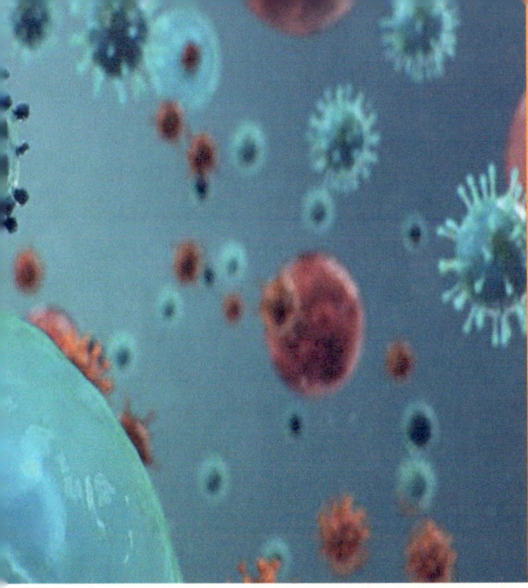

Chapter 3

MICROBIAL PHYSIOLOGY AND GENETICS

Contents

Introduction

Microbial physiology provides essential data on the fundamental processes that sustain microbial life, such as metabolism, growth, and reproduction. It explores the cellular machinery of microbes, detailing how microorganisms convert nutrients into energy and build necessary cellular components. Understanding these physiological processes is important not only for scientific research but also for practical applications in areas like medicine and biotechnology. When researchers investigate how microorganisms respond to environmental conditions, they uncover the various strategies microbes use to thrive in different settings. For instance, some bacteria resist extreme environments by modifying their metabolic pathways, demonstrating the complex relationship between microbial physiology and ecological adaptability. Additionally, the incorporation of genetic studies has made significant progress in microbial biotechnology. Using genetic techniques, scientists can engineer microbial genomes to enhance desirable traits, such as higher biomass yield or greater stress tolerance. Advances in gene expression systems for Gram-positive bacteria, especially those with low guanine and cytosine content, exemplify this potential. The ability to use inducible expression systems enables scientists to employ these microbes as cell factories in medical and agricultural biotechnology. These developments highlight the importance of genetic modification in boosting microbial efficiency, offering innovative solutions to urgent problems in food production and medicine (de Vos et al., 1997). Moreover, studying how microorganisms interact with their environment provides valuable insights into ecosystem functions. Microbes play a key role in many biogeochemical cycles, particularly those of carbon and nitrogen. A well-known model organism in this context is Sphagnum, found in peatland ecosystems with high microbial diversity. The unique physiology of Sphagnum and its associated microbiome illustrates the intricate interactions between plant and microbial life that regulate large-scale carbon storage in soils. As climate change alters these interactions, it becomes increasingly important to investigate the physiological mechanisms of both Sphagnum and its microorganisms. Recent research emphasises the need for a comprehensive understanding of these relationships through genomic studies, ultimately helping us better comprehend ecosystem responses to environmental change (Weston et al., 2015).

Definition and Scope of Microbial Physiology

Microbial physiology constitutes a branch of microbiology that examines the functions, structures, and properties of microorganisms at the cellular level. It encompasses a broad spectrum of topics, including metabolism, growth, cell differentiation, and mechanisms of microbial adaptation to various environmental stresses.

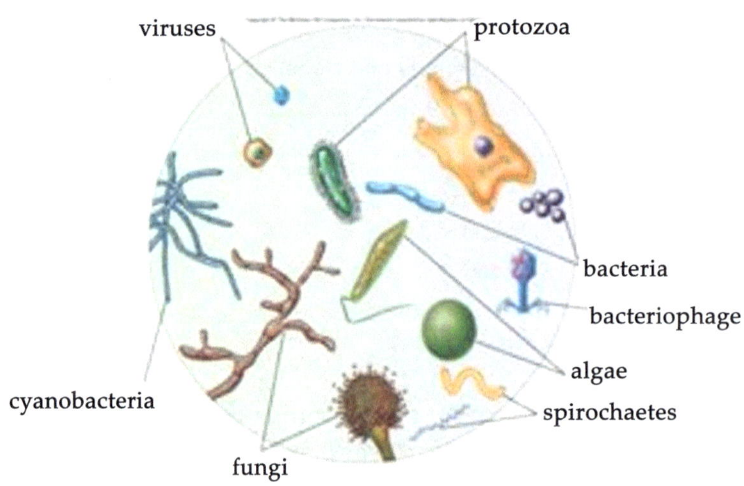

Figure 3.1. Microbial physiology.

Source: https://external-content.duckduckgo.com/iu/?u=https%3A%2F%2Ftse4.mm bing.net%2Fth%2Fid%2FOIP.sdzmtcMykbsdEOjMzGfY1gHaEK%3Fpid%3DApi&f=1&ipt =f1299934ec099dd309fff462beba45b92ab 35c132c936a0618339d72e47d7be5.

Central to microbial physiology is the comprehension of how microorganisms communicate with their environment, which involves the adsorption of nutrients and the removal of wastes.

Studying these processes not only enhances our understanding of the life cycles of archaea, bacteria, fungi, and viruses but also elucidates their crucial roles in ecosystems, human health, and disease. Therefore, the scope of microbial physiology extends beyond cellular mechanics to include the ecological and evolutionary significance of microorganisms in diverse environments. An examination of the methodological approaches employed in microbial physiology reveals its inherently interdisciplinary nature. Techniques such as genomics, metabolomics, and proteomics play vital roles in elucidating complex biochemical pathways that underpin microbial processes. These methods enable researchers to infer relationships between microbial activity and health outcomes, particularly within human microbiomes. A significant focus of current research is on understanding dysbiosis, a state of microbial imbalance associated with numerous disease conditions. Notably, discussions concerning the relationship between the gut microbiome and human health are exemplified by workshops aimed at establishing quantifiable characteristics of the gut microbiome as markers of well-being (McBurney et al., 2019) (Figure 3.1).

This emphasises the significance of a collaborative, interdisciplinary research endeavour to elucidate such complex interactions. Furthermore, microbial physiology is continually transformed by technological innovations and evolving conceptual frameworks. The traditional assumption that disease and health are confined within the organism has been challenged by the recognition of microbial communities as essential contributors to these states (Morar & Skorburg, 2018). This evolving perspective informs our understanding of how microbial physiology not only impacts individual organisms but also influences broader ecological processes and health outcomes. As scientists further investigate the physio-genetic dynamics of microorganisms, it becomes increasingly evident that a comprehensive understanding of microbial physiology is crucial for addressing major health challenges and advancing biotechnological applications. Consequently, the discipline of microbial physiology exemplifies a genuine integration of the biological sciences, wherein an understanding of microbial complexity is vital for fostering both theoretical and applied microbiology, as well as genetic research.

Importance of Studying Microbial Physiology

The research into microbial physiology is of paramount importance in understanding the fundamental principles that govern existence at the microscopic level. Microbial physiology examines the biochemical and physiological processes undertaken by microorganisms, offering insights into their metabolic activities, reproductive mechanisms, and responses to environmental stimuli. The knowledge gained from microbial physiology has broad applications, especially in the fields of biotechnology and medicine. By studying microbial processes, researchers can utilize such microorganisms beneficially, for example, in bioremediation, wherein microorganisms aid in the remediation of contaminated environments, and in pharmaceutical production. Additionally, studying microbial physiology is crucial in developing strategies to combat infectious diseases, as it allows researchers to target specific microbial functions or structures, leading to the development of more effective medicines and vaccines. Moreover, the interaction between microbial physiology and host health is significant, particularly concerning the human microbiome. Microbial communities residing within and on the human body are responsible for maintaining homeostasis, influencing processes ranging from digestion to immune responses. Dysbiosis, or imbalance of these microbial communities, has been associated with various diseases, including metabolic disorders, autoimmune conditions, and mental health issues. Scientific investigations have demonstrated that the gut microbiota, for instance, plays a role in the gut-brain axis, mediating interactions between the brain and the gastrointestinal system, thereby affecting behaviour and mood (Hou et al., 2022). Consequently, exploring microbial physiology provides essential insights into how these microbial populations influence health and disease and paves the way for novel treatments leveraging microbiota modulation for improved health outcomes. The relevance of microbial physiology extends beyond human health to encompass ecological and environmental considerations. Microorganisms are central to nutrient cycling, contribute to organic matter decomposition, and regulate greenhouse gas concentrations. They are crucial for activities such as nitrogen fixation, which underpins plant growth and agricultural productivity.

Furthermore, in light of global challenges such as climate change, understanding microbial physiology could inform strategies to mitigate environmental impacts. For example, some microorganisms can be engineered to enhance carbon sequestration or improve soil health, thereby addressing food insecurity and climate change simultaneously (Lin et al., 2021). In sum, the study of microbial physiology not only advances our fundamental understanding of living organisms but also equips us with the tools necessary to address pressing societal challenges.

3.1. Basic Cellular Structures of Microorganisms

The identification of the fundamental cell structures of microorganisms is crucial to understanding microbial physiology and genetics. Microorganisms, such as bacteria, archaea, fungi, and protozoa, have distinct cell architectures that determine their functions. For example, bacterial cells are usually characterised by a peptidoglycan-based rigid cell wall, which provides shape and structural strength. This cell wall also helps protect against environmental stresses and supports osmotic balance. Archaea, however, possess unique cell membranes composed of ether-linked lipids, distinguishing them from bacteria and reflecting their adaptation to extreme environments. These structural differences among prokaryotic microorganisms highlight the evolutionary diversity of microbial life and have important implications for understanding their roles in various biological processes. Beyond their membranes and cell walls, microbial cellular structures include the cytoplasm and various organelles, each contributing to the microbe's physiology. The cytoplasm is a gel-like substance where metabolism occurs, including ribosomes that are essential for protein synthesis. Prokaryotes, such as bacteria, lack membrane-bound organelles but carry out necessary cellular functions through simpler structures. For instance, bacterial ribosomes are vital for transforming genetic information into proteins, demonstrating efficient functioning within compact cellular systems. Significantly, the process of evolutionary divergence of cells, as outlined in the Omnis cellula e cellula dogma, indicates a common lineage for all cellular organisms and suggests that microbial structures evolved under similar constraints and opportunities, providing further evidence of their biological importance (Baluška et al., 2023). The study of microbial cell structures also extends to their genetic components, emphasising the close relationship between cellular physiology and genetics. Microorganisms exhibit remarkable genetic variability, including chromosomal DNA, plasmids, and transposable elements, which contribute to their adaptability and evolution. This genetic diversity enables microorganisms to thrive in diverse environments and develop resistance to antibiotics and other stresses. Moreover, understanding microbial genetics underscores the role of horizontal gene transfer — gene exchanges between organisms outside of normal reproduction—in shaping microbial communities and their evolution. As ongoing research uncovers more about microbial life, concepts such as the 'homeostatic reprogramming hypothesis' reveal how microbial functions and structures are interconnected, enhancing our understanding of microbial communities (Ma et al., 2024).

3.1.1. Prokaryotic versus Eukaryotic Cells

The distinction between prokaryotic and eukaryotic cells constitutes a fundamental principle of microbial physiology and genetics. Prokaryotic cells, characterised by their simple structures, lack a nucleus and membrane-bound organelles.

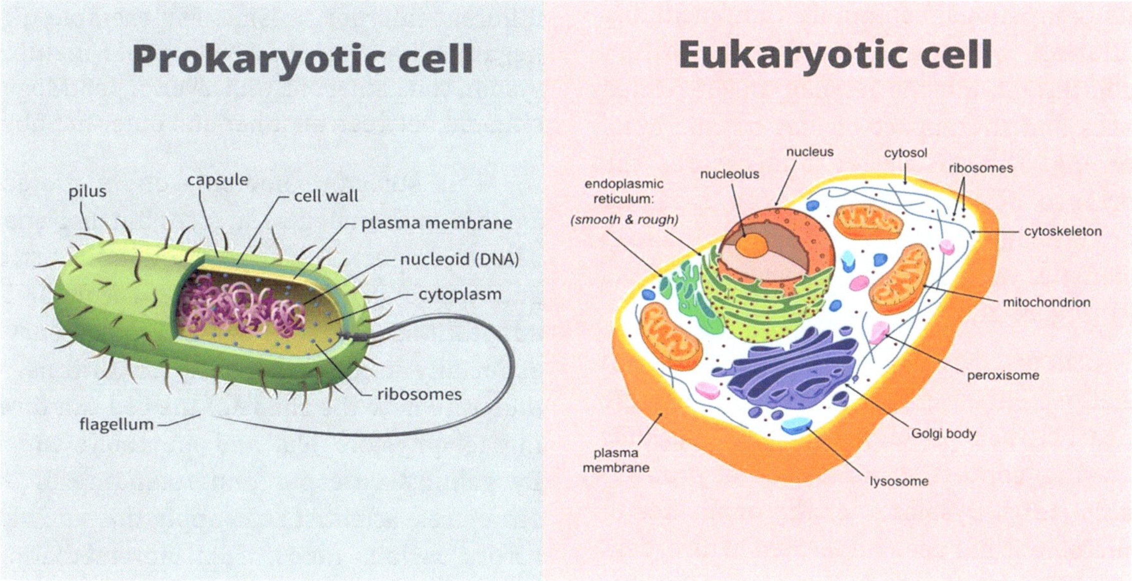

Figure 3.2. Prokaryotic cell versus eukaryotic cell.

Source: https://external-content.duckduckgo.com/iu/?u=https%3A%2F%2Fdashamlav.com%2Fwp-content%2Fuploads%2F2021%2F12%2Fprokaryotic-eukaryotic-cells-dashamlav.jpg&f=1&nofb=1&ipt=b53d8c647fa24791b38abb75cd78f46079b8f6792e3b77867e7732db111bc570.

This organisational simplicity facilitates ease of cell division and adaptability, which accounts for the ability of prokaryotes, such as bacteria, to thrive in diverse habitats. Conversely, eukaryotic cells possess a permanent nucleus and specialized organelles, enabling a higher degree of cellular organisation and specialisation. Such cellular complexity permits eukaryotes, including fungi, plants, and animals, to perform more advanced physiological functions. These structural differences not only influence metabolic pathways but also guide the evolutionary trajectories of these groups. Understanding these distinctions provides a foundational basis for examining cellular interactions within ecosystems, as well as in health and disease contexts. Beyond structural variations, the functional importance of prokaryotic and eukaryotic cells has significant implications for microbial ecology. For example, the gut microbiota predominantly comprises prokaryotic organisms that play vital roles in digestion, immunity, and overall health. The communication networks between eukaryotic and prokaryotic cells, such as the microbiota-gut-brain axis, exemplify the extensive influence these cells exert on physiological processes. Prokaryotes produce a diverse array of metabolites, from neurotransmitters that can influence host behaviour and mood to factors affecting numerous other host functions, demonstrating a complex interkingdom interaction. An understanding of this bidirectional communication, including modulation by neurotransmitters, offers valuable insights into the aetiology of gut-related illnesses and the impact of diet on microbial patterning. This discussion underscores the importance of analysing both cell types to explore the complexities of microbial physiology and genetics in health and disease (Baj et al., 2019) (Figure 3.2. 2).

Recent discoveries regarding gut microbial populations enhance the understanding of the balance between prokaryotes and eukaryotes within the context of inflammatory bowel diseases (IBD). Dysbiosis, or the imbalance of gut microbiota, has been implicated in disorders such as IBD, with a notable increase in specific prokaryotic taxa frequently documented. Advances in high-throughput sequencing technologies have elucidated significant alterations in microbial populations, and the intricate interactions among bacteria, fungi, and viruses in the gut have been characterised.

The interplay between prokaryotic and eukaryotic cells in the pathogenesis of IBD underscores that these microbial communities play not only a passive but also an active role in disease processes. This insight opens new avenues for therapeutic strategies aimed at microbial manipulation to restore homeostasis within the gut microbiota and potentially mitigate IBD symptoms. It highlights the critical importance of adopting an integrated approach in microbiological investigations of human health (Zuo et al., 2018).

3.1.2. Unique Structures in Microbial Cells

Microbial cells exhibit a remarkable diversity of characteristic structures that allow them to survive in various habitats and carry out specialized functions. A clear example of this is the presence of specialized outer cell walls and membranes, which differ significantly among different microorganisms. For example, Gram-negative bacteria have a double-membrane system consisting of a thin layer of peptidoglycan situated between an inner and outer membrane.

This structure not only offers protection against environmental stresses but also enables selective permeability, allowing nutrients and waste products to pass through. Such adaptations are vital for microbial survival, especially under changing conditions, and illustrate how the shape of the cell can directly impact physiological and metabolic capacity. By gaining a deeper understanding of these structures, scientists can apply this knowledge across various fields, from bioremediation to biotechnology. Another intriguing aspect of microbial cell architecture is the presence of specialized organelles that differ from eukaryotic cell organelles. Many bacteria, for instance, possess intracytoplasmic membranes, which provide additional surface area for metabolic processes, especially in environments rich in substrates like organic carbon. These membranes can house numerous enzymatic pathways responsible for energy production in bacteria, such as those used by photosynthetic cyanobacteria or chemolithotrophic organisms capable of converting inorganic compounds into energy (Figure 3.3).

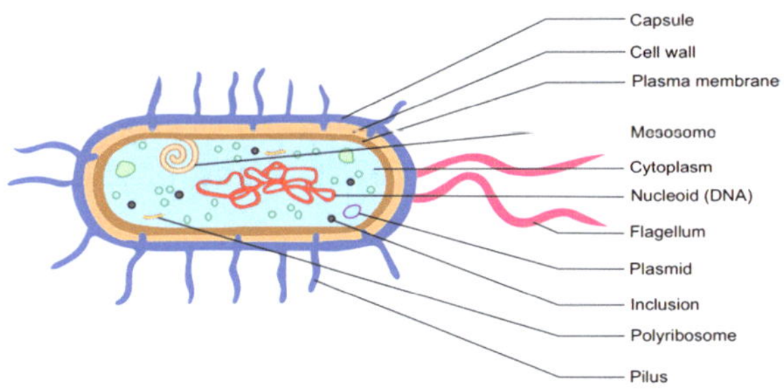

Figure 3.3. Ultrastructure of a bacterial cell.

Source: https://external-content.duckduckgo.com/iu/?u=https%3A%2F%2Fimg.brainkart.com%2Farticle%2Farticle-Ultrastructure-of-a--jhj.png&f=1&nofb=1&ipt=c5b360062ab4d0c08c9379bb5d823b0d0cf0acf74a79839a72234f7365a12631.

Moreover, some archaea have specialized cells known as gas vesicles, which enable them to float in aquatic environments, thereby enhancing light exposure and nutrient uptake. This inventive structural feature of microbial cells provides strong evidence for the complex relationship between form and function, which underpins their ecological diversity across a remarkably wide range of habitats. The functions of new microbial structures also reflect their adaptive strategies for surviving extreme conditions. For example, polar microbial communities feature specialized biochemical pathways and cell structures that allow them to endure cold, saline environments observed during seasonal changes in sea ice. Studies show that community composition subtly shifts under different temperature and salinity conditions, demonstrating the dynamic nature of microbial physiology. During such transitions, bacteria and algae exhibit distinct metabolite profiles tailored to their specific environments, highlighting the link between specialized cell forms and environmental adaptation. Additionally, the accumulation of compatible solutes like proline and glycine betaine exemplifies how these microorganisms maintain cellular integrity and function under stress. Understanding these processes is essential for evaluating microbial roles in ecosystem functioning and biogeochemical cycles, especially as climate warming continues to affect polar ecosystems (Dawson et al., 2023). This foundational knowledge of microbial structures greatly enriches the broader fields of microbial physiology and genetics.

3.1.3. Role of Cell Membranes in Microbial Function

The role of cell membranes in microbial life is vital because they both protect and support the numerous cellular functions necessary for growth and survival. Mainly composed of phospholipids, membranes form a compartmentalised space that helps preserve the cell's structure. This is especially important for microbial cells like bacteria, which depend on their membranes to separate metabolic processes from the external environment. The structural integrity of cell membranes not only shields microorganisms from harmful environmental factors but also controls the entry and exit of nutrients and waste, thereby influencing their physiological state and gene expression. The function of cell membranes is therefore central to microbial metabolism and plays a key role in enabling microorganisms to adapt to changing environmental conditions. Additionally, microbial cell membranes are dynamic and exhibit considerable flexibility in function and composition, depending on environmental and metabolic needs. In the case of pathogens such as *Escherichia coli*, the outer membrane contains essential components like lipopolysaccharides and phospholipids that help defend against external stressors, including antibiotics. These membrane-associated molecules also affect the cell's shape, growth, and ability to adapt to stress. Furthermore, disruptions in membrane composition can impair cellular functions, potentially increasing their vulnerability to environmental factors. Understanding these interactions enhances our knowledge of metabolic pathways used by microorganisms and provides a basis for developing engineering strategies to optimise microbial production processes, particularly within the field of synthetic biology, as discussed in recent reviews of microbial genetics and physiology (Wang et al., 2021) (Figure 3.4).*Escherichia coli*

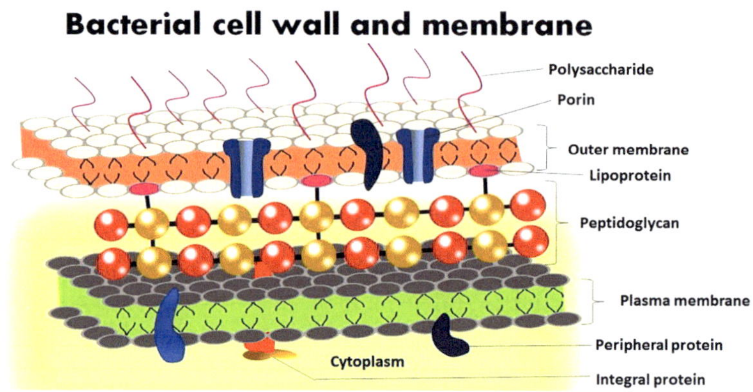

Figure 3.4. Bacterial cell wall and membrane.

Source: https://external-content.duckduckgo.com/iu/?u=https%3A%2F%2Fwww.biologybrain.com%2Fwp-content%2Fuploads%2F2021%2F06%2FBacterial-cell-membrane-768x387.jpg&f=1&nofb=1&ipt=5037ba95fa22a781e9ded02c8d560aaf62abbaefbc10c288e1f76afbf0dfac79.

Notably, the interaction between host-derived factors and microbial cell membranes is a growing area of interest, especially in the context of health and disease. To illustrate, changes in cell membrane lipid structure have been linked to inflammatory conditions such as inflammatory bowel disease (IBD), where the gut microbiota plays a crucial role. Disruption of lipid regulation has been shown to impact microbial physiology as well as the immune function of the host, highlighting the central interface in the function of the intestinal epithelial barrier. Microbial and host lipid interactions can also influence not only disease development but also the overall health of the gut ecosystem. By exploring these interactions, researchers aim to identify new biomarkers and therapeutic targets that will enhance understanding of microbial dynamics and intestinal inflammation (Kayama & Takeda, 2023). Consequently, studying cell membranes in microbial processes helps us understand the complex biological interdependencies that underpin health and disease states.

3.2. Metabolic Pathways in Microorganisms

Understanding metabolic pathways in microorganisms is essential for grasping their genetic adaptations and physiological functions. Microorganisms are highly versatile in their metabolic processes, enabling them to thrive in diverse habitats and metabolise various substrates for energy and growth. Processes like fermentation, respiration, and biosynthesis are carefully regulated based on genetic makeup, environmental conditions, and nutrient availability. For example, different bacterial species may generate energy through alternative biochemical pathways such as anaerobic respiration or photosynthesis, highlighting the evolutionary significance of metabolic diversity among microbial lineages. Not only does this diversity ensure survival amid environmental changes, but it also plays a crucial role in host microbiomes, demonstrating the mutualistic relationship between host health and microbial metabolism. The interactions between microorganisms and their hosts emphasise the importance of microbial pathways on larger scales than individual cells. Studies have shown that specific gut microbiota communities in humans metabolise diet-derived nutrients in ways that influence host metabolism and immune responses. For instance, research on a high-protein, high-fat Western diet indicates it leads to a unique microbiome composition in primates, characterised by a rise in Firmicutes and a decrease in *Prevotella*. Conversely, in a primate model such as the vervet, the trend reverses, revealing significant diversity in metabolic pathways across species. These findings suggest that gut microbiota not only respond to nutritional inputs but can also impact the host's metabolic health and disease susceptibility, making the understanding of metabolic pathways vital for elucidating these complex interactions (Amato et al., 2015). Furthermore, the regenerative capabilities of microorganisms hint at intricate relationships between metabolic pathways and tissue maintenance mechanisms. For example, the adult intestinal epithelium undergoes rapid turnover and possesses regenerative capacity primarily supported by stem cell activity. In microbial populations, metabolic routes are also vital for repair and regeneration, especially when responding to environmental stresses like nutrient deprivation or injury. Research on the *Drosophila melanogaster* midgut has demonstrated that stem cells contribute to intestinal homeostasis, revealing regenerative processes analogous to those in microbial communities. By understanding how cell growth and repair are influenced by metabolic pathways, scientists can uncover broader implications for tissue regeneration and homeostasis across various organisms and deepen our understanding of microbial physiology and genetics (Nászai et al., 2015).

3.2.1. Overview of Catabolic and Anabolic Pathways

An understanding of catabolic and anabolic activities is fundamental to microbial physiology and genetics because these activities determine how microorganisms acquire, utilize, and store energy.

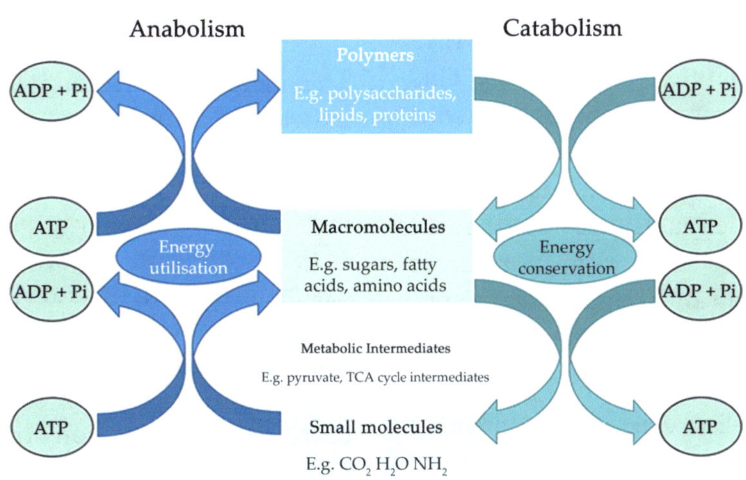

Figure 3.5. Catabolic and anabolic pathways.

Source: https://external-content.duckduckgo.com/iu/?u=https%3A%2F%2Fsciencevivid.com%2Fwp-content%2Fuploads%2F2022%2F08%2FCoupling-of-anabolic-and-catabolic-pathways.png&f=1&nofb=1&ipt=cb4d0ce1beb72d5a3678865f8bf97e6ba4c085b2e6f2ed57eb60b4c4d60012a1.

Catabolic activities, primarily involving the breakdown of complex molecules into simpler forms, are a vital source of energy production through processes such as glycolysis and the citric acid cycle. These biochemical reactions not only generate the energy necessary for various cellular functions, stored within cells, but also produce metabolic intermediates that can be directed into anabolic processes. By degrading carbohydrates, proteins, and fats, microorganisms effectively obtain the energy essential for survival, growth, and reproduction, thereby enabling them to inhabit diverse ecological niches. This essential distinction between energy release and its utilization forms the basis of microbial metabolism, influencing processes from growth regulation to gene expression in response to environmental stimuli. Conversely, anabolic pathways are critically involved in biosynthesis and cellular repair, responsible for constructing macromolecules requisite for microbial structure and activity. Through mechanisms such as protein synthesis and nucleotide biosynthesis, anabolic processes harness energy and precursors derived from catabolic activities, assembling them into larger and more complex biomolecules. This is particularly significant for microorganisms, which are frequently subjected to fluctuating nutrient availability and environmental stresses. For example, the capacity to synthesize nucleotides and amino acids from more basic precursors can directly affect a microorganism's genetic stability and resilience (Figure 3.5).

Interestingly, the balance between catabolism and anabolism can change depending on metabolic needs or external conditions, highlighting the complex regulatory mechanisms that control microbial life and survival strategies under various circumstances. The reliance of catabolic and anabolic processes on each other is further underlined by their ability to enable metabolic diversification in microorganisms. As these organisms must adapt to changing environments, they can easily switch between energy production and biosynthesis to optimise their growth and efficiency, a sensitivity that is vital for survival. These metabolic pathways not only reflect cellular energy management but also impact broader biological processes such as disease development. For instance, the structure and function of gut microbiomes can influence diseases like colorectal cancer, where metabolic interactions between microbial communities are key (Reber, 2021). Moreover, research into immunometabolism shows that there are specific metabolic pathways involved in immune cell differentiation and function, thereby emphasising the interconnected nature of metabolism across different biological systems (Makowski et al., 2020). Understanding these pathways is crucial for biotechnological applications and for advancing therapeutic strategies in health care.

3.2.2. Energy Production in Microbial Cells

The metabolic diversity of microbial cells is instrumental in energy production and their capacity to adapt to various environmental conditions. Microorganisms utilize diverse mechanisms for energy generation, including respiration and fermentation, which are essential for their survival and ecological roles. Electrochemically active bacteria (EAB) are particularly significant in facilitating contemporary energy conservation through extracellular electron transfer (EET). For example, *Shewanella oneidensis* MR-1 has been extensively studied as a model organism to investigate the physiological and genetic mechanisms underpinning its metabolic diversity. A comprehensive understanding of the catabolic processes of *S. oneidensis* MR-1 allows researchers to enhance energy production methods, notably in microbial fuel cells (MFCs), where microbial activities convert organic substrates into electrical energy, thereby advancing biotechnological applications (Hirose et al., 2019) (Figure 3.6).

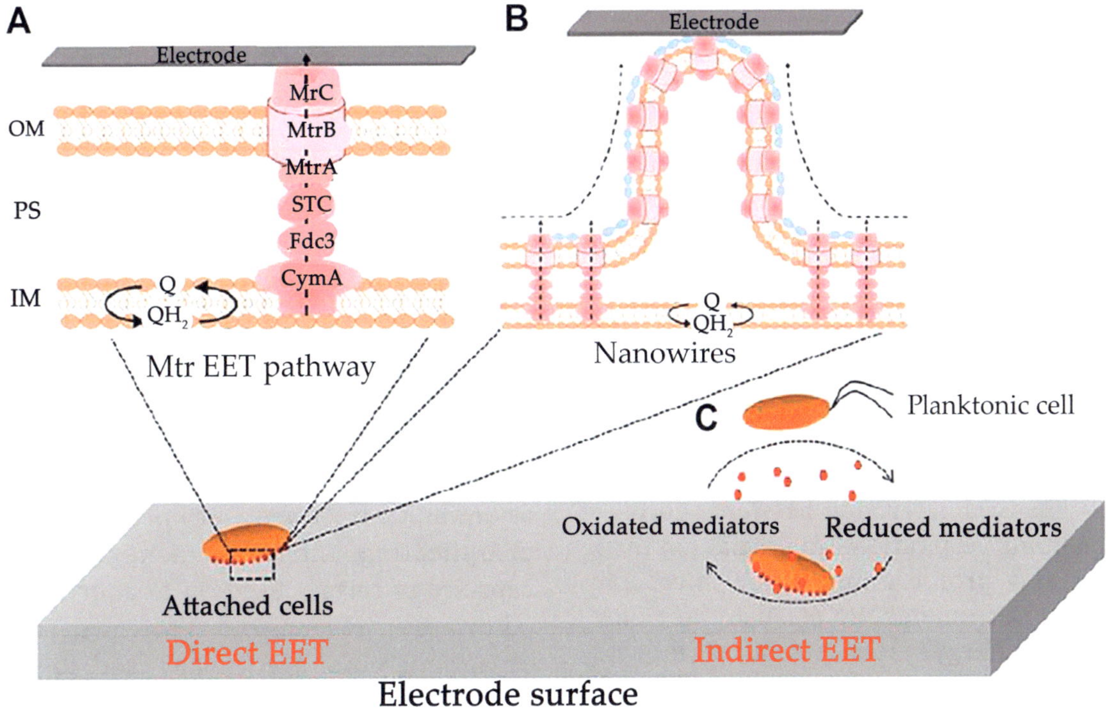

Figure 3.6. Extracellular electron transfer (EET) pathways of *Shewanella oneidensis* MR-1 to electrodes.

Source: https://www.researchgate.net/figure/Extracellular-electron-transfer-EET-pathways-of-Shewanella-oneidensis-MR-1-to_fig1_356756405.

Microbial electrochemical technologies (METs) represent a new convergence of electrochemistry and microbiology, harnessing microorganisms' unique traits to generate energy. Over the past two decades, METs have been widely used in electricity production through interactions between microorganisms and electrodes. They not only serve as a prominent alternative energy source but also contribute to sustainable technologies such as wastewater treatment and biofuel synthesis. Research has shown that METs could facilitate a circular economy by reusing carbon, thereby integrating microbial metabolism into sustainable energy generation. Additionally, combining synthetic biology with METs is opening innovative pathways for designing microbial systems with high energy efficiency, supporting the growth of renewable energy sources (Sarah, 2019). Advances in genetic modification of microbial cells have further expanded the potential for targeted energy production, particularly through EET pathways. Genetic engineering enables the optimisation of microbial metabolism for increased energy capture and product synthesis in microbial electrosynthesis. These modifications enhance power output from MFCs and improve waste-to-energy conversion processes. The intersection of microbial physiology and molecular genetics paves the way for developing novel microbial strains for improved bioelectrochemical systems. As research progresses into genetic engineering and synthetic biology, it becomes increasingly clear that microbial cells could play a pivotal role in future sustainable energy solutions (Hirose et al., 2019; Sarah, 2019).

3.2.3. Importance of Metabolic Flexibility

Metabolic flexibility constitutes a vital facet of microbial physiology, enabling organisms to adapt to fluctuating environmental conditions and substrate availability. It is particularly essential for microorganisms that prosper in diverse ecological niches, where nutrient and oxygen supplies significantly influence metabolic pathways. For example, the biochemical mechanisms through which certain bacteria alternate between aerobic and anaerobic respiration are crucial for their survival and proliferation under microoxic conditions. Such metabolic plasticity not only maximises energy yield but also impacts microbial interactions within ecosystems, contributing to nutrient cycling and ecological stability. An understanding of the intricacies of metabolic flexibility in microorganisms can substantially enhance insights into broader implications concerning microbial genetics and physiology, emphasising the evolutionary processes underpinning microbial viability in complex environments- as demonstrated in recent research on microbial behaviour under various oxidative conditions (Prakash et al., 2025). The relevance of metabolic flexibility extends beyond ecological considerations, encompassing significant implications for agricultural management, particularly in the domain of animal husbandry. Investigations have established that rumen bacterial metabolism, exemplified by the NK 3 A 20 group, plays a pivotal role in hydrogen and methane production, thereby influencing greenhouse gas emissions from ruminants (Rachel et al., 2023). By elucidating the metabolic processes of these microorganisms, scientists can develop strategies to inhibit methane formation and optimise feed utilisation. The regulation of hydrogen production based on substrate availability underscores the adaptability of ruminal microbial communities. It highlights the importance of metabolic flexibility in promoting animal health while minimising environmental impact. These findings emphasise the significance of metabolic plasticity in microbial biology and its potential to address sustainability challenges in agriculture.

Furthermore, the function of metabolic flexibility is integral to the resolution of microbial resistance to environmental stresses and therapeutic interventions. In clinical contexts, pathogenic microbes exhibiting metabolic plasticity can respond to hostile conditions such as antibiotic treatments or immune responses, complicating infection management. The capacity of certain bacteria to alter metabolic pathways in response to nutrient deprivation or antimicrobial agents may lead to chronic infections and the development of antibiotic resistance. An understanding of the genetic foundations of metabolic plasticity, supported by ongoing research, has the potential to facilitate the development of targeted therapeutics aimed at disrupting microbial adaptation, thus improving treatment outcomes. Therefore, the study of metabolic flexibility not only augments knowledge of microbial physiology but also fosters innovative approaches in medicine and agriculture, emphasising the interconnectedness of microbial genetics and physiology across various disciplines.

3.3. Microbial Growth and Reproduction

The process of microbial development and propagation is inherently linked with a complex, multilateral relationship involving both genetic and environmental factors. Microorganisms such as bacteria and fungi primarily develop and propagate through asexual means, including binary fission, wherein a cell divides into two genetically identical daughter cells. This reproductive method is straightforward yet highly efficient, facilitating rapid population increase under optimal conditions and resulting in exponential growth patterns. Factors such as nutrient availability, temperature, and pH significantly influence microbial growth dynamics. For instance, particular species exhibit resilience and thrive in extreme environments, demonstrating adaptive traits that enhance their reproductive success across diverse habitats. Accordingly, understanding the genetic basis governing these reproductive strategies is essential for elucidating microbial physiology, offering insights into their evolutionary trajectories and ecological roles. At the genetic level, microbial growth is regulated by specific genes controlling cell cycle timing, including genes involved in chromosome duplication and the synthesis of cell wall components necessary for maintaining structural integrity during division. Notably, studies involving probiotic strains such as *Bifidobacterium animalis* subsp. *lactis* illustrates how targeted microbial introduction can modulate growth patterns and gene diversity within indigenous gut microbiota. By analysing single-nucleotide polymorphism variations and growth rates, researchers have demonstrated adaptive responses to environmental cues, such as probiotic supplementation. This reflects the intricate mechanisms through which microorganisms alter their reproductive and growth behaviours in response to environmental dynamics, underscoring the importance of genetic considerations in microbial adaptability and community dynamics (Shen et al., 2024). Furthermore, microbial reproduction, its regulation, and timing are not solely physiological processes but are also influenced by evolutionary forces shaping microbial lifecycles. For example, in various ecosystems, the coordinated reproductive cycles of certain microorganisms have evolved to synchronise with seasonal changes, thereby optimising survival and reproductive opportunities. Drawing inspiration from avian migratory studies, researchers have also examined the extent to which genetic variation in clock genes can regulate reproductive timing among microorganisms, despite a less well-defined relationship. Exploring genetic constraints on adaptive evolution in microorganisms provides insight into their responses to ecological stress and offers potential implications for microbial evolution and ecology. Therefore, the intersection of microbial growth, reproduction, and genetics remains a fertile area for further investigation, considering these processes are embedded within broader ecological frameworks (Louis-Stéphane et al., 2023).

3.3.1. Factors Affecting Microbial Growth

Understanding how environmental factors influence microbial growth is essential for grasping their physiology and genetics. The most critical factor is often the presence or absence of nutrients, which directly impacts microbial metabolism and growth. Macronutrients such as carbon, nitrogen, and phosphorus are vital for cellular functions like energy metabolism, biosynthesis, and repair. Trace elements like iron and zinc are also crucial, serving as cofactors in enzymatic reactions. When these nutrients are plentiful, microbial populations flourish, resulting in high biomass and metabolic activity. Conversely, nutrient scarcity can cause low growth rates or even cell death. Therefore, understanding nutrient cycling within microbial communities is vital for agricultural management and environmental regulation. Optimising these processes allows for manipulation of microbial communities to enhance crop yields and sustainability. Temperature also significantly influences microbial growth by affecting enzymatic activity and membrane fluidity. Each species has an optimal temperature range for growth, metabolism, and reproduction. Psychrophiles thrive in cold conditions, while thermophiles prefer warm environments. Temperatures outside these optimal ranges inhibit growth by denaturing proteins and disrupting cellular functions (Figure 3.7).

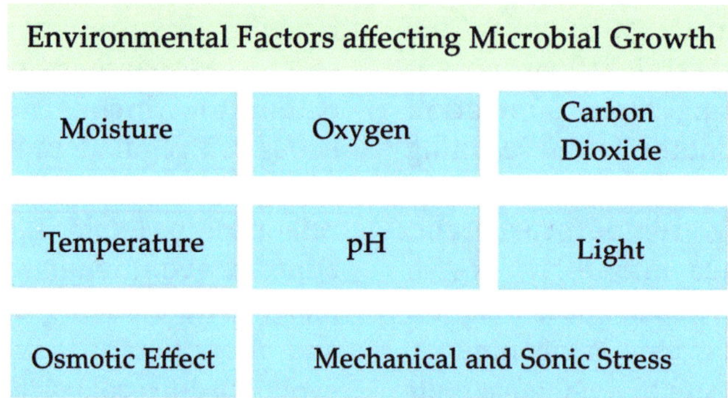

Figure 3.7. Environmental factors affecting microbial growth.

Source: https://microbenotes.com/environmental-factors-affecting-microbial-growth/.

Furthermore, temperature plays a crucial role in delineating microbial community structures, as different species exhibit varying temperature tolerances. Adaptation to temperature has become increasingly significant as a factor during global climate change, during which shifting temperatures have the potential to redefine microbial dynamics within ecosystems. This consideration is particularly pertinent when examining microbial nutrient mobilization in soil, a vital component for maintaining agricultural productivity and ecosystem functionality. Consequently, understanding the thermal effects on microbial growth is essential for predicting changes in microbial populations under global climatic conditions. Another critical factor influencing microbial growth is pH, which regulates enzyme activity, nutrient availability, and overall cellular performance. Various microorganisms display different affinities for pH, with some adapted to thrive in acidic environments and others in alkaline conditions. The pH level in a given environment can profoundly impact nutrient and toxin solubility, thereby determining microbial community composition. For instance, extremophiles such as acidophiles and alkaliphiles have evolved specialized mechanisms to sustain cellular functions under extreme pH conditions. Additionally, the interaction of ph with other environmental factors, such as water availability and temperature, adds complexity to microbial growth. Advances in metagenomics, as highlighted by Zarraonaindia & Gilbert (2015), emphasise the importance of pH in shaping microbial communities within their natural habitats. Ongoing research into the interactions between pH, microbial physiology, and genetics will increasingly contribute to enhancing agricultural productivity and the efficient management of microbial ecosystems, consistent with findings from the Human Microbiome Project as reported by Juengst & Huss (2009).

3.3.2. Modes of Reproduction in microorganisms

Microbial existence exhibits remarkable diversity in reproductive modes, which are crucial for thriving and adapting to various environments. Asexual reproduction through binary fission is one of the main methods in microorganisms, where a cell divides into two identical progeny cells. This mechanism enables rapid population growth and is common in bacteria. Furthermore, the simplicity of binary fission allows for quick adaptation to environmental changes, enabling microorganisms to utilize resources efficiently. Besides asexual reproduction, some microorganisms also engage in genetic recombination through methods such as conjugation, transformation, or transduction.

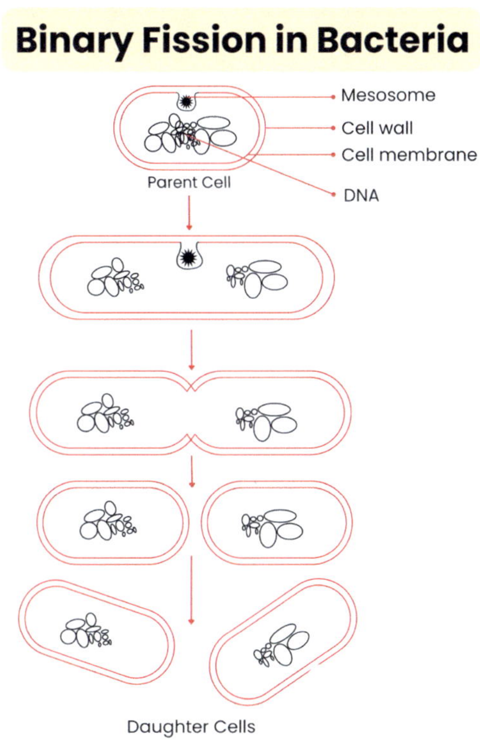

Figure 3.8. Binary fission in bacteria.

Source: https://www.vedantu.com/biology/reproduction-in-bacteria.

The recombination increases genetic diversity, making it possible for new traits to emerge and confer advantages in competitive environments. The holobiont theory further complicates understanding microbial reproduction by highlighting the relationship between host organisms and their microbiomes. The holobiont concept suggests that the combined behaviour of a host and its microbial community provides a better basis for selection at the holobiont level rather than at the level of individual microbes. This perspective opens avenues for exploring vertical and horizontal microbial community transmission, where the former involves offspring inheriting microorganisms from their parents, and the latter pertains to acquiring microorganisms from the environment. These processes can significantly influence microbial community structure and function, implying that reproductive modes may extend beyond traditional definitions to include the transmission of symbiotic associations between hosts and microbiomes, as observed in contemporary holobiont selection models (Roughgarden, 2020) (Figure 3.8).

The interactions among environmental parameters also influence microbial reproductive activities. Environmental factors such as nutrient availability, temperature, and the presence of toxic substances may cause microbial populations to modify their reproductive patterns. For example, under conditions of environmental stress, some microorganisms may enter the spore formation stage, thereby enhancing their ability to survive adverse conditions before resuming metabolic activity once stability is restored. This adaptability is supported by data linking microbial fitness to metal resistance genes, thereby offering insights into the connection between reproduction and survival across various ecological niches (Carlson et al., 2017). A comprehensive understanding of microbial reproduction is therefore essential for understanding larger-scale ecological interactions, evolutionary processes, and the potential for engineering microbial systems for beneficial applications in biotechnology and ecological management.

3.3.3. Growth Curve Phases and Their Significance

The microbial growth curve is typically divided into four distinct phases: lag, log, stationary, and death. Each phase represents a specific response of microbial populations to environmental conditions and nutrient sources. During the lag phase, cells adapt to their new environment and produce the necessary enzymes and molecules essential for growth. This adaptive stage is vital because it prepares microorganisms for the subsequent exponential growth observed during the log phase. The quick adjustment of microorganisms to environmental changes influences metabolic activities and generally impacts growth dynamics. Understanding these growth stages is therefore important in microbial physiology and genetics, as they ultimately guide research into microbial adaptability and survival strategies under various conditions. Once microorganisms enter the log phase, they begin to grow rapidly, leading to a geometric increase in cell numbers. This phase involves continuous cellular division and occurs under optimal environmental conditions, with minimal waste accumulation and abundant resources. It is a crucial phase, as it can be used to study metabolic activity, such as the rate of substrate consumption and product formation. For example, research on various microbial activities at this stage can shed light on cellular respiration and fermentation processes (Figure 3.9).

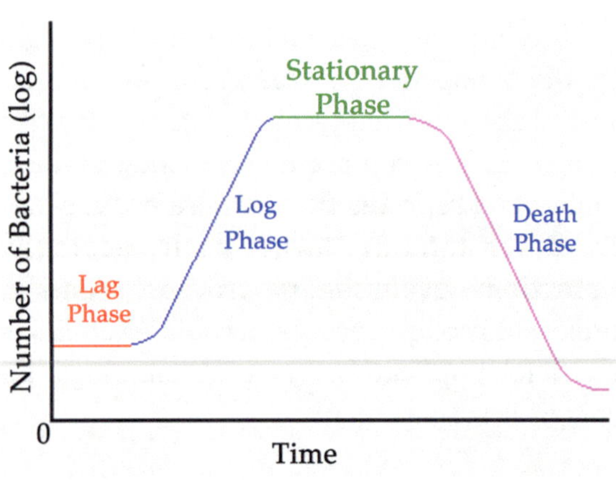

Figure 3.9. Phases of the bacterial growth curve.

Source: https://homework.study.com/cimages/multimages/16/curve4629487187208285227.gif.

The growth kinetics that occur have significant implications in biotechnology, where optimising microbial growth is essential for successful product formation. Understanding this phase guides genetic manipulation research and metabolic engineering applications aimed at enhancing microbial function for industrial purposes. As microbial populations approach the stationary phase, there is a sharp decline in growth rate, and population size stabilises due to resource scarcity and waste product accumulation. Competition for nutrients intensifies, and cells may enter a state where survival mechanisms become crucial. This is when microbial tolerance to stressors, such as high pH or osmotic stress, becomes most effective. The physiological responses of microorganisms, including metabolic and gene expression changes, play a vital role in maintaining viability under stressful conditions. For example, Lijklema (1971) demonstrated how biochemical processes and oxygen consumption reflect the adaptive responses of microorganisms when interacting with their environment. Additionally, this phase significantly impacts microbial ecology and biotechnology research grounded in understanding microbial stability and resilience, such as the influence of diet on microbial populations discussed by Beever et al. (2008). Such dynamics are central to both academic research and applied sciences in microbial management.

3.4. Genetic Material in Microorganisms

Microbial genetic material analysis provides valuable insights into microbial genetics, physiology, and the strength of interactions between microbial genomes and host environments. Microorganisms, especially bacteria, have unique genetic structures that enable their adaptability and survival. This plasticity is particularly evident in the gut microbiota of warm-blooded animals, where microbial cells can outnumber host cells by up to 100 times. Microorganisms are essential for numerous physiological functions, including metabolism and immune system regulation. Understanding microbial population genetic diversity helps explain how these microorganisms influence health and disease, highlighting the need for further exploration of their genetics to comprehend their complex interactions with host systems, as shown in recent reports on gut microbiota and genetic makeup (Fathima et al., 2022). The role of genetic material in microorganisms extends beyond individual species to include interactions within microbial communities. Dysbiosis, or microbial imbalance, can lead to serious health issues, impacting the immune system and overall metabolism. The gut microbiome develops from its sterile state at hatching through an evolutionary process shaped by environmental, dietary, and genetic factors. These interactions underline the importance of genetic material not only for microbial survival but also for maintaining homeostasis in the host. Disruption of this balance may result in various diseases, including cardiovascular disorders and cancers, further underscoring the complex connection between microbial genetic material and host health (Hou et al., 2022). Advances in genetic and microbial manipulation have opened new opportunities for managing dysbiosis-related health problems. Probiotics, prebiotics, and synbiotics are strategies used to modify the gut microbiota, promoting balance and health. The heterogeneity and intricacy of microbial populations often hinder straightforward correlations between specific microbial compositions and health outcomes. Consequently, more research is required into the genetic factors that influence microbial interactions, community structure, and their effects on host biology. Ultimately, increasing knowledge of microbial genetic material offers the potential to develop innovative clinical approaches, such as targeted microbiota modulation and fecal microbial transplants, aiming to promote health and reduce microbiota-related diseases (Fathima et al., 2022; Hou et al., 2022).

3.4.1. Structure and Function of Microbial DNA

Microbial DNA exhibits distinctive structural characteristics tailored to meet the specific requirements of microbial organisms. Microbial genomes are generally composed of circular DNA molecules, which are more efficient and compact compared to linear DNA found in eukaryotes. The circular morphology facilitates rapid replication and efficient gene expression, features that are crucial for microorganisms inhabiting unpredictable environments. This compactness is further supported by nucleoid-associated proteins that organise the DNA within the microbial cell. These structural attributes enhance the organism's ability to respond swiftly to environmental changes by ensuring that essential processes such as replication, transcription, and translation are carried out effectively, thereby promoting microbial survival and growth. Additionally, the potential for microbial DNA to be involved in horizontal gene transfer increases genetic diversity, allowing microorganisms to evolve rapidly in response to new challenges or to acquire advantageous traits, such as antibiotic resistance, which are critical factors in microbial evolution. The functions of microbial DNA extend beyond mere gene coding; they encompass a range of biochemical processes integral to cellular physiology. For example, microbial genomes contain genes encoding proteins involved in energy metabolism, nutrient uptake, and stress response. These functions are vital for microbial survival amidst fluctuating environmental conditions characterised by diverse resources and stressors. The characterisation of microbial DNA can determine the metabolic capabilities of microbial populations and enable researchers to assess their roles in ecological processes such as biogeochemical cycling. Furthermore, the study of plasmids, or extrachromosomal DNA molecules, underscores the significance of DNA-mediated horizontal gene transfer, which enhances adaptability to extreme environments and contributes to the formation of microbial communities with specialized functional roles (Zhai et al., 2024) (Figure 3. 10).

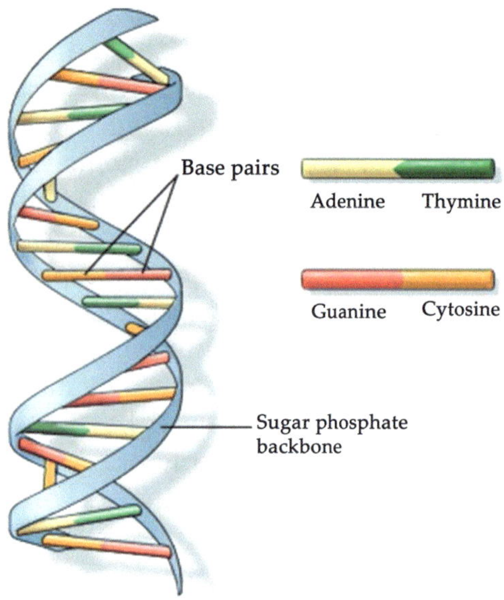

Figure 3.10. DNA molecules.

Source: https://medlineplus.gov/images/PX000098_PRESENTATION.jpeg.

Investigating microbial DNA structure and function highlights its crucial role in maintaining microbial physiology and genetics. Studying circulating microbial DNA (cmDNA) in peripheral blood underscores the dynamic interactions between host and microbes. The study shows that cmDNA has a distinct composition compared to gut microbial DNA and suggests a selective mechanism that regulates its presence in the bloodstream. Additionally, the reduced diversity of cmDNA indicates a more advanced interaction between microbial communities and the host immune system, shedding light on how such dynamics could impact overall health. Advanced genomic tools, such as genome-resolved metagenomics, deepen our understanding of microbial traits and ecological significance. These studies explain the dynamic relationships between microorganisms and their environments, ultimately enhancing our knowledge of microbial ecology and its relevance to human health and ecosystem function (Greenlon et al., 2022).

3.4.2. Plasmids and Their Role in Genetic Diversity

Plasmids are diminutive circular DNA molecules that are devoid of chromosomal DNA and are vital to microbial genetic diversity. Their independent replication and transfer between bacteria render them an optimal mechanism for horizontal gene transfer (HGT), the primary driver of evolutionary adaptation. Plasmids possess the capacity to encode various genes, including those conferring antibiotic resistance and metabolic functions, thereby enabling bacteria to respond more swiftly to environmental stresses. Unlike chromosomal mutations, which occur over extended periods, HGT via plasmids can transpire within populations in mere hours, significantly augmenting genetic variability.

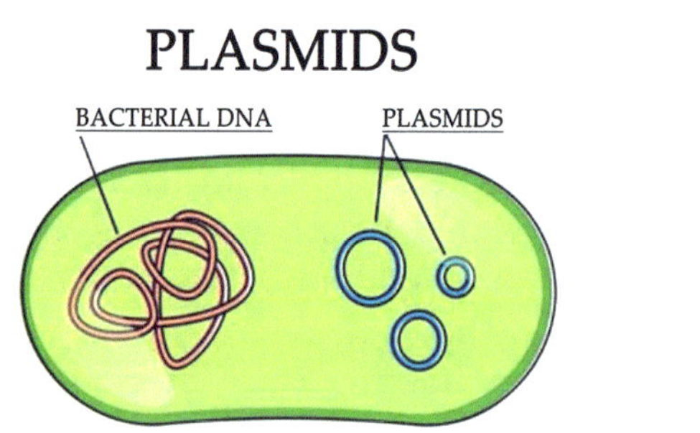

Figure 3.11. Plasmid DNA.

Source: https://geneticeducation.co.in/wp-content/uploads/2019/11/plasmid-DNA-.001-e1573187155268.jpeg.

Furthermore, plasmids can harbour a wide range of traits that are environmentally linked to the host bacterium's surroundings, underscoring their dynamic role in adaptation to specific ecological niches, as evidenced by experiments with Curtobacterium (Finks et al., 2024) (Figure 3.11).

The diversity of plasmids and their associated genes is not only extensive but also exhibits significant variation across different bacterial species. Plasmids are prevalent within certain bacterial groups, although their presence and genetic composition can be highly heterogeneous, even among closely related strains. This lack of phylogenetic conservation indicates that plasmids are typically transmitted horizontally, thereby introducing novel genetic elements into bacterial populations. Such a process enhances microdiversity within microbial communities and plays a vital role in niche differentiation. For example, plasmids conferring antibiotic resistance are particularly important, as their dissemination within natural ecosystems poses serious public health challenges due to the rapid evolution of resistance (Tokuda et al., 2024).

Moreover, understanding how plasmids contribute to genetic diversity and facilitate adaptation is critical in addressing emerging issues within microbial communities. The mechanisms of plasmid transfer and their survival in diverse environments underscore the significance of mobile genetic elements in microbial evolution. By enabling the exchange of traits such as antibiotic resistance genes, plasmids influence the overall competitive fitness of microbial populations. Consequently, plasmid-mediated horizontal gene transfer is fundamental to microbial physiology and is integral to efforts aimed at preventing the spread of antimicrobial resistance. A comprehensive understanding of these processes is essential, not only for microbiology but also for public health, as it supports the development of effective interventions against the escalating threat posed by resistant microorganisms (Finks et al., 2024; Tokuda et al., 2024).

3.4.3. Horizontal Gene Transfer Mechanisms

Horizontal gene transfer (HGT) constitutes a fundamental biological process through which microorganisms acquire genetic material from other organisms. Unlike vertical gene transfer, which occurs during reproductive processes, HGT facilitates the dissemination of DNA between unrelated organisms, thereby promoting rapid genetic adaptation. It serves as a significant catalyst in microbial evolution, particularly in response to environmental stressors. For example, specific atomic structures such as the ATPases present in *Thaumarchaeota* have expanded their ecological niches via horizontal transfer mechanisms. These adaptive features, coupled with environmental responses, underscore the dynamic interplay of microbial physiology and genetic flexibility, emphasising the critical role of HGT in microbial diversity and survival amid changing environments, including extreme conditions like acidic soils and oceanic depths (Wang et al., 2019). The implications of HGT extend beyond individual survival, influencing broader ecological interactions and microbial community adaptations. Microbial symbionts, which are integral components of larger biological entities, significantly benefit from the genetic diversity conferred by HGT. Notably, in coral reef ecosystems, the switching and shuffling of symbionts in response to environmental pressures demonstrates the potential for substantial reorganisation of host functions. This genetic exchange enables holobionts to adapt rapidly, highlighting HGT's role not only in immediate survival but also in long-term adaptive strategies. Microbial strains subjected to high environmental pressures evolve to better fit their habitats, with the evolutionary process markedly accelerated, illustrating a dynamic relationship wherein HGT acts as a driving force for diversification and resistance within microbial communities (Webster & Reusch, 2017) (Figure 3.12).

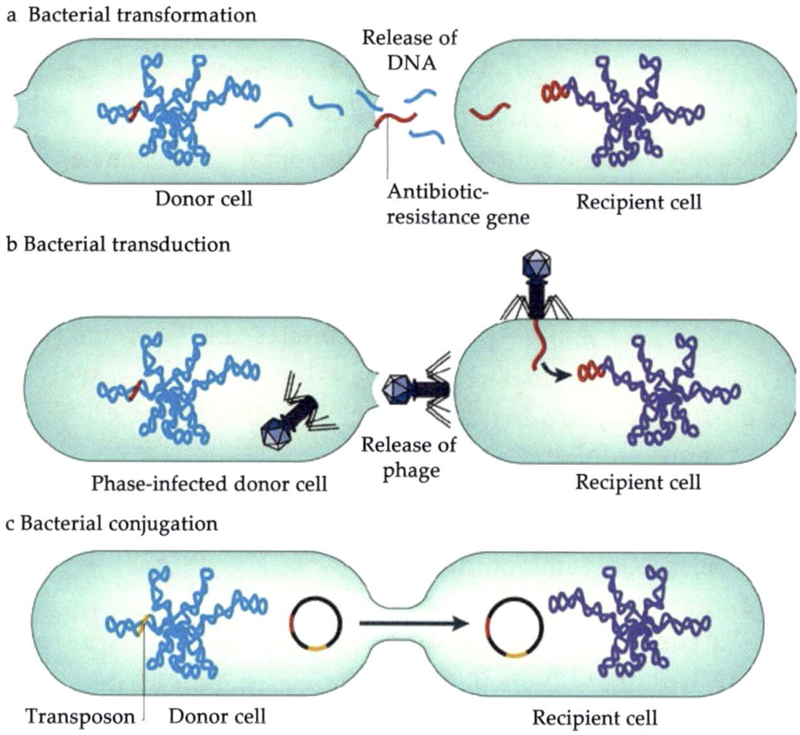

Figure 3.12. Major pathways in horizontal gene transfer (HGT).

Source: https://www.researchgate.net/figure/Major-pathways-in-Horizontal-Gene-Transfer-HGT-a-Bacterial-transformation-b-Bacterial_fig2_325495945.

Furthermore, the implications of mechanisms for horizontal gene transfer extend significantly into critical discussions regarding microbial adaptation to global environmental change. The capacity of microbial organisms to rapidly acquire advantageous genes enhances their resilience to stressors linked to climate change, pollution, and habitat destruction. As microbial populations migrate and evolve, the horizontal transfer of beneficial genetic traits becomes a fundamental component of transgenerational acclimatisation across diverse species. The potential influence of HGT on public health must also be acknowledged, particularly within the context of antibiotic resistance. As bacteria exchange genes that confer resistance to pharmaceuticals, addressing such issues necessitates a comprehensive understanding of the mechanisms underlying HGT. Ultimately, the role of horizontal gene transfer in microbial genetics and physiology highlights the importance of ongoing research into microbial adaptation mechanisms, given their vital functions in ecological stability and human health (Webster & Reusch, 2017; Wang et al., 2019).

3.5. Gene Expression and Regulation in Microorganisms

Gene regulation in microorganisms is essential for their survival in changing environments. Microorganisms, ranging from bacteria to yeast, often face fluctuating conditions that require immediate physiological responses. As a result, they have developed sophisticated regulation mechanisms to control gene transcription, enabling them to thrive both in nutrient-rich and nutrient-limited conditions. For instance, transcription factors play vital roles by binding to specific DNA sequences and regulating the activity of RNA polymerase, thereby controlling gene transcription. In addition to transcriptional regulation, post-transcriptional processes such as RNA splicing and degradation further refine gene expression, allowing microorganisms to swiftly adjust their metabolic pathways according to environmental cues, which is crucial for their survival and competitiveness. The coordination of gene expression and microbial physiology is also influenced by the importance of epigenetic modifications. Although epigenetic processes like DNA methylation and histone modification were once thought to be exclusive to multicellular organisms, they have now been identified in various microbial species. Such modifications can alter gene expression patterns without changing the DNA sequence, thus enabling microorganisms to efficiently adapt to environmental stresses. For example, when subjected to abiotic stresses, microbial cells may undergo changes in chromatin structure that increase the accessibility of genes responsible for stress responses (Figure 3.13).

Understanding these epigenetic regulatory mechanisms is of paramount importance as it provides valuable insights into the complexity of microbial adaptation and survival under stress conditions, thereby enhancing our knowledge of microbial genetics and physiology (Cadavid et al., 2023). Moreover, small RNA molecules and their functions in gene regulation have become a focal point of research within microbial genetics.

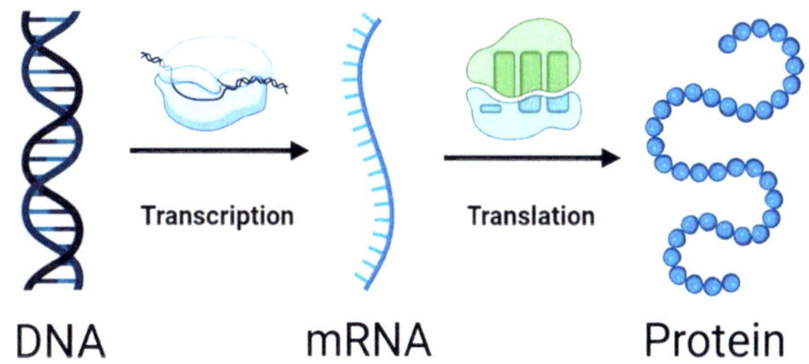

Figure 3.13. Gene expression.

Source: https://microbenotes.com/wp-content/uploads/2023/10/Gene-Expression.jpeg.

These concise RNA fragments (sRNAs) possess the capacity to modulate gene expression by targeting mRNA and proteins, thereby regulating various cellular processes such as metabolism, stress response, and virulence. Recent investigations indicate the involvement of sRNAs in the regulatory networks responsible for adaptive responses to fluctuating nutrient availability, as evidenced in Fed-Fast-Refed cycles documented in other organisms (Ji et al., 2023). This complex network of sRNA-mRNA interactions underpins the adaptive versatility of microbial metabolic pathways, which demonstrate significantly different levels of expression in response to environmental stimuli. Exploring these small RNA networks not only enhances our understanding of microbial gene regulation but also paves the way for biotechnological advancements, including the development of novel therapeutic antimicrobial strategies and the optimisation of industrial fermentation processes.

3.5.1. Transcription and Translation Processes

Transcription and translation are fundamental processes in microbial physiology and genetics, serving as the primary mechanisms through which genetic information is expressed. Transcription entails the synthesis of RNA from a DNA template, initiated by the binding of RNA polymerase to specific promoter sequences. This enzyme unwinds the DNA double helix, creating space for the synthesis of an RNA strand complementary to the DNA template. In prokaryotes, both transcription and translation occur concurrently, facilitating an immediate response to environmental stressors and thereby supporting survival across diverse habitats. Beyond regulating messenger RNA (mRNA) synthesis, transcription also influences gene expression regulation, which is crucial for microbial adaptability and pathogenicity. This sophisticated sequence of molecular events exemplifies how microorganisms can rapidly alter their physiological states in response to environmental changes, demonstrating their success in niche adaptation. Translation subsequently converts mRNA into proteins, which serve as the ultimate effectors of cellular function. This process occurs within the ribosome, a highly intricate molecular machine that interprets mRNA sequences into a polypeptide chain. It begins with the assembly of ribosomal subunits around the mRNA start codon, wherein transfer RNA (tRNA) molecules deliver amino acids to the elongating peptide chain through codon-anticodon interactions. In microorganisms, efficient translation is vital, as it enables rapid protein synthesis and the immediate production of functional proteins necessary for cellular activities such as metabolism, replication, and defence against competitors or host immune responses.

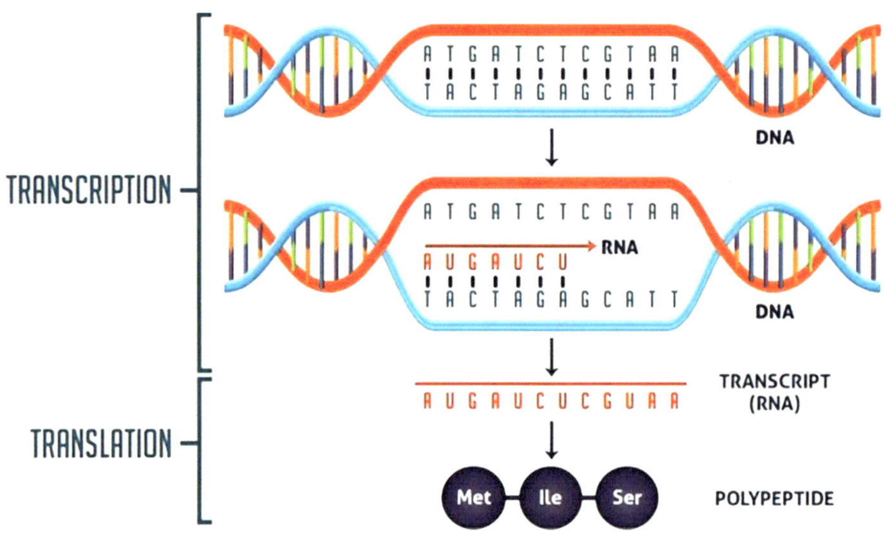

Figure 3.14. Transcription and translation processes.

Source: https://assets.technologynetworks.com/production/dynamic/images/content/323080/transcription-vs-translation-worksheet-323080-640x360.jpg.

Regulation of translation also influences microbial growth and virulence rates, making it an important focus in the study of microbial genetics and physiology. The complex connection between transcription and translation further highlights their significance in microbial biology. For example, global regulatory mechanisms can coordinate these processes when microorganisms face stressors, helping them adapt their metabolic pathways to improve survival in harsh conditions. Recent studies have uncovered how gene expression control interacts with signalling mechanisms, showing how microbes use these processes to respond to their environment. For instance, the role of specific transcription factors, such as MYC2 in mediating responses to jasmonic acid, demonstrates the complexity of gene regulation during environmental stress (Li et al., 2024). Similarly, thc concept of the 'germ-free syndrome' has initiated discussions on transcriptional responses to microbial presence, which in turn impacts human health and the necessity for various microbial interactions (Ma et al., 2024). These findings highlight the crucial role that transcription and translation play in developing microbial resilience and adaptability.

3.5.2. Regulatory Mechanisms in Microbial Gene Expression

The regulatory mechanisms responsible for controlling microbial gene expression are fundamental components in the adaptation and survival of microorganisms under diverse environmental conditions. These mechanisms enable microorganisms to optimize their genetic responses to emergent challenges for efficient resource utilization. Central to this process are transcription factors, which bind to specific DNA sequences to induce or repress the transcription of target genes. Various environmental signals, such as nutrient availability and stress, influence the activity of these transcription factors, thereby modulating gene expression patterns.

Furthermore, the roles of signaling pathways, including those mediated by protein kinase A and protein kinase B, have been acknowledged in regulating core metabolic processes, as delineated by the complex interplay between environmental stimuli and microbial gene expression (Wang et al., 2024). Beyond transcriptional regulation, post-transcriptional mechanisms also play a vital role in microbial gene expression, encompassing RNA stability, translational efficiency, and the functions of regulatory RNAS. Small non-coding RNAs (sRNAs), for example, can modulate gene expression through interactions with target mRNAs, affecting their stability and translation. These interactions allow sRNAs to respond swiftly to environmental changes, facilitating dynamic and rapid regulation of gene expression without the time lag typically associated with protein synthesis. Additionally, mechanisms governing mRNA decay can regulate protein levels in response to environmental cues, illustrating a multi-layered gene regulatory system within microorganisms. This intricate complexity underscores the importance of continued research into the molecular foundations of microbial physiology and genetics (Chen et al., 2024) (Figure 3.15).

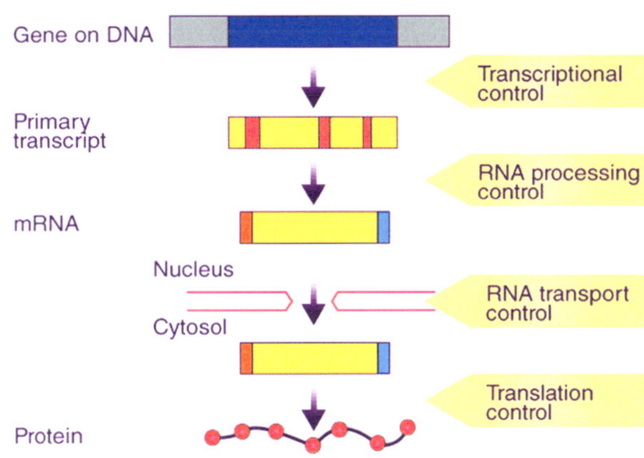

Figure 3.15. Regulation of microbial gene expression.

Source: https://cdn1.byjus.com/wp-content/uploads/2018/01/Gene-Regulation-3.png.

Metabolic pathways, such as gluconeogenesis in specific microbial organisms, also demonstrate the intricate processes of gene regulation in microbial gene expression. Key gluconeogenesis enzymes, such as phosphoenolpyruvate carboxykinase and glucose-6-phosphatase, are regulated with extreme accuracy by both transcriptional and translational mechanisms. The expression of the rate-determining enzymes is regulated by particular signal molecules and nutrients, illustrating how microbial metabolism is optimised for utilising different substrates. Recent research has emphasised the role of transcription factors in integrating gluconeogenic gene responses to dietary signals and suggests that targeted nutrient supplementation may enhance metabolic efficiency. The complex interrelationship between gene regulation and metabolic adaptation highlights the significance of insights gained from microbial gene expression research in both foundational science and practical applications (Wang et al., 2024).

3.5.3. Impact of Environmental Factors on Gene Regulation

Gene regulation in microorganisms is significantly influenced by various environmental parameters, which can determine microbial physiology and adaptability. These parameters include temperature, water availability, and nutrient resources, collectively creating a dynamic environment that necessitates rapid microbial adaptation for survival. For example, temperature changes can result in alterations in microbial metabolic processes, thereby impacting the expression profiles of stress resilience genes. Empirical research indicates that environmental variability may stimulate stress responses and promote the upregulation or downregulation of specific genes to facilitate survival and adaptation. This underscores the complex relationship between environmental fluctuations and genetic responses in microbial organisms. Understanding these interactions enables scientists to elucidate how microbial communities evolve and adapt to changing environments.

Additionally, management practices within agricultural systems exert considerable influence over soil and plant-associated microbial communities. Different cultivation approaches, such as conventional versus traditional farming, introduce distinct stressors capable of modifying microbial diversity and composition. A study involving *L. angustifolia* demonstrated that conventional farming practices resulted in a measurable decline in beneficial microbial taxa, illustrating the profound impact of human intervention on gene regulation within microbial populations. Environmental factors like precipitation patterns and temperature variations have been identified as correlated with microbial community structures, confirming that these factors interact with management strategies to modulate gene expression in soil microorganisms. Consequently, an integrated approach considering both environmental and management factors is essential for promoting sustainable crop cultivation while maintaining healthy microbial communities.

These communities are vital for soil fertility and nutrient cycling. Equally important is the effect of individual pollutants, such as heavy metals, on microbial gene regulation and community dynamics. Research on cadmium soil pollution has revealed that even minimal pollution levels induce significant structural changes in microbial communities, notably affecting gene expression and metabolic activity. Cadmium exposure not only modifies microbial diversity but also promotes the selective proliferation of taxa such as *Firmicutes* and *Actinobacteria*, likely due to their stress resistance capabilities.

Furthermore, these modifications elevate the potential for pollutants to inhibit metabolic processes crucial for organism survival and adaptation at the community level. These findings highlight the importance of monitoring and regulating environmental pollution to preserve the delicate balance of microbial communities, thereby ensuring that gene regulation remains responsive to natural ecosystem processes rather than being suppressed by anthropogenic stressors. Such insights are highly relevant to the broader fields of Microbial Physiology and Genetics.

3.6. Applications of Microbial Physiology and Genetics

The convergence of microbial genetics and physiology underscores pioneering applications across various industries, particularly in medicine and pharmaceutical research. The complex mechanisms within microbial cells provide valuable insights into their metabolic networks, which can be harnessed to develop strains for biofuel production, pharmaceutical development, and other bioproduct synthesis. Techniques such as CRISPR-Cas9 enable precise modifications of microbial genomes, allowing scientists to enhance desirable traits, such as increased tolerance to environmental stresses or improved substrate utilisation. Such advancements not only optimise production systems but also promote the development of sustainable practices within industries reliant on microbial fermentation. Furthermore, the interplay between microbial physiology and genetic engineering is fostering innovative biotechnological applications, significantly contributing to economic and environmental sustainability. Another vital application involves understanding and managing antimicrobial resistance. As pathogens increasingly develop resistance to existing drugs, there exists an urgent necessity for novel antimicrobial agents. The study of genetic resistance pathways facilitates the identification of new drug targets and the development of innovative therapies. Microbial genetics also plays a crucial role in the discovery of novel antibiotics, particularly through the investigation of natural products and synthetic biology. The current landscape of antimicrobial research highlights the critical challenge posed by drug-resistant bacteria, necessitating coordinated efforts among academia, industry, and policymakers to invigorate the pursuit of new medicines. Interdisciplinary collaboration remains essential in addressing the complex issue of antibiotic resistance, requiring the formulation of robust strategies to safeguard public health (Miethke et al., 2021). Organ-on-a-chip technology exemplifies an innovative application of microbial physiology and genetics. These systems replicate human organ functions based on living cells, enabling high-fidelity simulations of diseases and physiological states. By integrating microbial communities, researchers can examine host–microbiome interactions and their impact on human health. This novel approach offers insights into complex disease mechanisms and drug responses, thus playing a vital role in personalised medicine. Despite several challenges to large-scale implementation, organ-on-a-chip devices have the potential to revolutionise drug discovery and safety testing by providing responses that more closely mimic human physiology than traditional animal models. As research advances, the prospects for improving therapeutic efficacy and safety assessments in clinical settings become increasingly promising (Donald, 2022).

3.6.1. Role in Biotechnology and Genetic Engineering

Microbial physiology and genetics are key areas in biotechnology and genetic engineering, especially through the use of various microorganisms in industrial processes. Choosing the right microbial hosts is crucial for successful bioprocesses, with factors like metabolic capacity, substrate use, and genetic compatibility being important considerations. For example, *Yarrowia lipolytica* is a promising chassis strain because it can produce high levels of valuable bioproducts from a wide range of substrates. This yeast is stable, robust, and has stable genetic modifications that improve its use in the production of chemicals, fuels, and pharmaceuticals, showing its value in industrial biotechnology (Park et al., 2022). Moreover, metabolic engineering has progressed, allowing microbial processes to be designed to be more efficient and sustainable for bioproduction.

Additionally, new applications of engineered microorganisms highlight the significant role of genetic engineering in modern biotechnology. Synthetic biology, for example, has been used to modify microbial strains so they can produce complex molecules that are difficult to make using traditional chemical methods (Figure 3.16).

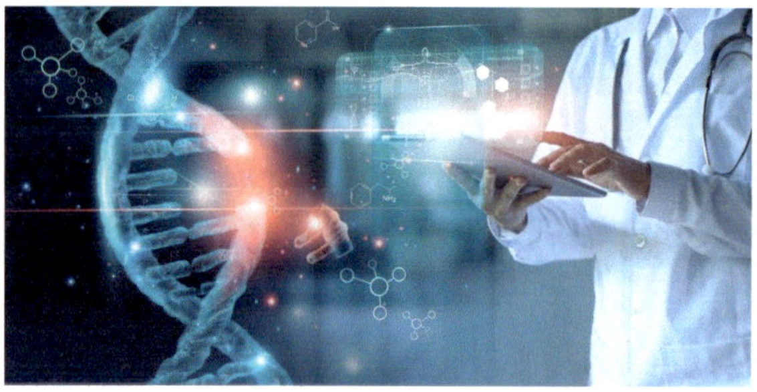

Figure 3.16. Roles in biotechnology and genetic engineering.

Source: https://www.azolifesciences.com/images/Article_Images/ImageForArticle_745_16457952738893668.jpg.

For instance, the genetic transformation of *Yarrowia lipolytica* to produce omega-3 fatty acids exemplifies how genetic modification can enhance yield and streamline production processes, thereby rendering biobased manufacturing economically feasible. This exemplifies a broader trend where microorganisms are utilized not only as models for fundamental biological research but also as production organisms for bioactive metabolites in industrially relevant applications. Such bioprocesses tend to provide sustainable alternatives to traditional methods, aligning increasingly with the global emphasis on sustainability (Park et al., 2022). In addition to strain optimisation for production, the growing adoption of organ-on-a-chip technologies opens new avenues for drug research and development. These microfluidic devices can replicate human organ physiology and disease states, thereby overcoming the limitations of conventional animal models, which often fail to accurately predict human outcomes. By cultivating living cells within these devices, researchers can develop sophisticated models that more closely resemble human biology than traditional approaches. This progression indicates a potential shift towards highly personalised medical practices, as organ-on-a-chip systems can also facilitate individual-specific drug responses, significantly advancing the understanding of therapeutic efficacy and safety. Consequently, the integration of microbial genetics and advanced modelling techniques exemplifies the innovative potential of biotechnology in research and clinical practice, offering substantial prospects for future advancements.

3.6.2. Importance in Medicine and Antibiotic Resistance

The role of microbial physiology and genetics in medicine is increasingly prominent, particularly concerning antibiotic resistance. The rising issue of antibiotic-resistant bacteria presents a significant public health challenge, as it transforms many infections once easily treatable into more complicated and costly conditions. Understanding the genetic underpinnings of antibiotic resistance is imperative for developing effective treatment strategies. Studies in microbial genetics elucidate the mechanisms by which bacteria acquire resistance genes through horizontal gene transfer, mutations, and selection processes- mechanisms that have led to the emergence of superbugs resistant to conventional therapies. This knowledge is vital in the development of new antibiotics and the enhancement of existing treatment protocols, highlighting the importance of integrating microbial genetics with medical technology. Furthermore, the exploration of microbial interactions within the human microbiome warrants critical attention. The Human Microbiome Project has elucidated the complex interplay between human cells and microbial communities, indicating that health outcomes are influenced not only by genetics but also by microbiota dynamics. This interaction between human genes and microbiota may affect disease progression and the efficacy of drug therapies. Consequently, understanding these interactions is essential for preventive care and effective treatment. The integration of microbial physiology and genetics into clinical practice offers a comprehensive perspective on patient health, especially amidst the escalating challenge of antibiotic resistance, necessitating novel approaches to managing bacterial infections across diverse populations. Additionally, the ongoing evolution of bacteria in response to antibiotic pressure emphasises the importance of adaptive processes in medicine. Organisms such as *Helicobacter pylori* exemplify the complexities of microbial interactions and disease outcomes, as they can oscillate between pathogenic and symbiotic states, complicating treatment efforts. Consideration of these evolutionary adaptations is crucial in the development of pharmaceuticals aimed at combating antibiotic resistance, as they significantly influence disease incidence and progression. By focusing on preventive strategies and innovative therapies informed by microbial genetics, we can improve patient outcomes and safeguard the effectiveness of current antibiotics, thereby strengthening public health resilience against resistant bacterial populations (Juengst & Huss, 2009; Koskella et al., 2014).

3.6.3. Contributions to Environmental Microbiology

The interface between genetics and microbial physiology has markedly advanced research in environmental microbiology, particularly in understanding the complex ecosystems inhabited by microorganisms. Current initiatives, such as the Human Microbiome Project, exemplify how microbiological flora in various environments give rise to higher-order ecological and physiological processes. This research has not only led to the sequencing of diverse microbial genomes but also established the symbiotic relationships between human hosts and their microbiota. Considering the human body as an ecosystem where various symbiotic organisms coexist, researchers have elucidated how such associations can influence health and disease states, thereby underscoring the central role of microorganisms in environmental conditions such as gut health, nutrient cycling, and pathogen resistance. This perspective necessitates a reevaluation of how microbial contributions are perceived at both community and individual levels in environmental microbiology (Juengst &Huss , 2009).

Furthermore, the application of microbial genetics in environmental microbiology extends to bioremediation, wherein microorganisms are utilized to restore polluted environments. The ability of microbes to decompose pollutants exemplifies the significant genetic diversity present within microbial communities. These organisms exhibit a high degree of adaptability, which has evolved in response to environmental pressures, thereby underscoring the imperative for ongoing research into microbial physiology. Such research proves invaluable for controlling environmentally induced human stress, highlighting the importance of genetic information in identifying novel microbial strains with bioremediation potential. In light of persistent environmental challenges, understanding the genetic mechanisms underlying microbial resilience and metabolic activity is essential for developing sustainable strategies in agriculture and waste management (Maloy & Schaechter, 2006).

Additionally, advances in microbial genomics continue to elucidate microbial interactions within the environment, revealing the critical role these organisms play in maintaining ecological stability. With the progress in microbiology, the integration of advanced genomic tools enables scientists to investigate how microbial communities respond to environmental perturbations such as global warming and ecosystem degradation. By deciphering the genetic blueprints of diverse microbial assemblages, researchers can assess their functional contributions to ecosystem services, including carbon sequestration and nutrient cycling. This knowledge is vital not only for predicting microbial responses to environmental stresses but also for guiding conservation efforts to preserve biodiversity. Establishing an extensive foundation of microbial genetic knowledge will empower future microbiologists to address urgent environmental issues effectively, ensuring that their work remains vital to the health of natural ecosystems and human well-being (Maloy & Schaechter, 2006).

SUMMARY

In synthesising the research in microbial physiology and genetics, it is increasingly evident that the complex relationship between microbial communities and their human host is fundamental to understanding health and disease. The research underscores the vital role of microbiota in maintaining homeostasis, including immune regulation and metabolism. Dysbiosis, or the imbalance of microbial communities, has been associated with a wide range of diseases, from cardiovascular conditions to cancers, thereby reinforcing the importance of microbiome balance for optimal health. Scholars have called for further investigation into how specific mechanisms of microbiota influence host physiology and the progression of pathological conditions, as reviewed in the literature on microbiota-host interactions (Hou et al., 2022). The emerging concept of the microbiota-gut-brain axis highlights a significant pathway through which microorganisms affect neurological function and mental health. Interactions mediated by microbial metabolites and the immune system exert substantial influence on disorders such as anxiety, depression, and neurodegenerative diseases. This relationship underscores the potential for developing innovative therapeutic strategies aimed at modulating the microbiome to enhance mental health outcomes. As research methodologies advance, both in human clinical studies and animal models, new insights into the complexity of the gut-brain axis are continually emerging (John et al., 2019). These findings elevate the importance of microbial physiology beyond environmental adaptation, positioning it as a critical factor in human development and disease management. Ultimately, the fields of microbial physiology and genetics are central to modern biomedical research, bearing significant implications for health, disease prevention, and therapeutic interventions. Overcoming challenges associated with dysbiosis and harnessing the potential of microbiota-based therapies will be essential for advancing healthcare. Future research should focus not only on examining the interactions between specific microbial communities and host health but also on elucidating the genetic foundations of these interactions. By fostering a more integrated understanding of microbial communities, researchers can better inform clinical practices, leading to innovative solutions for disease prevention and control, reducing microbial imbalances, and thereby improving health outcomes across diverse populations (Hou et al., 2022).

Knowledge of microbial physiology and genetics is increasingly advancing, particularly as discoveries in the microbiome continue to emerge. The focus is primarily on exploring the structure of microbial networks, which typically involves analysing aggregate statistics through comparative sampling. Traditional methods often examine one or two samples at a time, thus effectively assessing diversity or compositional dissimilarity. However, recent studies have highlighted the limitations of these classical approaches when attempting to quantify variability across multiple samples simultaneously. To attain a more accurate estimation of microbiome stability and diversity, especially within dynamic ecosystems, a novel framework has been proposed. This model, known as the FST-based analysis of variability between vectors of relative abundances (FAVA), provides a robust method for quantifying compositional variation among several samples and enhances our understanding of microbial population processes over time and under different experimental conditions (Maike et al., 2025). The activities of the gut microbiota are multifaceted and have profound impacts on host physiology and health. Emerging research increasingly indicates that microbial-derived metabolites, particularly bile acids, play a central role in modulating health outcomes across various species, such as cats and dogs. Specifically, the gut microbiota metabolises primary bile acids produced in the liver into secondary bile acids, which exert typical physiological effects. These conversions are significant because they can activate host bile acid receptors, thereby influencing metabolic signalling pathways and immune responses. Incorporating knowledge of bile acid metabolism into veterinary practice is essential for practitioners interested in harnessing the therapeutic potential of microbial interactions. As recent reviews have emphasised, understanding microbiota-host interactions is key to developing evidence-based practices in veterinary medicine, equipping clinicians with the intellectual tools necessary to utilize this dynamic (Hou et al., 2022). Looking ahead, the intersection of microbial physiology, genetics, and health outcomes underscores the necessity for interdisciplinary research paradigms. Advances in multi-omic technologies represent significant breakthroughs in elucidating the complex nature of microbial interactions and their implications for host health. By integrating genomic, transcriptomic, and metabolomic analyses, researchers can better understand how microbial communities influence health and disease. This comprehensive approach not only facilitates the investigation of microbial functions but also enhances our ability to design targeted therapeutic interventions. As we continue exploring the vast potential inherent in microbiome studies, it is clear that fostering collaborations among veterinarians, microbiologists, and computational biologists will be crucial for advancing research in microbial physiology and genetics in meaningful ways (Hou et al., 2022; Maike et al., 2025).

CLOSER LOOK

MOLECULAR MECHANISMS OF GENETIC VARIATION

Genetic variation refers to differences in DNA sequences among individuals upon which evolution, diversity, and adaptation are founded. On a molecular level, there are several mechanisms causing variation in prokaryotic and eukaryotic organisms.

An important cause is mutation, which involves changes in the nucleotide sequence of DNA. Mutations may be pointing mutations (single nucleotide mutations), insertions, deletions, or duplications. Mutations may be spontaneous during DNA replication or induced by environmental agents like radiation or chemicals. Mutations can be silent, harmful, or beneficial based on their effect on gene function (Figure 3.17).

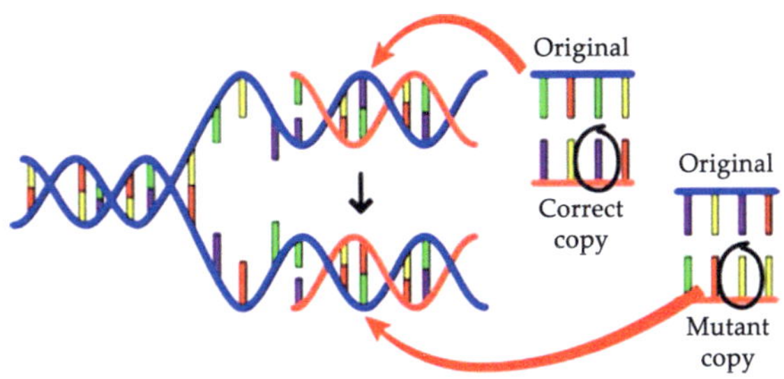

Figure 3.17. Illustration of DNA replication showing the formation of a correct copy and a mutant copy due to a replication error. Mutation occurs when an incorrect base is incorporated, altering the genetic sequence.

Source: https://external-content.duckduckgo.com/iu/?u=https%3A%2F%2Fwww.ebi.ac.uk%2Ftraining%2Fonline%2Fcourses%2Fhuman-genetic-variation-introduction%2Fwp-content%2Fuploads%2Fsites%2F76%2F2020%2F05%2FFIG1.png&f=1&nofb=1&ipt=f2b920e491d785aee9fec0d671a1e9efb11ccd8072365710d6592a8c655f2fb9.

Another key process is genetic recombination, particularly during sexual reproduction in eukaryotes. Homologous recombination during meiosis leads to the exchange of genetic material between homologous chromosomes and the creation of novel combinations of alleles. In prokaryotes, recombination occurs through processes like transformation (uptake of foreign DNA), transduction (bacteriophage-mediated transfer of DNA), and conjugation (direct cell-to-cell DNA transfer via pili). Mobile genetic elements, such as transposons (jumping genes), can also bring about genetic variation. These DNA pieces are able to move within the genome, disrupting or changing gene function and regulation. Retrotransposons, operating via RNA intermediates, are especially active in eukaryotic genomes. Gene and genome duplication are more advanced processes that bring in variation by adding duplicate genetic information with which new functions have the opportunity to evolve. Duplicated genes can ultimately gain mutations leading to neofunctionalization or subfunctionalisation. In addition, epigenetic modifications such as DNA methylation and histone modification do not alter DNA sequences but could affect gene expression and phenotypic variation. These molecular events collectively generate genetic diversity, required for population adaptation, natural selection, and the creation of new traits between generations.

REFERENCES

1. Amato, K. R., Cerda, G., Cramer, J. D., Gomez, et al. (2015). *Variable responses of human and non-human primate gut microbiomes to a Western diet.* https://core.ac.uk/download/142077405.pdf (accessed on 16th July 2025).
2. McBurney, M. I., Davis, C., Fraser, C. M., Schneeman, B. O., Huttenhower, C., Verbeke, K., Walter, J., & Latulippe, M. E. (2019). Establishing What Constitutes a Healthy Human Gut Microbiome: State of the Science, Regulatory Considerations, and Future Directions. *The Journal of nutrition, 149*(11), 1882–1895. https://doi.org/10.1093/jn/nxz154(accessed on 16th July 2025).
3. Baj, A., Moro, E., Bistoletti, M., Orlandi, V. T., Crema, F., & Giaroni, C. (2019). Glutamatergic signaling along the microbiota–gut–brain axis. *International Journal of Molecular Sciences, 20*, 1482–1482. https://doi.org/10.3390/ijms20061482 (accessed on 16th July 2025).
4. Baluška, F., Miller, W. B., & Reber, A. S. (2023). Sentient cells as basic units of tissues, organs and organismal physiology. *The Journal of Physiology, 602.* https://www.semanticscholar.org/paper/6be6bc5e34531696d2737791499607l6255909cb (accessed on 16th July 2025).
5. Wang, B., Qin, W., Ren, Y. *et al.* Expansion of *Thaumarchaeota* habitat range is correlated with horizontal transfer of ATPase operons. *ISME J* **13**, 3067–3079 (2019). https://doi.org/10.1038/s41396-019-0493-x (accessed on 16th July 2025).
6. Beever, D. E., Juniper, D. T., DePeters, et al. (2008). *Digestion, rumen fermentation and circulating concentrations of insulin, growth hormone and IGF-1 in steers fed diets based on different proportions of maize silage and grass silage.* https://core.ac.uk/download/12662.pdf (accessed on 16th July 2025).
7. Cadavid, I. C., Balbinott, N., & Margis, R. (2023). Beyond transcription factors: More regulatory layers affecting soybean gene expression under abiotic stress. *Genetics and Molecular Biology, 46.* https://www.semanticscholar.org/paper/55269e95f41c81656a21055b425f5c502b387ff6 (accessed on 16th July 2025).
8. Carlson, H., Coates, J., & Deutschbauer, A. (2017). *Microbial metal resistance and metabolism across dynamic landscapes: High-throughput environmental microbiology.* https://core.ac.uk/download/323062660.pdf (accessed on 16th July 2025).
9. Nászai, M., Carroll, L. R., & Cordero, J. B. (2015). Intestinal stem cell proliferation and epithelial homeostasis in the adult Drosophila midgut. *Insect biochemistry and molecular biology, 67*, 9–14. https://doi.org/10.1016/j.ibmb.2015.05.016(accessed on 16th July 2025).
10. Chen, Y., Sun, J., Tao, J., & Sun, T. (2024). Treatments and regulatory mechanisms of acoustic stimuli on mood disorders and neurological diseases. *Frontiers in Neuroscience, 17.* https://www.semanticscholar.org/paper/d103205135914efa1cb21148cb7d79be39740708 (accessed on 16th July 2025).
11. Contreras-Negrete, G., Valiente-Banuet, A., Molina-Freaner, F., Partida-Martínez, L., & Hernández-López, A. (2024). Agricultural practices and environmental factors drive microbial communities in the mezcal-producing *Agave angustifolia* Haw. *Microbial Ecology, 87.* https://www.semanticscholar.org/paper/40175dac7af2537b5dbbc6e6df1b7e6ef46a5f9c (accessed on 16th July 2025).

12. Cryan, J. F., O'Riordan, K. J., Cowan, C. S. M., Sandhu, K. V., Bastiaanssen, T. F. S., Boehme, M., Codagnone, M. G., et al. (2019). The microbiota–gut–brain axis. *Physiological Reviews, 99*, 1877–2013. https://doi.org/10.1152/physrev.00018.2018 (accessed on 16th July 2025).

13. Dawson, H. M., Connors, E., Erazo, N., Sacks, J. S., Mierzejewski, V., Rundell, S., Carlson, L. T., et al. (2023). Microbial metabolomic responses to changes in temperature and salinity along the western Antarctic Peninsula. *The ISME Journal, 17*, 2035–2046. https://www.semanticscholar.org/paper/c7de559e42a75f9ee130646be59ba8e8fff1ec9a (accessed on 16th July 2025).

14. Webster, N., Reusch, T. Microbial contributions to the persistence of coral reefs. *ISME J* **11**, 2167–2174 (2017). https://doi.org/10.1038/ismej.2017.66(accessed on 16th July 2025).

15. Fathima, S., Shanmugasundaram, R., Adams, D., & Selvaraj, R. K. (2022). Gastrointestinal microbiota and their manipulation for improved growth and performance in chickens. *Foods, 11*, 1401–1401. https://doi.org/10.3390/foods11101401 (accessed on 16th July 2025).

16. Finks, S. S., Moudgalya, P., Weihe, C., & Martiny, J. (2024). The contribution of plasmids to trait diversity in a soil bacterium. *ISME Communications, 4.* https://www.semanticscholar.org/paper/4023c3a69455c71bff0290a38d0d5f93f0653366 (accessed on 16th July 2025).

17. Zarraonaindia, I., & Gilbert, J. A. (2015). Understanding grapevine-microbiome interactions: implications for viticulture industry. *Microbial cell (Graz, Austria)*, *2*(5), 171–173. https://doi.org/10.15698/mic2015.05.204accessed on 16th July 2025).

18. Glaven, S. M. (2019). Bioelectrochemical systems and synthetic biology: More power, more products. *Microbial Biotechnology, 12*, 819–823. https://www.semanticscholar.org/paper/4271a0194fe376ea641b5a314d743a6ed8674a71 (accessed on 16th July 2025).

19. Greenlon, A., Sieradzki, E. T., Zablocki, O., Koch, B., Foley, M. M., Kimbrel, J. A., Hungate, B., et al. (2022). Quantitative stable-isotope probing (qSIP) with metagenomics links microbial physiology and activity to soil moisture in Mediterranean-climate grassland ecosystems. *mSystems, 7.* https://www.semanticscholar.org/paper/b3fed238c18c7b58e747add75e59188826369a94 (accessed on 16th July 2025).

20. Weston, D. J., Timm, C. M., Walker, A. P., Gu, L., Muchero, W., Schmutz, J., Shaw, A. J., Tuskan, G. A., Warren, J. M., & Wullschleger, S. D. (2015). Sphagnum physiology in the context of changing climate: emergent influences of genomics, modelling and host-microbiome interactions on understanding ecosystem function. *Plant, cell & environment*, *38*(9), 1737–1751. https://doi.org/10.1111/pce.12458(accessed on 16th July 2025).

21. Hirose, A., Kasai, T., Koga, R., Suzuki, Y., Kouzuma, A., & Watanabe, K. (2019). Understanding and engineering electrochemically active bacteria for sustainable biotechnology. *Bioresources and Bioprocessing, 6*, 1–15. https://www.semanticscholar.org/paper/aff8dd4733d83ee53dd0865442546198c6344c2a (accessed on 16th July 2025).

22. Hou, K., Wu, Z. X., Chen, X. Y., Wang, J. Q., Zhang, D., Xiao, C., Zhu, D., et al. (2022). Microbiota in health and diseases. *Signal Transduction and Targeted Therapy, 7.* https://doi.org/10.1038/s41392-022-00974-4 (accessed on 16th July 2025).

23. Eric Juengst & John Huss Juengst, Eric & Huss, John (2009). From metagenomics to the metagenome: Conceptual change and the rhetoric of translational genomic research. Genomics, Society and Policy 5 (3):1-19.(accessed on 16th July 2025).

24. Ingber, D. E. (2022). Human organs-on-chips for disease modelling, drug development and personalized medicine. *Nature Reviews Genetics, 23*, 467–491. https://doi.org/10.1038/s41576-022-00466-9 (accessed on 16th July 2025).

25. Ji, N., Xiang, L., Zhou, B., Lu, Y., & Zhang, M. (2023). Hepatic gene expression profiles during fed–fasted–refed state in mice. *Frontiers in Genetics, 14.* https://www.semanticscholar.org/paper/80f7bee57b77dc0c6611597af55b2aad9888b526 (accessed on 16th July 2025).

26. Kaminsky, R. A., Reid, P. M., Altermann, E., Kenters, N., Kelly, W., Noel, S. J., Attwood, G., et al. (2023). Rumen *Lachnospiraceae* isolate NK3A20 exhibits metabolic flexibility in response to substrate and coculture with a methanogen. *Applied and Environmental Microbiology, 89.* https://www.semanticscholar.org/paper/7228568793e9785d4175bc445b5e8ee2d3578ff1 (accessed on 16th July 2025).

27. Kayama, H., & Takeda, K. (2023). Emerging roles of host and microbial bioactive lipids in inflammatory bowel diseases. *European Journal of Immunology, 53.* https://www.semanticscholar.org/paper/1bb517703774446819fd90db95543c7ca6f720f0 (accessed on 16th July 2025).

28. de Vos, W. M., Kleerebezem, M., & Kuipers, O. P. (1997). Expression systems for industrial Gram-positive bacteria with low guanine and cytosine content. *Current opinion in biotechnology, 8*(5), 547–553. https://doi.org/10.1016/s0958-1669(97)80027-4(accessed on 16th July 2025).

29. Koskella, B., & Lin, D. (2014). Friend and foe: Factors influencing the movement of the bacterium *Helicobacter pylori* along the parasitism–mutualism continuum. https://core.ac.uk/download/323080778.pdf (accessed on 16th July 2025).

30. Le Clercq, L. S., Bazzi, G., Cecere, J., Gianfranceschi, L., Grobler, J. P., Kotzé, A., Rubolini, D., et al. (2023). Time trees and clock genes: A systematic review and comparative analysis of contemporary avian migration genetics. *Biological Reviews, 98.* https://www.semanticscholar.org/paper/d413d4999c71c7d485f614ef0394a6e51c5c647e (accessed on 16th July 2025).

31. Li, S., Ma, C., Li, S., Zhang, M., Zhang, C., Qi, J., Wang, L., et al. (2024). MPK4 phosphorylates MYC2 transcription factors to regulate jasmonic acid signaling and herbivory responses in maize. *Plant Physiology.* https://www.semanticscholar.org/paper/b2aa29ade9b978478ca0dd8056b80ea1e52d0899 (accessed on 16th July 2025).

32. Li, X., Li, C., Zhang, W., Wang, Y., Qian, P., & Huang, H. (2023). Inflammation and aging: Signaling pathways and intervention therapies. *Signal Transduction and Targeted Therapy, 8.* https://doi.org/10.1038/s41392-023-01502-8 (accessed on 16th July 2025).

33. Lijklema, L. (1971). *Factors affecting pH change in alkaline wastewater treatment – II: Carbon dioxide production.* https://core.ac.uk/download/pdf/11471763.pdf (accessed on 16th July 2025).

34. Lin, X., & Li, H. (2021). Obesity: Epidemiology, pathophysiology, and therapeutics. *Frontiers in Endocrinology, 12.* https://doi.org/10.3389/fendo.2021.706978 (accessed on 16th July 2025).

35. Ma, Z., Zuo, T., Frey, N., & Rangrez, A. (2024). A systematic framework for understanding the microbiome in human health and disease: From basic principles to clinical translation. *Signal Transduction and Targeted Therapy, 9.* https://www.semanticscholar.org/paper/80b7b73d4bb222eda75cfc27ef736bbb1915760f (accessed on 16th July 2025).

36. Makowski, L., Chaib, M., & Rathmell, J. C. (2020). Immunometabolism: From basic mechanisms

to translation. *Immunological Reviews, 295*, 5–14. https://doi.org/10.1111/imr.12858 (accessed on 16th July 2025).

37. Miethke, M., Pieroni, M., Weber, T., Brönstrup, M., Hammann, P., Halby, L., Arimondo, P. B., et al. (2021). Towards the sustainable discovery and development of new antibiotics. *Nature Reviews Chemistry, 5*, 726–749. https://doi.org/10.1038/s41570-021-00313-1 (accessed on 16th July 2025).

38. Morar, N., & Skorburg, J. A. (2018). *Bioethics and the Hypothesis of Extended Health.* https://core.ac.uk/download/287612197.pdf (accessed on 16th July 2025).

39. Morrison, M. L., Xue, K. S., & Rosenberg, N. A. (2025). Quantifying compositional variability in microbial communities with FAVA. *Proceedings of the National Academy of Sciences of the United States of America, 122.* https://www.semanticscholar.org/paper/2393ccacdbe7ebf7ef2411745b1252c43944269e (accessed on 16th July 2025).

40. Park, Y. K., & Ledesma-Amaro, R. (2022). What makes *Yarrowia lipolytica* well suited for industry? *Trends in Biotechnology, 41*, 242–254. https://doi.org/10.1016/j.tibtech.2022.07.006 (accessed on 16th July 2025).

41. Prakash, O., Chauhan, A., & Green, S. J. (2025). The study of microbial physiology under microoxic conditions is critical but neglected. *Environmental Microbiology Reports, 17.* https://www.semanticscholar.org/paper/ff67d16f35156877eab38b1ba810081c71c51617 (accessed on 16th July 2025).

42. Reberšek, M. (2021). Gut microbiome and its role in colorectal cancer. *BMC Cancer, 21.* https://doi.org/10.1186/s12885-021-09054-2 (accessed on 16th July 2025).

43. Roughgarden, J. (2020). *Holobiont evolution: Mathematical model with vertical vs. horizontal microbiome transmission.* https://core.ac.uk/download/287612317.pdf (accessed on 16th July 2025).

44. Rowe, J. C., & Winston, J. A. (2024). Collaborative metabolism: Gut microorganisms play a key role in canine and feline bile acid metabolism. *Veterinary Sciences, 11.* https://www.semanticscholar.org/paper/788bd0a828a7d06edd27222aa73d99645056ab7d (accessed on 16th July 2025).

45. Maloy, S., & Schaechter, M. (2006). The era of microbiology: a golden phoenix. *International microbiology : the official journal of the Spanish Society for Microbiology*, *9*(1), 1–7.(accessed on 16th July 2025).

46. Shen, X., Jin, H., Zhao, F., Kwok, L. Y., Zhao, Z., & Sun, Z. (2024). Short-term probiotic supplementation affects the diversity, genetics, growth, and interactions of the native gut microbiome. *iMeta, 3.* https://www.semanticscholar.org/paper/066144434cbfb68af1f443335bd75697aac2a1a1 (accessed on 16th July 2025).

47. Tokuda, M., & Shintani, M. (2024). Microbial evolution through horizontal gene transfer by mobile genetic elements. *Microbial Biotechnology, 17.* https://www.semanticscholar.org/paper/f1ee559ea8f608e2d5182ac74a0fee9af536b9b5 (accessed on 16th July 2025).

48. Wang, G., Zhu, Y., Feng, D., Yao, J., Cao, Y., & Deng, L. (2024). Hepatic gluconeogenesis and regulatory mechanisms in lactating ruminants: A literature review. *Animal Research and One Health.* https://www.semanticscholar.org/paper/f9ad78fa6a568433ddf13fa92b3e155e242397b9 (accessed on 16th July 2025).

49. Wang, J., Ma, W., & Wang, X. (2021). Insights into the structure of *Escherichia coli* outer membrane as the target for engineering microbial cell factories. *Microbial Cell Factories, 20.* https://www.semanticscholar.org/paper/5f637415f4dc658e4f126daf62f85140bc1330dc (accessed on 16th July 2025).

50. Yao, H., Xiao, J., & Tang, X. (2023). Microbial fuel cell-based organic matter sensors: Principles, structures and applications. *Bioengineering, 10.* https://www.semanticscholar.org/paper/decaac8d5b5f23817d79236e8a43cf2d040e35d7 (accessed on 16th July 2025).

51. You, R., Li, H., Li, X., Luo, L., Wang, P., Xia, H., & Zhou, Y. (2024). Ecotoxicological impacts of cadmium on soil microorganisms and earthworms *Eisenia foetida*: From gene regulation to physiological processes. *Frontiers in Environmental Science.* https://www.semanticscholar.org/paper/7407097bd140b66479c6468def3b7f1325a0694e (accessed on 16th July 2025).

52. Zhai, T., Ren, W., Ji, X., Wang, Y., Chen, H., Jin, Y., Liang, Q., et al. (2024). Distinct compositions and functions of circulating microbial DNA in the peripheral blood compared to fecal microbial DNA in healthy individuals. *mSystems, 9.* https://www.semanticscholar.org/paper/96cc0c18099f1213ef48ad9db6c60d7c7ce3e7c6 (accessed on 16th July 2025).

53. Zuo, T., & Ng, S. C. (2018). The gut microbiota in the pathogenesis and therapeutics of inflammatory bowel disease. *Frontiers in Microbiology, 9.* https://doi.org/10.3389/fmicb.2018.02247 (accessed on 16th July 2025).

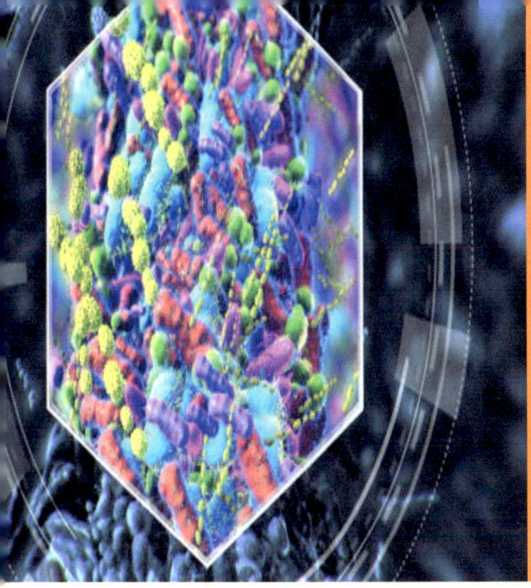

Chapter 4

HOST-MICROBE INTERACTIONS AND PATHOGENESIS

Contents

Introduction

The interaction between hosts and microbes constitutes a central focus within microbiological research, particularly in the study of pathogenesis. This dynamic process encompasses a range of mechanisms capable of resulting in either health or disease states, thereby underscoring the significance of microbial influence on host physiology. Recent scholarly endeavours highlight the critical role of microbial communities, or microbiomes, in maintaining host homeostasis and their potential to disrupt this balance, leading to pathological conditions. By investigating the molecular and cellular mechanisms underlying these interactions, researchers can attain a deeper understanding of the aetiology of diseases such as inflammatory bowel diseases and infections. Efforts to elucidate these relationships are evidenced by prominent conferences convening leading scientists to share advancements in the field, further affirming the importance of this area of study (Caly et al., 2012). The complexity of host- microbe interactions is demonstrated by the bidirectional effects microorganisms exert on immune responses within the host. Pathogenic microorganisms employ mechanisms to evade immune detection and eradication, ensuring their survival and proliferation within the host environment. Conversely, beneficial microorganisms bolster immune responses, thereby providing protection against infections and supporting overall health. An illustrative example is provided by inflammatory bowel disorders, such as ulcerative colitis and Crohn's disease, which result from dysregulated interactions between the gut microbiome and the host immune system. Current research employs systems biology approaches to elucidate the intricacies of these interactions, integrating data from various biological layers, including genetic and epigenetic regulators, with the aim of developing innovative therapeutic strategies to rectify dysregulations (Polytarchou et al., 2014). Host- microbe interactions are not solely academic pursuits but hold significant implications for health and disease management. Recent investigations have the potential to identify novel intervention pathways targeting microbial mechanisms, thereby advancing prevention and treatment strategies for infectious and chronic diseases. This calls for a multidisciplinary approach that combines microbiology, immunology, and computational biology to comprehensively understand these interactions and their broader implications. As technological innovations continue to shed light on the complex networks governing host- microbe dynamics, it becomes increasingly crucial to develop a more sophisticated understanding of these processes. Ultimately, unraveling the complexities of host- microbe interactions promises to transform our approaches to pathogenesis and therapeutic development in the future.

Definition of Host-Microbe Interactions

Understanding host- microbe interactions is essential for elucidating the intricate dynamics between microbial communities and their host organisms. These interactions encompass a broad spectrum, from mutualism- where both host and microbe benefit- to parasitism, wherein the microbe negatively impacts the host. Most of these interactions are closely associated with the host' s immune system and the metabolic activities of microorganisms, which can influence health and disease states. Current research underscores that microbial communities, particularly within the gut, have significant implications for various physiological processes, including digestion, immune modulation, and even psychological conditions. Through these functions, the microbiome can either promote homeostasis or contribute to pathological processes, highlighting the importance of a healthy microbial community in maintaining host health. Such host- microbe interactions are especially pertinent to pathogenesis, as pathogenic microorganisms exploit host mechanisms to infect and cause disease. An in- depth examination reveals that certain microorganisms have evolved sophisticated virulence factors enabling survival and proliferation within the host. For instance, microbes may manipulate host cell signaling pathways or evade immune detection, thereby causing harm and ensuring their persistence (Cadwell & Debnath, 2018). Furthermore, research into host-microbe interactions not only deepens understanding of infectious disease mechanisms but also informs therapeutic interventions, such as probiotics, which can be tailored to modulate the microbiome for pathogen resistance. This complex dynamic presents challenges to researchers seeking to delineate specific pathways involved in host-microbe interactions, thereby advancing the field of microbial pathogenesis. Additionally, the role of the gut microbiome in host health underscores the importance of microbial diversity and function in disease prevention. The gut microbiome comprises numerous microbial species, each contributing distinct functional roles that support host well- being (Sharpton et al., 2019). Disruptions in this microbial ecosystem may lead to dysbiosis, an imbalance associated with various chronic conditions, including autoimmune diseases, obesity, and nonalcoholic fatty liver disease (NAFLD). Advances in next-generation sequencing techniques have begun to elucidate the complexity of these microbial communities, particularly regarding their metabolic outcomes and contributions to health and disease. By illuminating the detailed mechanisms of host-microbe interactions, researchers can develop more targeted therapeutic strategies, bridging the gap between fundamental research and clinical application, thereby enhancing approaches to disease control linked to microbial imbalance (Figure 4.1 1).

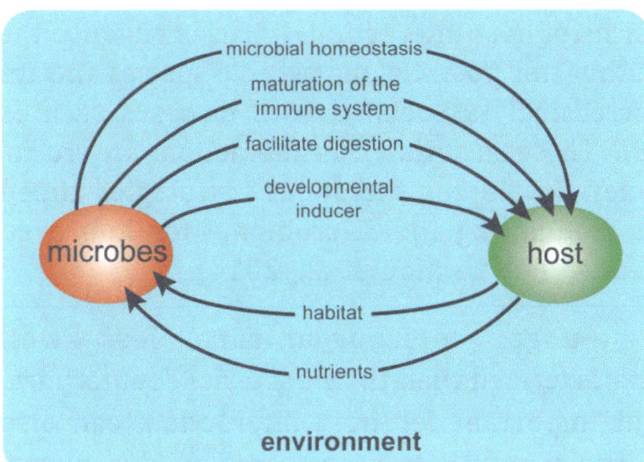

Figure 4.1. Schematic view of the interactions between host organisms and their microbiota.

Source: https://www.researchgate.net/profile/Sebastian-Fraune/publication/44669997/figure/fig6/AS:277155461255169@1443090419297/Schematic-view-of-the-interactions-between-host-organisms-and-their-microbiota.png.

Importance of Studying Pathogenesis

Pathogenesis studies are essential to understand the complex interactions between hosts and microorganisms, especially how different diseases develop and worsen. By examining how pathogens infect hosts, evade immune responses, and cause disease, researchers can identify targets for therapy. Pathogenesis involves not only the microorganisms themselves but also the host' s reaction to invaders, which adds complexity to the disease process. For example, Crohn's disease and ulcerative colitis are two forms of inflammatory bowel disease resulting from a complex interplay of genetic factors, immune responses, and interactions with the gut microbiome. Current research suggests that a systems biology approach to studying inflammatory bowel disease aims to integrate various omics data to unravel the molecular mechanisms underlying pathogenesis, with the goal of developing new therapies (Polytarchou et al., 2014). Additionally, investigating pathogen-host interactions enhances our understanding of public health issues and can inform better prevention strategies. The global spread of antibiotic- esistant microorganisms highlights the urgent need to develop new methods to fight infectious diseases. Studying the pathogenic processes by which pathogens like *Brachyspira hyodysenteriae* and *Lawsonia intracellularis* cause enteric disease enables the design of targeted interventions to disrupt these mechanisms. Effective prophylactic measures require a thorough understanding of the conditions that lead to disease, as demonstrated by studies of enteric infections in pigs. This research shows how changes in diet and group housing can predispose livestock to infection, with implications for broader animal and human health (Jacobson, 2003). Finally, advancements in diagnostic technologies underpin research in pathogenesis. Techniques such as polymerase chain reaction (PCR) have improved our ability to detect pathogens accurately and sensitively, facilitating more effective interventions. The development of models for disease monitoring provides deeper insights into the host response and microbial pathogenic strategies. Such research not only advances our understanding of individual diseases but also enhances microbiology by shedding light on the evolving nature of host-microbe interactions. The greater our knowledge of complexities, the more we will learn, leading to significant impacts on treatment development and public health improvements (Figure 4.2.).Jacobson, 2003

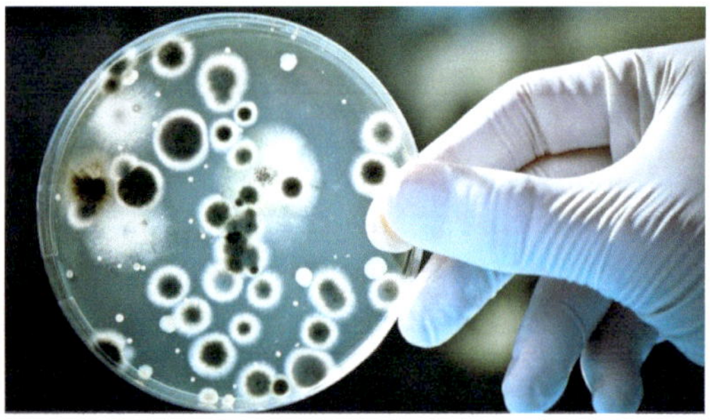

Figure 4.2. Microbial growth patterns used in studying pathogenesis.

Source: https://asm.org/getmedia/752a7290-80c0-417a-b816-16a6301e2d58/pathogenesis_feature.jpg?width=874&height=491&ext=.jpg.

4.1. Types of Microorganisms Involved in Host Interactions

The human microbiome is a complex community made up of many microorganisms, including bacteria, viruses, fungi, and archaea, all of which play vital roles in host interactions and can influence health and disease. Bacteria are the most numerous and diverse among them, with specific taxa occupying particular body regions such as the gut, skin, and mouth. The gut microbiota, in particular, has been the focus of extensive research due to its intricate link with various physiological processes, including digestion, metabolism, and immune function. These microorganisms are involved not only in nutrient absorption but also in interacting with the host's immune cells, creating a symbiotic environment essential for maintaining homeostasis. Dysbiosis, or microbial imbalance, can lead to pathologies like inflammatory bowel disease (IBD), where complex interactions among genetic, immune, and microbial factors contribute to disease development and severity, as recent studies have shown (Polytarchou et al., 2014). Besides bacterial communities, viruses—particularly bacteriophages—are recognised as key players in host-microbe interactions. Bacteriophages infect and regulate bacterial populations, influencing the overall microbial composition of the gut. This viral activity helps preserve stability and diversity within the microbiome, reflecting its delicate balance. Studies also reveal that these viral particles can exchange genes with bacteria through horizontal gene transfer, potentially improving microbial resilience or increasing virulence. In terms of host interactions, viruses enhance the pathogenic potential of bacterial species and are increasingly associated with diseases such as IBD. These bacteria-virus interactions are crucial when developing therapeutic strategies aimed at modulating the microbiome for improved health (Polytarchou et al., 2014).

Fungal microorganisms, less well characterized than their bacterial counterparts but important for host interaction, can also participate in host processes. The mycobiome, the term for the fungal component of the microbiome, can regulate the host immune response and play key roles in metabolic homeostasis. Recent studies have shown that some fungi can communicate with gut-residing bacteria, affecting their activity, growth patterns, and host signal modulation. This dialogue creates a multilayered communication network within the microbiome, with fungi acting as intermediaries of bacterial influence on host health. Similarly, the gut-brain axis—a two-way communication network between the central nervous system and the gut microbiota—demonstrates how changes in microbial composition can impact neurological and psychological health. As highlighted in research on this axis, disruptions to microbial balance are involved in many disorders, further emphasising the need to understand microbial roles in host interactions.

4.1.1. Bacteria

The intricate interaction between host and bacteria is fundamental to host-microbe relationships and pathogenic mechanisms. Bacteria such as *Yersinia pseudotuberculosis* possess specialized structures known as adhesins that facilitate adherence to host tissues. These virulence factors are not only instrumental in bacterial colonization but also influence the immune responses of the host. Research indicates that the multivalent adhesion molecule (MAM) of *Y. pseudotuberculosis* is essential for effective binding and host phagocytic uptake, particularly when interactions occur with immune cells such as hemocytes in the Galleria mellonella model. Most notably, disruption of this interaction has the unintended consequence of supporting pathogenic outcomes, as reduced phagocyte association results in increased bacterial clearance but may also provoke overwhelming immune responses that adversely affect host viability, thereby exposing a delicate balance between bacterial adhesion and host defense mechanisms (Krachler et al., 2021). The exploration of bacterial pathogenesis extends beyond adhesion to encompass broader implications of microbial interactions with host physiology. The *Vibrio* genus exemplifies this complex relationship, particularly through its type VI secretion system (T6SS). This system has been demonstrated to regulate intestinal motility in larval zebrafish and to elucidate the mechanisms by which bacterial activity induces cellular damage and activates immune responses. By causing tissue damage, *Vibrio* disrupts normal gut function, leading macrophages to migrate away from their usual midgut residence to injured tissues. Such cellular movements highlight the impact of bacterially induced pathology on host cellular dynamics, underscoring the necessity for further studies on how pathogenic bacteria regulate intestinal motility and overall gut health (Ngo, 2024).

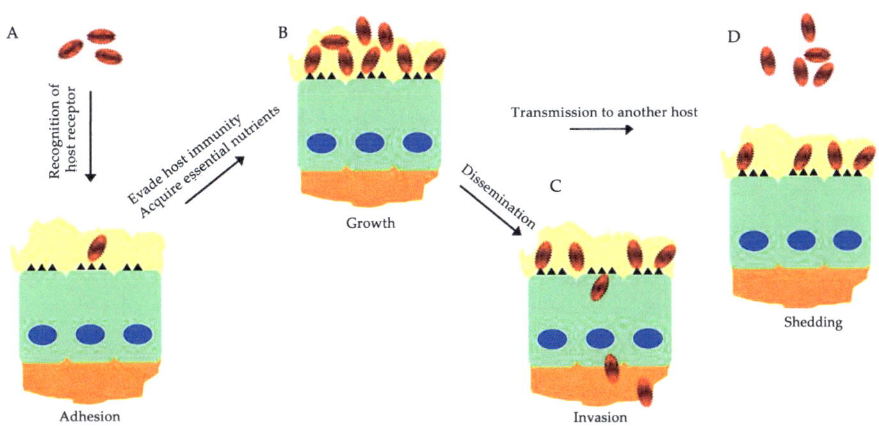

Figure 4.3. Major requirements for successful infection of human hosts by pathogenic bacteria. (A) Once bacteria enter the host, they need to adhere to mucosal surfaces by recognizing specific receptors on host cells. (B) The bacteria must be able to evade host immune mechanisms for survival (e.g., complement system, antibody) and acquire the necessary nutrients for the growth and expansion of the population (e.g., iron). (C) Once the population size has expanded to a certain level, bacteria can disseminate to other tissues/organs from the initial infection site by intracellular invasion through molecular interactions with host receptors or other means. (D) Some bacteria may be released into the surrounding environments and transmitted to another human host.

Source: https://www.researchgate.net/publication/277782368/figure/fig3/AS:271778094252054@1441808355789/Major-requirements-for-successful-infection-of-human-hosts-by-pathogenic-bacteria-A.png.

These complex interactions are central to developing strategies to mitigate bacterial infections and their pathological effects. The dual role of bacteria as both pathogens and immune modulators underscores the complexity of host-microbe interactions. Given the capacity of bacteria to significantly alter host physiological functions through the delivery of virulence factors, a comprehensive understanding of these processes is essential for the development of therapeutic strategies. Consequently, additional research into how bacterial components such as MAM and T6SS modulate host immunity and gut motility is imperative. Such investigations not only deepen our understanding of bacterial pathogenicity but also open new avenues for restoring host homeostasis compromised by pathogenic infections (Figure 4.3).

4.1.2. Viruses

Viruses constitute a distinctive category of pathogens that challenge conventional definitions of life owing to their reliance on host cells for replication and perpetuation. Unlike bacteria or fungi, viruses lack cellular structures and metabolic processes, rendering them entirely dependent on the activities of their hosts.

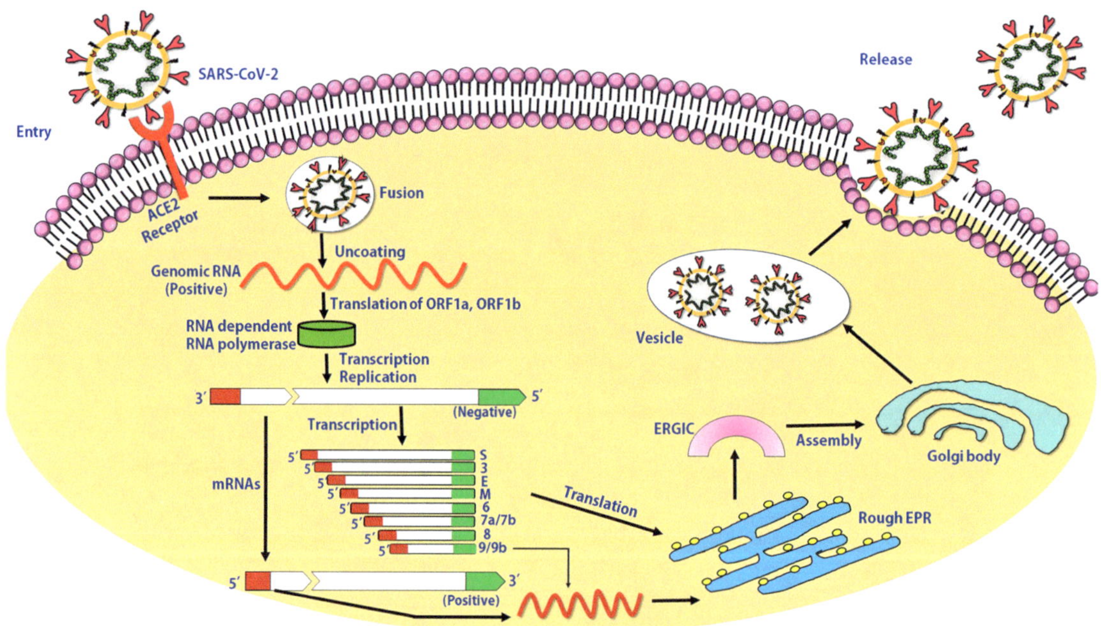

Figure 4.4. Pictorial representation of viral-host interaction and replication of the virus SARS-CoV-2.

Source: https://www.researchgate.net/profile/Ashish-Mishra-31/publication/344281686/figure/fig3/AS:936659797417985@1600328506238/Pictorial-representation-of-viral-host-interaction-and-replication-of-the-virus-SARS-CoV-2.png.

This dependence necessitates complex interactions between viruses and host organisms, which can result in outcomes ranging from harmless infection to severe disease. The host's immune response plays a pivotal role in dictating the progression of viral infections, often involving sophisticated mechanisms whereby the virus must evade innate and adaptive immune defences. An understanding of these interactions is vital for elucidating the mechanisms of viral pathogenesis, as viruses have evolved multiple strategies to manipulate host cellular processes and immune responses, leading to a spectrum of clinical manifestations and disease phenomena. The pathogenic potential of viruses is generally associated with their capacity to exploit host cellular machinery for replication and dissemination. Existing research has highlighted the role of autophagy, whereby viruses hijack autophagic machinery to promote their replication, as seen in recent studies involving autophagy-related proteins (ATGs). These proteins, besides aiding cellular material breakdown, are also involved in viral replication and egress.

These findings underscore the dual role of autophagy as both a cellular defence mechanism and a facilitator of viral pathogenesis. This intricate interplay emphasises the need for further detailed research to distinguish the mechanisms underlying these interactions, enabling a clearer understanding of how viruses manipulate host pathways to their advantage and paving the way for new therapeutic targets against viral infections. Furthermore, the understanding of viral interactions extends beyond replication to include their role in modulating the host immune response and the potential for establishing chronic infections. Certain viruses can induce immunomodulatory effects, thereby affecting the host's ability to mount a strong response to other pathogens. This influence is especially evident in viruses that employ immune evasion strategies or hijack immune signalling pathways, ultimately leading to chronic infection and possible sequelae such as autoimmune disease. With emerging evidence linking viral infections to chronic disease, it is evident that viruses are not merely transient invaders but can significantly impact host health and disease outcomes. As research continues to explore these dynamics, it becomes essential to adopt an integrative approach to better understand the implications of host-virus interactions within the broader context of pathogenesis (Figure 4.4).

4.1.3. Fungi

Fungi occupy pivotal roles in host-microbe interactions as both pathogens and beneficial symbionts. They have demonstrated remarkable versatility and evolutionary success in colonising diverse host environments, including those of plants and animals. Fungi exemplify strategies of immune response manipulation in hosts through the secretion of effector proteins that facilitate infection. This manipulation typically results from a complex interplay of host perception mechanisms, whereby specific fungal protein receptors detect specific fungal proteins. Recent research has advanced the concept of effector-triggered defence (ETD), distinguishing it from the conventional paradigms of pathogen-associated molecular pattern (PAMP)-triggered immunity (PTI) and effector-triggered immunity (ETI). Unlike PTI, which provides a broad-spectrum response to fungi, ETD constitutes a more sophisticated reaction initiated by the recognition of specific fungal effectors, thereby offering a more precise response to individual fungal pathogens (Stotz et al., 2014). The capacity of fungi such as the maize anthracnose pathogen *Colletotrichum graminicola* to secrete effectors that invade the host nucleus constitutes evidence of their pathogenic potential. Studies have identified a single effector protein, Cgep 1, which induces disease in maize and exhibits properties of nuclear localisation. This effector not only plays a crucial role in regulating host cellular processes but also represents an evolutionary adaptation that enhances fungal virulence. Gene analyses suggest that Cgep 1 likely evolved via gene duplications in ancestral lineages, reflecting the evolutionary dynamics of fungi over time. This positive selection, coupled with adaptive pressures, indicates that such effectors are vital for effective host-pathogen interactions across multiple species of *Colletotrichum* and underscores the role of fungi as agents of pathogenesis in agriculture (Vargas et al., 2016). Understanding the mechanisms underlying fungal pathogenesis is essential for developing effective control strategies in agriculture. The dual roles of fungi as both pathogenic and symbiotic organisms complicate this dynamic, as some fungi are integral to plant health and nutrient acquisition. Molecular investigations into fungal interactions provide insights into their capacity for survival within plant systems while concurrently inflicting damage. Ongoing research into effector proteins and their mechanisms of action holds the potential to facilitate the development of innovative biotechnological strategies to enhance host resistance. Furthermore, elucidating these interactions enhances understanding of fungi 's roles within ecosystem dynamics and their significance not only in disease development but also in maintaining ecosystem homeostasis. Accordingly, such research has the potential to inform future agricultural practices and management strategies (Stotz et al., 2014; Figure 4.5).

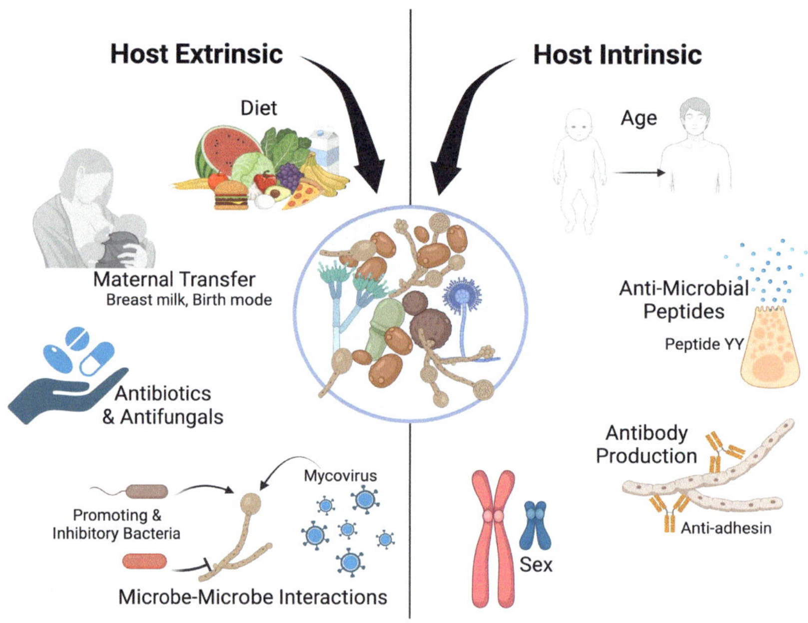

Figure 4.5. Host intrinsic and extrinsic factors that can influence fungal composition and function.

Source: https://www.cell.com/cms/10.1016/j.chom.2024.09.010/asset/724ce5e8-5339-4038-80b6-1d39e07d21d1/main.assets/gr2_lrg.jpg.

4.2. Mechanisms of Pathogenesis

Ngo, 2024Pathogenesis involves complex processes delineating how pathogens interact with host organisms to induce infection and disease. Central to these interactions is the capacity of pathogenic microorganisms to exploit host cellular mechanisms for their benefit. For example, it has been demonstrated that certain bacteria, such as *Vibrio*, utilize specialized secretion systems like the type VI secretion system (T6SS) to inject effector proteins into host cells. These proteins are capable of inducing cell death or disrupting normal cellular functions, thereby facilitating the colonization of the host environment. Specifically, the VgrG-1 protein's actin cross-linking domain (ACD) is responsible for impairing intestinal motility in larval zebrafish, exemplifying how bacterial pathogenicity can induce significant physiological alterations in the host. This phenomenon ultimately contributes to disease development and underscores the complexity of host-microbe interactions (Ngo, 2024). Furthermore, the metabolic activities of symbiotic microorganisms likewise play a crucial role in influencing host health and disease dynamics. *Bacteroides thetaiotaomicron* (*B. theta*), a prominent gut symbiont in humans, exemplifies such symbiosis through its metabolic end products. *B. theta* secretes amino acids and organic acids that modulate host nutrition and immune responses. Metabolomic research has demonstrated that metabolites such as acetate and formate exhibit dose-dependent signalling capabilities, which influence the secretion of other metabolites involved in pathogenesis as well as nutrient acquisition. This metabolic interaction clarifies the manner in which the host microbiota can regulate and modulate its own processes in response to microbial presence, illustrating a dynamic interaction where both host and microorganisms continuously adapt to each other's metabolic requirements (Catlett et al., 2020).

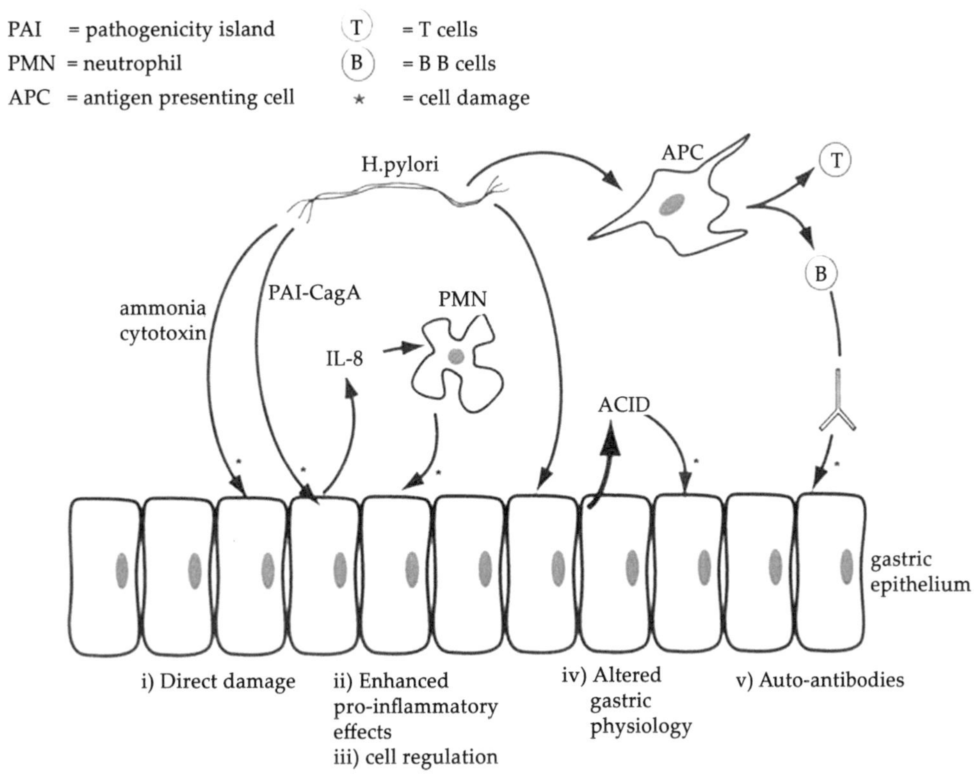

Figure 4.6. Overview of mechanisms of pathogenesis of disease caused by *Helicobacter pylori.*

Source: https://www.researchgate.net/publication/11399401/figure/fig4/AS:642485286080512@1530191837175/Overview-of-mechanisms-of-pathogenesis-of-disease-caused-by-Helicobacter-pylori.png.

A comprehensive understanding of these pathogenic mechanisms is essential for the development of targeted therapeutic strategies aimed at mitigating infectious diseases. Interventions that interfere with microbial adhesion, effector delivery, or host responses to microbial metabolites may constitute novel therapeutic approaches. As scientific knowledge progresses, elucidating the specific pathways and interactions within the host-microbe environment will facilitate precision medicine strategies to enhance our capacity to restore balance in disease states driven by pathogenic microbes. By deciphering the mechanisms utilized by commensal microorganisms and pathogens, future research can lead to innovative intervention tools that leverage the natural processes of the microbiome to improve host health and resilience (Catlett et al., 2020; Ngo, 2024) (Figure 4.6).Ngo, 2024

4.2.1. Adherence and Colonization

Adhesion and colonization are fundamental mechanisms in the development of host-microbe interactions, profoundly impacting the pathogenesis of infectious diseases. Pathogens utilize specialized structures such as pili, fimbriae, and adhesins to adhere to host tissues, a critical step for survival and subsequent colonization. Effective adherence not only ensures microbial persistence within niches but also enables pathogens to counteract host defences, thereby resisting clearance mechanisms.

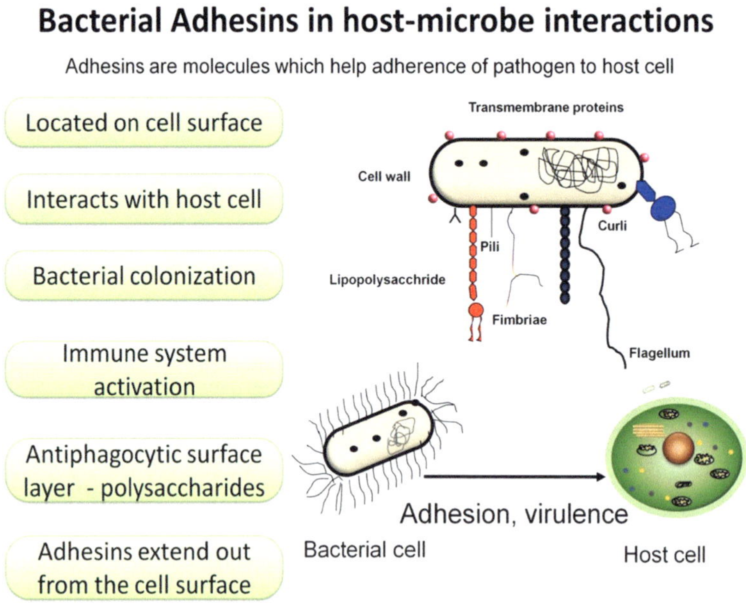

Figure 4.7. Bacterial adhesins in host-microbe interactions.

Source: https://www.researchgate.net/profile/Sanjiv-Kumar-25/publication/319710923/figure/fig1/AS:614112463708160@1523427229104/Bacterial-Adhesins-in-host-microbe-interactions.png.

Of particular importance are the competitive interactions during microbial colonization, which influence the balance between pathogenic and commensal microorganisms. Nonpathogenic microbes can inhibit the growth and colonization of pathogens through mechanisms such as competition for nutrients and the production of inhibitory compounds. Understanding microbial adherence is therefore vital, as it can inform therapeutic interventions aimed at restoring healthy microbiota and preventing pathogenic infections. Beyond attachment, microbial adherence plays a role in modulating host immune responses. Commensal bacteria are notably involved in immune regulation and maintaining homeostasis. For example, the skin microbiome comprises complex microbial communities that interact with the host to inhibit colonization by pathogenic microorganisms, such as *Staphylococcus aureus*, which is particularly relevant in conditions like atopic dermatitis (AD). Research indicates that a loss of microbial diversity correlates with increased disease severity and pathogen colonization. Notably, therapies involving commensal bacteria, such as *Staphylococcus hominis*, show promise in reducing *S. aureus* load and alleviating AD. This emphasises the importance of promoting microbial diversity as a preventive strategy against disease progression linked to pathogen colonization (Paller et al., 2019). Recent advancements in host-microbe interaction research, particularly through human intestinal organoid (HIO) cultures, have shed light on the complexities of microbial adherence and colonization. These models enable a detailed study of enteropathogen and commensal microbe pathogenesis under conditions that accurately mimic physiological processes. HIOs allow researchers to precisely understand how individual microbial interactions influence health and disease, insights unattainable with traditional cell lines or animal models. Moreover, HIO technology facilitates the exploration of therapeutic options targeting microbial pathogenesis and enhances prospects for vaccine and targeted therapy development. Consistent with ongoing research, HIOs are poised to deepen our understanding of microbial colonization strategies and their implications for host health (Adeniyi-Ipadeola et al., 2023) (Figure 4. 4.7).*Staphylococcus aureus*

4.2.2. Invasion of Host Tissues

Invasion of host tissues by pathogenic microorganisms constitutes a critical aspect of host-microbe interactions and pathogenesis research. Successful invasion typically initiates with the adherence of pathogens to host cells, mediated by virulence factors known as adhesins. These adhesins are structural proteins that facilitate bacterial attachment to epithelial surfaces, thereby invading the mucosal lining' s mechanical defences. For example, *Yersinia pseudotuberculosis* employs a multivalent adhesion molecule (MAM) that binds to host cells, supporting its colonization ability. The capacity of microbes to secure a niche within host tissues provides a foundation for subsequent pathogenic processes, such as immune evasion and the promotion of further tissue damage, underscoring the importance of adhesion in overall pathogenicity. Following adhesion, pathogenic microorganisms utilize various mechanisms for tissue invasion and exploit cellular machinery for replication. During this process, pathogens like *Yersinia pseudotuberculosis* actively interact with host immune cells, such as phagocytes, to infiltrate internal tissues. The interaction of microbial adhesins with host phagocytes can lead to phagocytosis for immune evasion or incite inflammatory responses that result in tissue destruction. Interestingly, the loss of essential adhesins, such as the MAM of *Y. pseudotuberculosis,* does not invariably compromise pathogenicity. In some instances, the absence of phagocyte attachment has been associated with enhanced bacterial clearance, yet paradoxically, it may also provoke excessive immune activation leading to increased mortality. This complex dynamic illustrates that microbial adhesion and immune system activation at their interface are principal determinants of the success or failure of host-pathogen interactions.

Furthermore, tissue invasion influences not only infection progression but also significantly impacts the host's immune response. The mechanisms by which microorganisms invade and interact with the immune system can cause deleterious effects, including uncontrolled inflammation and tissue destruction. Notably, the induction of humoral immune responses, such as melanin production, has been observed when the pathogen evades phagocytosis. In *Y. pseudotuberculosis*, elevated melanin levels have been correlated with reduced pathogen clearance and increased phagocyte death due to hyperactivation of the host immune system. These complex interactions demonstrate the dual role of microbial invasiveness as a driving force of pathogenicity, highlighting the need for further research into the host and microbial factors that synergistically regulate infection outcomes and influence overall disease progression (Brown et al., 2014; Krachler et al., 2021) (Figure 4.8).

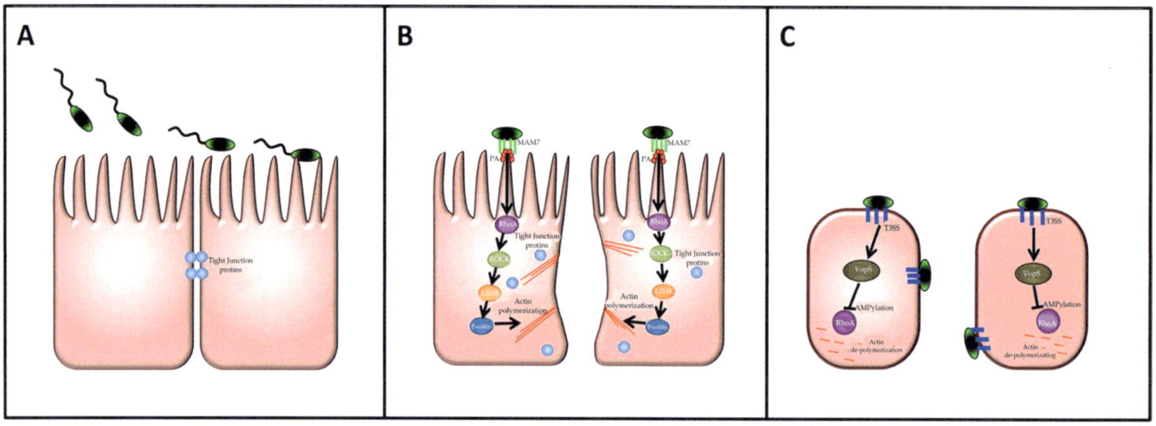

Figure 4.8. Adhesion molecule compromises epithelial barrier integrity and accelerates T3SS effector-mediated tissue damage during infection. (A) Flagella-driven, highly motile V. parahaemolyticus (green) reach the gut epithelium and attach to the cell surface. (B) MAM7 (green) binding to PA (red) on the epithelial surface leads to RhoA activation (purple). (C) These MAM7-mediated events increase the surface area accessible to V. parahaemolyticus, thus increasing the efficacy of T3SS (dark blue) effector transfer.

Source: https://www.researchgate.net/profile/Anne-Marie-Krachler/publication/279919274/figure/fig1/AS:616376960024577@1523967127241/Multivalent-Adhesion-Molecule-7-compromises-epithelial-barrier-integrity-and-accelerates.png.

4.2.3. Evasion of the Immune Response

The interaction between host and microbial pathogen is characterised by a complex interplay of immune evasion mechanisms that are vital for microbial survival and virulence. For instance, *Plasmodium falciparum*, the parasite responsible for malaria, utilizes antigenic variation as a method to evade the host's adaptive immune response. This mechanism permits the parasite to modify its surface proteins, thereby avoiding immune detection by antibodies generated during prior infections. Recent advancements in genome sequencing have shed light on the evolutionary dynamics of *P. falciparum*, illustrating how selective pressures interact with its genetic architecture to enhance immune resistance. As scientists delve into population genomics, they identify specific regions within genes that are subject to strong selective forces, providing insights into their functional roles in immune evasion and potential implications for developing tailored therapies and vaccines (Kirchner et al., 2016). Additionally, certain pathogens such as flaviviruses exhibit sophisticated mechanisms to counteract host immune defences, particularly the type I interferon response. Members of the *Flaviviridae* family, including dengue and Zika viruses, have evolved mechanisms that actively suppress interferon signalling pathways, thereby diminishing the host's antiviral responses. This suppression facilitates robust viral infections, often associated with severe disease manifestations. The ability to inhibit interferon-mediated immune responses reflects an advanced understanding of host cellular processes, influencing the pathogenic potential of these viruses. Investigations into these molecular mechanisms are now imperative, especially given the current absence of effective antiviral treatments for many flaviviral infections. Such research is critical not only for elucidating viral pathogenesis but also for informing the development of novel therapeutic strategies to counteract these evasion tactics (Clark et al., 2017). In summary, immune evasion constitutes a fundamental aspect of host-microbe interactions, playing a significant role in the pathogenesis of infectious diseases. Pathogens such as *P. falciparum* and flaviviruses exemplify the complex and dynamic strategies employed to circumvent host immunity. A comprehensive understanding of these processes is essential for advancing medical research aimed at improving disease management and therapeutic interventions. As insights into the genetic and molecular bases of immune evasion continue to expand, the prospects for the development of more effective vaccines and therapeutic agents become increasingly promising. Focusing on host-pathogen interactions not only enhances our understanding of pathogen biology but also emphasises the importance of sustained surveillance and research to address global health challenges posed by infectious diseases.

4.3. Host Immune Response to Microbial Infections

The host immune response to microbial infection involves a complex interplay among various components of both the innate and adaptive immune systems. The initial contact between pathogens and the host triggers innate immune responses, which serve as the body's immediate defence mechanisms. This response encompasses the activation of phagocytic cells such as macrophages and neutrophils, as well as the release of pro-inflammatory cytokines that recruit additional immune cells to the site of infection. These responses not only facilitate the elimination of pathogens but also serve to alert the adaptive immune system, which mounts a more specific response. Enhanced interactions among immune cells during this phase are critical for establishing an effective defence that reduces microbial load and ultimately eradicates the infection. As the immune response progresses, adaptive immunity becomes predominant, involving the activation of T and B lymphocytes. T cells differentiate into cytotoxic cells that directly eliminate infected host cells, while B cells produce antibodies that bind to specific pathogens, neutralising them and marking them for destruction by other immune cells. This adaptive response is essential for establishing immunological memory, which persists well beyond the clearance of the infection and provides rapid and robust protection against future encounters with the same pathogen. The coordination between innate and adaptive immunity ensures the presence of both immediate and long-term defence mechanisms, underscoring the importance of a robust host immune system in controlling microbial infections. Understanding these interactions also informs new therapeutic strategies aimed at enhancing immune function. Microbial dysbiosis, or imbalance, can significantly modulate the host immune response and predispose individuals to various infections and diseases. For example, the loss of diversity in commensal organisms, as observed in conditions such as atopic dermatitis (AD), has been associated with increased susceptibility to pathogenic infections, particularly by organisms such as *Staphylococcus aureus*. Commensal microbes play a regulatory role in maintaining immune homeostasis in healthy individuals and inhibit colonization by pathogens through competition for nutrients and modulation of immune functions. Research has demonstrated that restoring microbial balance through the use of probiotics can mitigate the severity of immune-compromised conditions such as AD. A comprehensive understanding of host-microbe interactions may therefore be pivotal in developing novel therapies aimed at modulating microbial communities to enhance host defences and improve resistance to infection (Paller et al., 2019).*Staphylococcus aureus*

4.3.1. Innate Immunity

Innate immunity constitutes the body's initial line of defence against invading pathogens, characterised by non-specific and rapid responses that play a vital role in infection control. It comprises physical barriers such as the skin and mucosal membranes, along with cellular components including phagocytes and natural killer (NK) cells. The skin is not merely a passive barrier; it also harbours a complex microbiome engaged in dynamic interactions with host immune processes. For example, beneficial skin commensals are instrumental in limiting the overgrowth of pathogenic bacteria, thereby confining potential infections. By establishing a balanced microbiome on the skin surface, innate immunity exemplifies intricate host-microbe interactions, which inhibit colonization by pathogens such as *Staphylococcus aureus* and prevent disease initiation (sPaller et al., 2019).

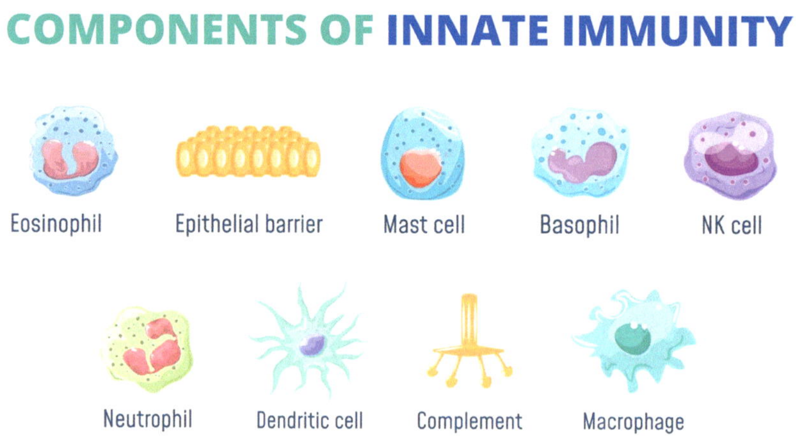

Figure 4.9. Components of innate immunity.

Source: https://www.biocode.org.uk/wp-content/uploads/2021/11/Blog-Thumbnail-Components-of-Innate-Immunity.png.

Consequently, understanding the interactions between microbial communities and innate immune responses is crucial for developing effective strategies for infectious disease control. Moreover, the study of innate immunity also involves examining its role in regulating inflammatory responses and its interactions with the adaptive immune system. Components of innate immunity are equipped with pattern recognition receptors (PRRs) that identify pathogen-associated molecular patterns (PAMPs), thereby eliciting a potent immune response. This recognition process activates various immune cells, including dendritic cells and macrophages, leading to inflammation and subsequent recruitment of adaptive immune elements. These interactions are of paramount importance, particularly in the modulation of immune responses during the initial stages of pathogen exposure. The balance between commensal organisms and innate immunity also exemplifies how microbial influence is utilized to modulate infant immune development and susceptibility to conditions such as asthma and atopic dermatitis in adulthood (Paller et al., 2019). Such relationships enable researchers to design interventions that bolster innate immunity while maintaining the stability of the microbiome. Moreover, the function of innate immunity extends beyond mere defence against pathogens; it is crucial in maintaining homeostasis within the host organism. As an integral component of the immune system, innate responses aid in preserving tissue integrity and facilitating wound healing following injury or infection. The coordinated activity of immune cells, including neutrophils and macrophages, effectively eliminates damaged tissue and pathogens, thereby promoting tissue repair and regeneration. In conditions such as atopic dermatitis, research has demonstrated that imbalance within the cutaneous microbiome can impair innate immune functions, which contribute to disease manifestations (Paller et al., 2019). The delicate equilibrium between sustaining microbial diversity and fostering effective innate immune activity highlights the therapeutic potential of targeting strategies aimed at restoring microbial homeostasis to mitigate inflammatory conditions. Finally, advancing the understanding of innate immunity within host-microbe interactions is essential for developing innovative approaches to combat various pathologies (Figure 4.9).

4.3.2. Adaptive Immunity

Adaptive immunity is a vital part of host defence that operates through a highly specialized response capable of distinguishing self from non-self antigens. Unlike the innate immune system, which offers an immediate but non-specific response, adaptive immunity develops over time to establish immunological memory. Activation of lymphocytes, notably T and B cells — key players in identifying specific pathogens — contributes to this maturation process. It begins with antigen presentation, where antigen-presenting cells (APCs) ingest and display foreign antigens. This process activates T helper cells, which then stimulate B cells to produce highly specific antibodies. These antibodies neutralise microorganisms and mark them for destruction by other immune cells, demonstrating the synergistic relationship between adaptive immunity and microbial encounters faced by the host. Moreover, the role of adaptive immunity is highlighted in microbial infections, such as in atopic dermatitis and asthma, which can potentially be influenced by microbial interactions. The skin, as a vast interface between host and environment, hosts a complex microbiome that can modulate both innate and adaptive immune responses. Evidence indicates that crosstalk between skin commensals and the immune system significantly affects disease severity. For instance, reduced diversity of the cutaneous microbiota is linked to increased levels of pathogenic bacteria like *Staphylococcus aureus*, which may exacerbate adaptive immune responses. Understanding these dynamics is crucial for therapeutic interventions aimed at restoring microbiome balance, thereby fostering a more effective immune response and preventing chronic inflammatory diseases associated with dysregulated adaptive immunity (Paller et al., 2019). Additionally, knowledge of adaptive immunity extends beyond human medicine, notably in veterinary contexts, especially regarding enteric diseases in livestock. Studies on adaptive immune mechanisms in pigs offer insights into pathogens such as *Lawsonia intracellularis* and *Brachyspira hyodysenteriae*, which are known to trigger complex host responses. The development of diagnostic tools, such as PCR, has improved pathogen detection and facilitated the assessment of their interactions with the host immune system. Host-microbe interactions in swine also illustrate how external factors like diet and living conditions influence disease susceptibility. Research into the immune responses of pigs can further enhance understanding of adaptive immunity related to gastrointestinal health and support the development of improved prophylactic measures against such pathogens (Jacobson, 2003) (Figure 4.10).Jacobson, 2003

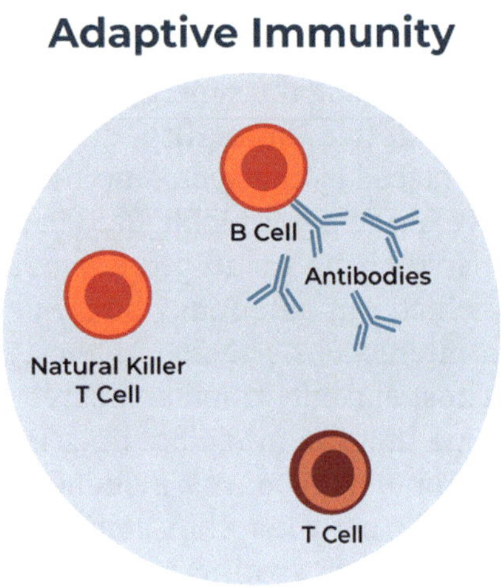

Figure 4.10. Adaptive immunity.

Source: https://media.geeksforgeeks.org/wp-content/uploads/20240220100851/Adaptive-Immunity.png.

4.3.3. Role of Inflammation

Inflammation constitutes an indispensable protective response to host-microbe interactions, functioning both as a defence mechanism against pathogens and as a potential contributor to pathogenesis. Upon exposure to microbial pathogens, the immune system triggers inflammatory responses aimed at excluding and eliminating the invading microorganisms. This process involves the activation of immune cells at the site of infection, the production of pro-inflammatory cytokines, and the activation of multiple molecular signalling cascades. However, chronic inflammation may produce detrimental effects, as prolonged exposure to pro-inflammatory mediators can lead to tissue injury and disease progression. In conditions such as atopic dermatitis and asthma, an overactive inflammatory response is observed, exemplifying the double-edged nature of inflammation in host-microbe interactions. Therefore, understanding the balance between protective and pathological inflammation is essential for the development of therapeutic interventions that can modulate immune responses without compromising host defences. The role of the microbiome in modulating inflammation offers an additional dimension to our understanding of host-microbe interactions. The cutaneous microbiome, composed of complex microbial communities residing on the skin, plays a vital role in maintaining immune homeostasis by inhibiting colonization by pathogenic bacteria such as *Staphylococcus aureus* and by preserving epidermal barrier integrity. Dysbiosis, characterised by disruption of the balance within these microbiota populations, results in inflammatory skin diseases, with decreased microbial diversity correlating with increased severity of conditions such as atopic dermatitis.

Indeed, the reconstitution of microbial homeostasis through therapeutic means, such as the application of beneficial commensal microorganisms, has been shown to reduce inflammation and confer clinical benefits. These findings underscore the critical function of the microbiome in modulating inflammatory processes and open potential avenues for novel therapeutic strategies in treating inflammatory disorders (Paller et al., 2019). Recent research has also elucidated the symbiotic relationship between autophagy and inflammation, further emphasising host-microbe interactions. Autophagy, a cellular process responsible for the degradation and recycling of intracellular components, influences inflammatory pathways, and vice versa. The identification of autophagy-related proteins (ATGs) has been instrumental in uncovering their multifunctional roles beyond classical autophagy, including modulation of immune signalling, phagosome transport, and viral particle replication. The interaction between autophagy and inflammation is particularly significant, as enhanced autophagic flux can suppress immune pathology by mitigating excessive inflammatory signals. Conversely, impaired autophagic regulation may lead to pathogenic inflammation and an increased risk of diseases such as autoimmunity. A deeper understanding of these complex molecular interactions holds promise for guiding approaches aimed at targeting inflammatory pathways to treat disease (Cadwell & Debnath, 2018).*Staphylococcus aureus*

4.4. Factors Influencing Host-Microbe Interactions

The identification of determinants underlying host-microbe interactions is essential for elucidating the mechanisms of microbial pathogenesis. Among these determinants, microbiota composition varies significantly according to individual host characteristics such as immunity and genetics. The host immune system influences whether the microbiome is established, promoting the proliferation of commensal microorganisms while inhibiting the growth of pathogenic microbes. This relationship becomes particularly evident in infections where pathogens have evolved sophisticated means to evade immune responses. For example, intracellular pathogens can manipulate host cell functions to create environments conducive to their survival and proliferation, thereby complicating the host's immune response. Given the dynamic nature of these interactions, it is crucial to study not only the pathogens but also the context of the host immune environment (Soni & Pandey, 2024). Environmental factors — including diet, drug intake, and pathogen exposure — also significantly affect host-microbe interactions. The use of antibiotics, for instance, can disrupt normal microbiota, leading to dysbiosis and potential opportunistic infections or chronic diseases. Similarly, dietary components can modulate the composition and density of gut microbiota, thereby impacting the host's immunological responses. In high-risk populations, such as very preterm infants, colonization of the gastrointestinal tract and skin begins in utero and is profoundly influenced by environmental exposures and gestational age (Underwood & Sohn, 2017). These environmental determinants play a role in modulating immune responses and have long-term implications for health, increasing susceptibility to conditions such as necrotising enterocolitis and sepsis. Recognising these factors underscores the importance of therapeutic interventions aimed at restoring or enhancing a healthy microbiota within vulnerable populations.

Moreover, the specific anatomical location of microorganisms within the host markedly influences the outcome of host-microbe interactions. Various tissues present unique microenvironments that can either support or hinder microbial survival and activity. For example, intracellular pathogens have evolved strategies to infect specific cell types, enabling them to evade immune detection while exploiting host machinery for replication. Such specificity is vital for pathogenic success but poses challenges for diagnosis and treatment. Addressing the complexity of these interactions necessitates advanced methodologies, such as integrated host microbiome single-cell genomics, to thoroughly understand the significance of microbial persistence within the host (Soni & Pandey, 2024). Ultimately, investigating these intricate host-microbe networks may lead to more targeted therapies and preventative measures, thereby improving clinical outcomes for infectious diseases and other microbial-related disorders. However, these potential benefits must be balanced with cautious consideration of associated risks.

4.4.1. Host Genetics

The dynamic interaction between host genetics and interactions with microorganisms is crucial to the susceptibility or resistance of an individual to disease caused by a variety of pathogens. Variations in host genes can significantly influence immune responses and the overall composition of the microbiome. Single-nucleotide polymorphisms (SNPs) in genes that regulate immune responses, for example, determine the effectiveness with which an organism can inhibit infection. Consequently, certain genetic signatures may confer increased susceptibility to diseases that would otherwise be controlled or mitigated by a healthy microbial burden. Genetic diversity within host populations is a key factor that influences the course of pathogenesis and may elucidate why some individuals develop severe illness from microbial infections while others remain unaffected or recover rapidly. Furthermore, understanding the genetic foundations of host-pathogen interactions enables the identification of biomarkers for disease outcomes. Host genetics can inform therapeutic treatment strategies, particularly within the framework of personalised medicine. For instance, identifying specific alleles that enhance immune responses can guide clinicians in selecting appropriate vaccines or treatment protocols tailored to individual genetic profiles. Additionally, research into the genetic determinants of microbiome composition indicates that certain microorganisms are more likely to thrive in hosts with specific genetic predispositions, thereby creating environments that are either conducive or hostile to pathogenic organisms.

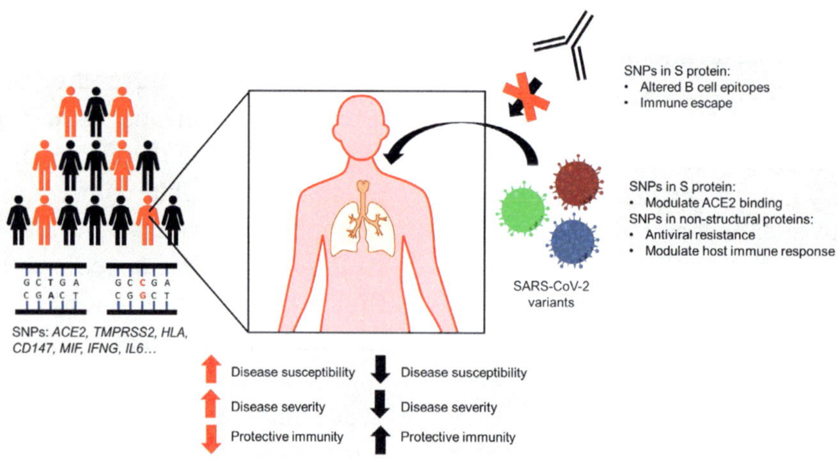

Figure 4.11. The impact of host genetics and viral variation on SARS-CoV-2 infection and COVID-19 severity.

Source: https://www.researchgate.net/profile/Stephen-Crooke/publication/342906119/figure/fig1/AS:11431281464884048@1748267655436/The-impact-of-host-genetics-and-viral-variation-on-SARS-CoV-2-infection-and-COVID-19.png.

Therefore, the intersection of host genetics and microbial dynamics opens new avenues for intervention in infectious disease management, offering the potential to improve public health outcomes. Recent advancements in genomic technologies have further enriched our understanding of the genetic complexities underlying microbial interactions. Genome-wide association studies (GWAS) and high-throughput sequencing enable researchers to investigate host genetic variation and its impact on microbiome assembly and function. Consequently, this emerging field offers promising opportunities to explore how microbial communities influence host gene expression, immune responses, and disease susceptibility. With these technological developments, researchers can elucidate the intricate networks regulating host-microbe interactions and better understand the mechanisms underlying pathogenesis. The prospect of applying these genetic insights to develop beneficial interventions underscores the importance of continued investigation into host genetics as a fundamental aspect of host-microbe interactions and disease development, as demonstrated by recent research addressing critical issues in modern health systems (Perez-Nadales et al., 2014; Jiang & Wang, 2018) (Figure 4.11).

4.4.2. Microbial Virulence Factors

Microbial virulence determinants play a fundamental role in elucidating the intricate host-microbe interactions and pathogenesis. The virulence factors, including toxins, adhesins, and invasion proteins, facilitate pathogens in establishing a niche within the host environment, ultimately leading to disease manifestation. For instance, toxins disrupt cellular processes and induce lysis of host tissues, thereby enabling pathogen proliferation within the host.

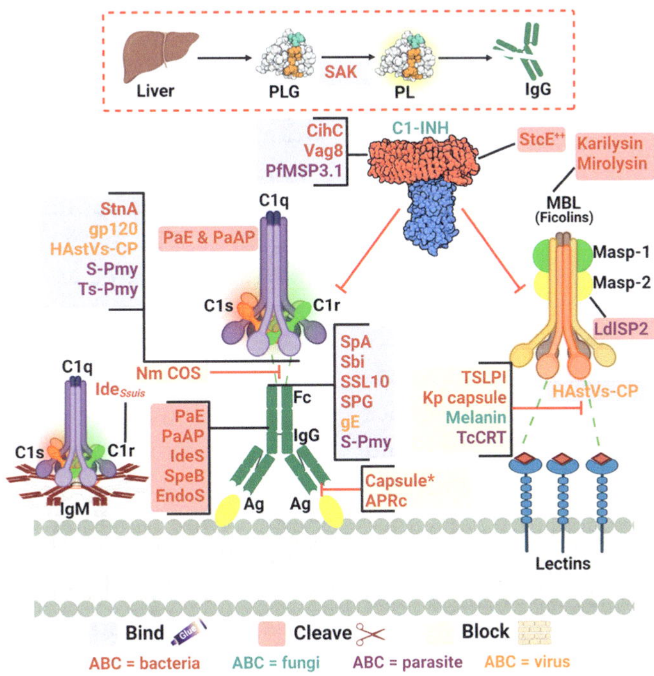

Figure 4.12. A schematic diagram showing microbial virulence factors involved in targeting the initiation phase of the complement system.

Source: https://www.researchgate.net/publication/377528084/figure/fig2/AS:11431281254832017@1719306791433/A-schematic-diagram-showing-microbial-virulence-factors-involved-in-targeting-the.tif.

Adhesins are integral in mediating the adhesion of microorganisms to epithelial surfaces, a crucial step in the colonization process. These virulence factors are not only vital for microbial survival but also serve to evade host immune responses, underscoring the necessity of comprehending these processes to develop effective therapeutic interventions (Jiang & Wang, 2018). In recent decades, advancements in microbiological sciences have elucidated the complex signaling pathways and gene regulatory systems that control virulence factor expression. These processes are modulated by the host environment, with microorganisms responding to host signals to optimise their pathogenicity. For example, the upregulation of specific virulence genes in response to host factors allows pathogens to adapt and survive within various tissues.

The interaction between microbial virulence factors and host defences highlights the dynamic nature of disease pathophysiology, implying that successful infections result from highly adapted interactions between pathogen and host (Caly et al., 2012). Furthermore, understanding microbial virulence factors is crucial for identifying potential therapeutic targets. By elucidating their mechanisms of operation, researchers can innovate novel strategies for combating infections. Vaccines that elicit strong immune responses against certain virulence factors are particularly promising, as they may effectively prevent infection by eliminating pathogens before causing disease. Additionally, therapeutics designed to inhibit specific virulence factors hold the potential to disarm pathogens, enabling the host immune system to respond more efficiently. Ultimately, expanding our knowledge of microbial virulence factors is essential for advancing public health initiatives and improving clinical outcomes in infectious diseases (Jiang & Wang, 2018) (Figure 4.12).

4.4.3. Environmental Factors

Environmental factors significantly influence host-microbe interactions, especially concerning pathogen emergence and disease susceptibility. In various agricultural settings, cases of enteric illness in growing pigs have risen sharply, underscoring the need to understand how environmental conditions predispose humans and animals to infections. For instance, the presence of group-housing systems and dietary factors, such as the soybean meal content in feed, can affect the intestinal ecosystem, thereby increasing the risk of pathogen-related diseases like *Lawsonia intracellularis* and *Brachyspira hyodysenteriae*. These observations highlight the importance of understanding environmental stressors to prevent disease outbreaks in livestock, which ultimately improves animal health and agricultural productivity (Jacobson, 2003). In human health, the role of environmental influences on host susceptibility, such as in inflammatory bowel disease (IBD), has drawn particular interest. Current research indicates that dietary exposures are vital environmental triggers that interact with gut microbiota, especially in genetically predisposed individuals. The rising prevalence of IBD can partly be linked to diet, making further research into how specific nutrients influence host responses to microbial communities highly significant. Such research concentrates on three key aspects: diet as a causative factor, its role in disease regulation, and nutritional status assessment. Understanding these elements can enhance our comprehension of host-microbe interactions and improve preventive and therapeutic strategies for managing IBD (Sigall-Boneh et al., 2017). Moreover, the complex interaction between environmental conditions and microbial populations can initiate disease processes in other contexts. For example, the microbiome composition can be influenced by environmental factors such as pollution, antibiotic use, and dietary habits- all critical in unravelling disease mechanisms. Environmental stressors can disturb microbial balance, leading to dysbiosis, characterised by an overgrowth of pathogenic microorganisms and ensuing disease. This underscores the need for an integrated approach to understanding pathogenesis, where environmental, microbial, and host factors intersect. Recognising the importance of environmental impacts on host-microbe relationships enables scientists to develop more effective public health initiatives and therapeutic strategies to reduce the burden of infectious and chronic diseases alike (Jacobson, 2003). Jacobson, 2003Jacobson, 2003

4.5. Therapeutic Approaches to Combat Pathogenesis

Host-microbe interactions are complex and often lead to pathogenesis that requires new therapies. A key focus is the development of drugs that can selectively target and neutralise the activity of pathogenic agents. With advances in understanding the molecular mechanisms of pathogens such as viruses and bacteria, researchers have begun designing therapies that not only inhibit the growth of these organisms but also enhance the host's immune response. Therapeutic strategies targeting exosomes in HIV pathogenesis, for example, have gained interest. Studies indicate that HIV utilizes exosomal mechanisms for spread and the induction of neurocognitive diseases associated with the infection. A method that disrupts the viral RNA sorting into exosomes can inhibit this disease spread, demonstrating the therapeutic potential of selective exosomal therapy against complex infectious diseases (Patters, 2018). The advent of nanotechnology has opened new possibilities for effective antimicrobial drug delivery. Nanoparticles (NPs) possess unique properties that enable targeted delivery of therapeutic agents without increasing side effects in healthy tissues. Of particular interest are chitosan-alginate nanoparticles, which have been reported to be highly effective against cutaneous pathogens such as *Propionibacterium acnes*, an agent of acne pathogenesis. These NPs not only disrupt the bacterial cell membrane through direct antimicrobial action but also exhibit anti-inflammatory effects, which can enhance the inflammatory response caused by infection. Encapsulating existing drugs like benzoyl peroxide within these nanoparticles improves their efficacy, yielding superior results compared to conventional formulations. This new delivery system demonstrates the potential of nanotechnology to transform treatment options for dermatoses caused by pathogenic microorganisms (Friedman et al., 2013). Exploring therapeutic alternatives to reverse pathogenesis also involves re-evaluating established treatment protocols and optimising their efficacy through combination therapy. For instance, antiretroviral therapy (ART) for HIV infection has proven essential in controlling viral loads, though many patients still face chronic conditions such as HIV-associated neurocognitive disorders. Exosome-mediated pathology research highlights the need for multifactorial approaches that address both the virus and secondary infection effects. Developing adjunctive treatments that target exosomal transport and its effects offers the potential to significantly improve patient outcomes. By bridging traditional pharmacological approaches with innovative technologies like nanotechnology and targeted molecular strategies, researchers can create holistic therapeutic paradigms better equipped to address the pathogenesis of most infectious diseases (Friedman et al., 2013; Patters, 2018).

4.5.1. Antibiotics and Antimicrobial Agents

The intricate relationship between host and microbe plays a central role in determining the success of antimicrobial agents and antibiotics. The formation of biofilms, especially within pathogens like *Pseudomonas aeruginosa*, presents a significant challenge in medical practice. These biofilms can attach to biotic surfaces such as lung epithelial cells, effectively resisting conventional treatments. Research has shown that antibiotics tend to lose potency against biofilms in complex environments compared to in vitro experiments. More specifically, the biofilm-inhibitory activity of various antibiotics is regulated by host factors and microenvironmental conditions, requiring the inclusion of host-microbe interactions in evaluating drug efficacy (Crabbé et al., 2017). Understanding these interactions is vital for developing more effective antimicrobial strategies to combat recurrent infections caused by biofilm formation. Additionally, the respiratory microbiota of chronically infected patients, such as those with cystic fibrosis (CF), demonstrates how community interactions can alter antibiotic effectiveness. In CF, lung tissues are typically colonised by diverse microbial communities, including both pathogenic and commensal organisms. Conventional antibiotics often fail to produce positive outcomes due to the complex interactions among bacteria within the lung microbiome.

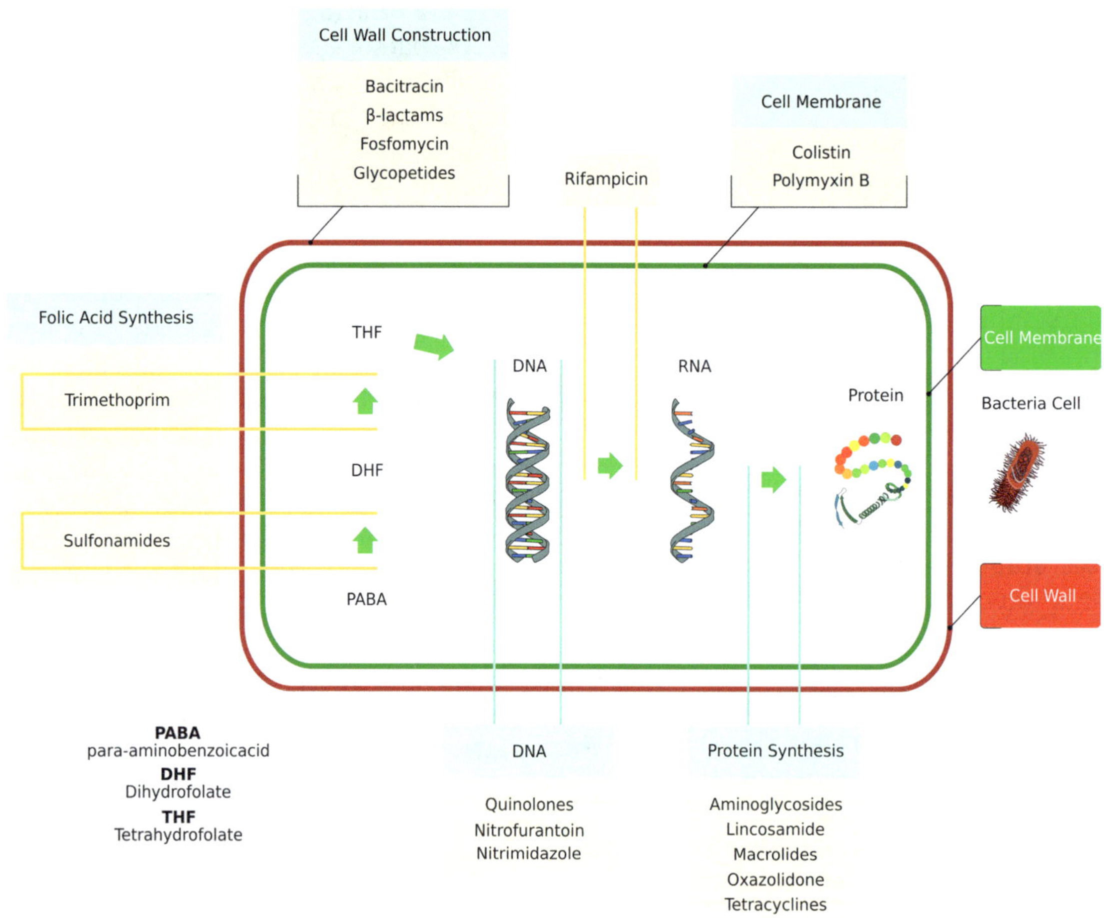

Figure 4.13. Molecular targets of antibiotics on the bacteria cell.

Source: https://upload.wikimedia.org/wikipedia/commons/thumb/0/08/Antibiotics_action.svg/1024px-Antibiotics_action.svg.png.

Mechanisms such as antibiotic degradation, modification of bacterial cell wall composition, and synthesis of matrix components play key roles in influencing drug penetration (Coenye et al., 2019). These species interactions can either form a barrier to antibiotics or render bacteria more vulnerable. Such insights into microbial dynamics are essential for designing customised treatment regimens that maximise the efficacy of antibiotics. Due to the challenges associated with traditional antibiotic therapy, researchers are increasingly exploring alternative methods and novel antimicrobial compounds. One promising approach involves synergy-based treatments combining antibiotics with anti-biofilm peptides or other adjunctive agents. For example, studies have confirmed that when used together with anti-biofilm peptide DJK-5, the antibiotic tobramycin significantly enhances the inhibition of *Pseudomonas aeruginosa* adhesion to both biotic and abiotic surfaces (Coenye et al., 2017). This combination not only targets the bacteria but also overcomes the protective barrier provided by biofilms. Given the continual evolution of microbial resistance, integrating such advanced techniques could greatly improve therapeutic success rates in chronic infections and further advance understanding of host-microbe interactions in disease pathogenesis (Figure 4.13).

4.5.2. Vaccination Strategies

Exploration of vaccination strategies is essential for understanding host-microbe interactions and disease development. Vaccines provide a preventative immune response, enabling the body to recognise and eliminate pathogens. These immunological therapies utilize the body's ability to develop immunity using live attenuated, inactivated microorganisms, or subunit vaccines containing key antigens. It is not only in the design of the vaccine but also in how they influence the host's microbiome that they significantly contribute to immune response development. Research has shown that an imbalanced microbiome can enhance vaccine effectiveness by affecting immune pathways and cytokine production, resulting in a stronger adaptive immune response. These findings highlight the importance of understanding microbiome dynamics when developing and implementing vaccination strategies, especially in diverse groups with varying microbiome profiles. The addition of advanced vaccination approaches includes consideration of new concepts like disease tolerance mechanisms alongside traditional immune responses. Disease tolerance refers to the host's ability to withstand the harmful effects of infection without necessarily eradicating the pathogen. This approach opens new avenues in vaccine development, aiming not only to kill pathogens but also to boost the host's capacity to limit disease severity. For example, studies propose that disease tolerance and immune-mediated resistance mechanisms may work together to improve cure rates in vulnerable individuals.

By understanding and manipulating these mechanisms, researchers can develop vaccines that offer not only temporary protection but also long-term resistance against a wide range of infectious agents, representing an integrated approach to managing host-microbe interactions within the context of pathogenesis. Recent advances, particularly involving cytokines like interferon-lambda (IFN-λ), illuminate new vaccination strategies against enteric viruses. IFN-λ is a vital component of the innate immune system, exhibiting potent antiviral activity, and can be exploited for vaccine development. Its role in modulating disease through virus-host interaction control underscores the importance of host-derived factors in vaccine design. Recombinant IFN-λ has therapeutic potential by modulating pathogen levels and maintaining intestinal health, and could be incorporated into vaccine platforms targeting chronic viral infections. As ongoing research continues to reveal the complex interactions between the immune system, microbiome, and pathogen behaviour, designing vaccines that harness these interactions — such as cytokine modulation — can considerably enhance our capacity to combat infectious diseases more effectively (Baldridge et al., 2017; Soares et al., 2014).

4.5.3. Probiotics and Microbiome Modulation

The modern understanding of probiotics goes beyond their traditional role as dietary supplements; they are increasingly seen as capable of modulating the gut microbiome, thereby influencing host health and disease susceptibility. Probiotics, defined as live microorganisms that, when consumed in adequate amounts, provide health benefits, can help restore or support gut microbiota diversity and function. Numerous studies have demonstrated that probiotics can reverse symptoms of gastrointestinal conditions such as irritable bowel syndrome and nonalcoholic fatty liver disease (NAFLD) by altering microbiome composition. Since the gut microbiome contains many more functional genes than the human genome, its interaction with the host and metabolic by-products plays a crucial role in maintaining homeostasis. This complex interaction between probiotics and the microbiome is central to understanding various pathologies, with disruptions potentially leading to adverse health effects (Sharpton et al., 2019).

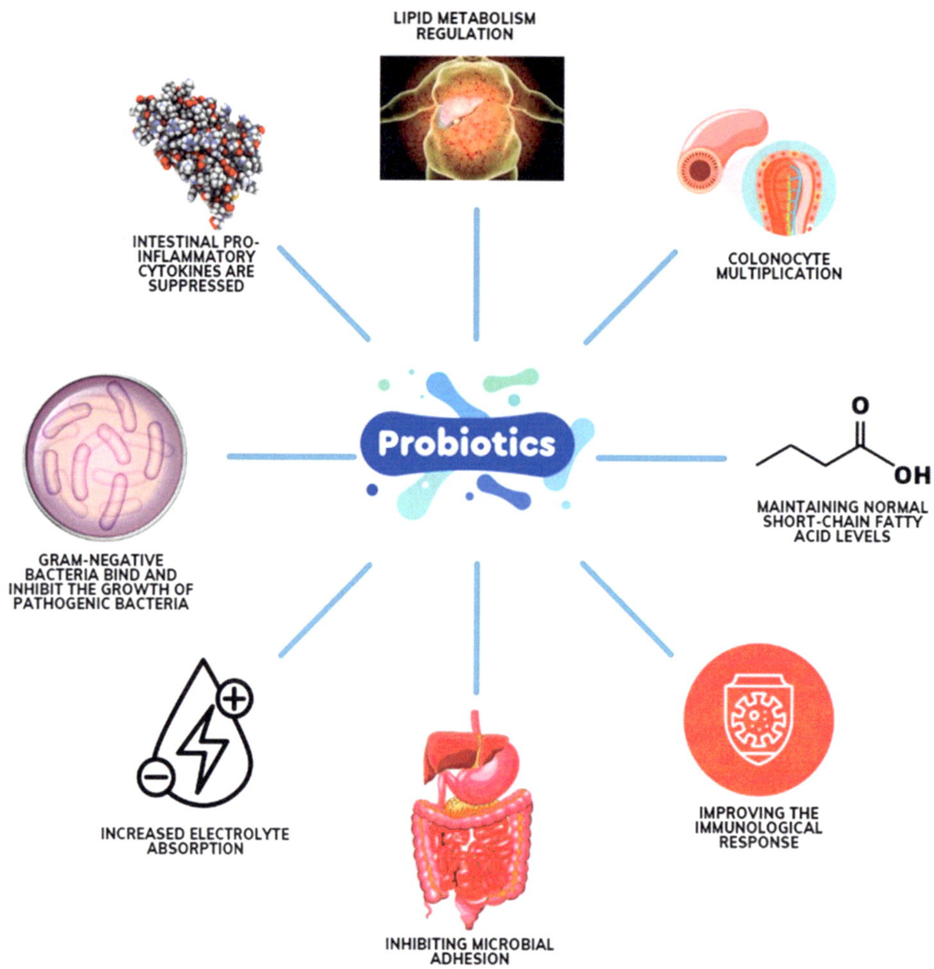

Figure 4.14. Action mechanisms of probiotics.

Source: https://www.mdpi.com/microorganisms/microorganisms-12-00234/article_deploy/html/images/microorganisms-12-00234-g001.png.

In addition to their role in intestinal health, probiotics also influence the brain-gut-microbiome axis — a complex network linking gut microbiota and nervous system activity. It has been shown that gut bacteria can affect brain function through immune, endocrine, and neural pathways, creating a bidirectional communication system between the central nervous system and the microbiota. This interaction can be disturbed in conditions like obesity and psychiatric disorders, where changes in the gut flora worsen symptoms and disease processes. Therefore, probiotic-induced modulation of the microbiome offers potential therapeutic benefits for restoring effective communication along the gut-brain axis and improving metabolic health (Martin et al., 2018). Recognising that probiotics can alter gut microbiota and, consequently, brain and behavioural health points to their potential in disease prevention and management. The impact of probiotic therapy on microbiome modification underscores the need for rigorous clinical trials to identify effective strains and appropriate dosages for specific health conditions. Despite the promise of probiotics, variability in patient responses and the complexity of microbiome physiology challenge their widespread application. Differences among individuals — regarding diet, lifestyle, genetics, and underlying health conditions — significantly influence the capacity of probiotics to modify gut microbiota populations. Consequently, future research should focus on personalised approaches that incorporate these variables to optimise therapeutic outcomes. As our understanding of host-microbe interactions deepens and the mechanisms of probiotic action become clearer, researchers will be better equipped to harness their full potential in restoring microbiome equilibrium, ultimately advancing the management of various diseases and overall health (Martin et al., 2018; Sharpton et al., 2019) (Figure 4.14).

SUMMARY

The complex dynamics of host-microbe interactions are central to understanding the intricacies of pathogenesis. Using systems biology approaches, researchers can unravel the multi-directional interactions between pathogens and host components, shedding light on disease mechanisms such as inflammatory bowel disease (IBD). By integrating data across genetic, epigenetic, and microbial axes, it is now possible to identify key regulators within the IBD interactome. This perspective emphasises that therapeutic strategies should not focus solely on pathogens but also consider the host's molecular environment, paving the way for personalised treatments tailored to an individual's biological landscape, as recent insights into IBD pathogenesis highlight (Polytarchou et al., 2014). Additionally, research into autophagy-related proteins (ATGs) has revealed new signalling pathways connecting host defence and microbial interactions. Emerging studies confirm that ATGs have broader roles beyond traditional autophagy mechanisms, encompassing critical functions such as immune signalling and inflammation. These findings offer vital insights into how the host can regulate microbial populations and maintain homeostasis. Understanding these interactions will deepen our knowledge of inflammatory and other diseases, highlighting that resolving these interactions is essential for designing site-specific therapies capable of counteracting the harmful effects of pathogenic host-microbe interactions (Cadwell & Debnath, 2018). Ultimately, research into host-microbe interactions is fundamental to advancing our understanding of pathogenesis and developing novel therapeutic approaches. Recognising the extraordinary complexity of these interactions, both host and microbial residents actively influence disease development and overall health. Future research must therefore continue to prioritise integrating diverse biological data to create a more comprehensive picture of pathogenesis. As scientists leverage these findings, they can identify biomarkers and treatments applicable across diseases, potentially unlocking solutions for some of the most challenging medical conditions (Polytarchou et al., 2014; Cadwell & Debnath, 2018).

Understanding host-microbe interactions is crucial for comprehending mechanisms of pathogenesis. Current research highlights the complexity of these interactions, particularly in conditions such as inflammatory bowel disease (IBD), which includes ulcerative colitis (UC) and Crohn's disease (CD). IBD affects millions of individuals in the United States and results from intricate interactions between the host's genetic and epigenetic profiles and the microbiome. Employing a systems biology approach allows researchers to integrate molecular and cellular data, thereby enhancing the understanding of IBD pathogenesis. Identifying key regulators or hubs within the IBD interactome can reveal therapeutic targets, facilitating the design of improved treatments tailored to specific patient profiles (Polytarchou et al., 2014). Of particular interest is the interaction between viral infections and host metabolism, as exemplified by studies on the Cricket paralysis virus (CrPV) in silkworm and Drosophila cells. The contrasting metabolic profiles observed between persistent and acute phases of infection offer valuable insights into host-microbe interactions. Persistently infected Bm5 cells exhibit high levels of glucose and glutamine, which decline sharply under pathogenic conditions. Conversely, acute infections in S2 cells show a decrease in essential metabolites preceding their subsequent restoration at the onset of pathogenesis. This inverse pattern underscores the importance of investigating metabolic changes resulting from different types of infections and highlights the significance of infection stages in influencing host-microbe interactions (Meeus et al., 2020). Collectively, these findings underscore the importance of detailed research into the nuanced mechanisms governing host-microbe interactions and their roles in pathogenesis. Integration of data from viral pathogenesis and microbiome studies enables the development of more comprehensive models that illuminate potential therapeutic targets. Incorporating high-throughput data not only enhances our understanding but also presents opportunities for novel therapeutic strategies aimed at regulating and potentially mitigating the deleterious effects of pathogenic microorganisms. As research advances, deciphering these complex interrelationships will be vital for developing effective interventions and improving patient outcomes in infectious and inflammatory diseases alike.

CLOSER LOOK

MICROBIAL EVASION OF HOST IMMUNITY

Microorganisms have evolved sophisticated mechanisms to evade the host immune system, allowing them to live, replicate, and infect. These evasion mechanisms target both innate and adaptive immunity, impairing the host's ability to recognize and eliminate the pathogens.

Antigenic variation is one common strategy by which microorganisms modify surface proteins in order to escape the detection of host antibodies. This is seen in *Neisseria gonorrhoeae* and *Trypanosoma brucei*, which alter the surface antigens through gene rearrangement, rendering immunity memory irrelevant.

Others create capsules—polysaccharide coverings that shield from phagocytosis by immune cells. *Streptococcus pneumoniae*, for example, uses its capsule to avoid engulfment by macrophages and neutrophils.

The majority of pathogens produce proteases to degrade antibodies, such as *Haemophilus influenzae* IgA proteases. A few interfere with complement activation, either by imitating host proteins or by binding complement inhibitors to their surface, thereby evading lysis.

Intracellular pathogens like *Mycobacterium tuberculosis* and *Listeria monocytogenes* survive in macrophages by preventing phagosome-lysosome fusion or evading into the cytosol. This enables them to counter extracellular immune defense.

Viruses also employ several different evasion strategies. Some, such as herpesviruses, produce proteins that suppress MHC class I expression so the infected cell cannot present viral antigens to cytotoxic T cells. Others, such as HIV, rapidly mutate to escape neutralizing antibodies.

Moreover, some microorganisms hijack host immunity by releasing immunomodulatory molecules that suppress inflammation or stimulate regulatory T cells to inhibit immune attack. Such tactics are used by *Helicobacter pylori* to survive in the gastric mucosa.

These microbial evasive tactics enhance microbial virulence and survival, making infections refractory to control. Understanding these mechanisms is necessary to create effective vaccines, therapies, and diagnostic agents to fight infectious diseases.

REFERENCES

1. Adeniyi-Ipadeola, G., Nwanosike, H., & Ramani, S. (2023). *Human intestinal organoids as models to study enteric bacteria and viruses.* https://core.ac.uk/download/643777105.pdf (accessed on 16th July 2025).
2. Sigall-Boneh, R., Levine, A., Lomer, M., Wierdsma, N., Allan, P., Fiorino, G., Gatti, S., Jonkers, D., Kierkus, J., Katsanos, K. H., Melgar, S., Yuksel, E. S., Whelan, K., Wine, E., & Gerasimidis, K. (2017). Research Gaps in Diet and Nutrition in Inflammatory Bowel Disease. A Topical Review by D-ECCO Working Group [Dietitians of ECCO]. *Journal of Crohn's & colitis*, *11*(12), 1407–1419. https://doi.org/10.1093/ecco-jcc/jjx109(accessed on 16th July 2025).
3. Amos, A., Anyanful, A., Barber, M., Barnich, N., Beutin, L., Blango, M., et al. (2018). Virulence behavior of uropathogenic *Escherichia coli* strains in the host model *Caenorhabditis elegans*. https://core.ac.uk/download/188826801.pdf (accessed on 16th July 2025).
4. Vargas, W. A., Sanz-Martín, J. M., Rech, G. E., Armijos-Jaramillo, V. D., Rivera, L. P., Echeverria, M. M., Díaz-Mínguez, J. M., Thon, M. R., & Sukno, S. A. (2016). A Fungal Effector With Host Nuclear Localization and DNA-Binding Properties Is Required for Maize Anthracnose Development. *Molecular plant-microbe interactions : MPMI*, *29*(2), 83–95. https://doi.org/10.1094/MPMI-09-15-0209-R(accessed on 16th July 2025).
5. Stotz, H. U., Mitrousia, G. K., de Wit, P. J., & Fitt, B. D. (2014). Effector-triggered defence against apoplastic fungal pathogens. *Trends in plant science*, *19*(8), 491–500. https://doi.org/10.1016/j.tplants.2014.04.009 (accessed on 16th July 2025).
6. Perez-Nadales, E., Nogueira, M. F., Baldin, C., Castanheira, S., El Ghalid, M., Grund, E., Lengeler, K., Marchegiani, E., Mehrotra, P. V., Moretti, M., Naik, V., Oses-Ruiz, M., Oskarsson, T., Schäfer, K., Wasserstrom, L., Brakhage, A. A., Gow, N. A., Kahmann, R., Lebrun, M. H., Perez-Martin, J., ... Wendland, J. (2014). Fungal model systems and the elucidation of pathogenicity determinants. *Fungal genetics and biology : FG & B*, *70*(100), 42–67. https://doi.org/10.1016/j.fgb.2014.06.011(accessed on 16th July 2025).
7. Baldridge, M. T., & Lee, S. (2017). *Interferon-Lambda: A Potent Regulator of Intestinal Viral Infections.* https://core.ac.uk/download/84911326.pdf (accessed on 16th July 2025).
8. Caly, D. L., Coulthurst, S. J., Geoghegan, J. A., Malone, J. G., & Ryan, R. P. (2012). Socializing, networking and development: a report from the second 'Young Microbiologists Symposium on Microbe Signalling, Organization and Pathogenesis'. *Molecular microbiology*, *86*(3), 501–512. https://doi.org/10.1111/mmi.12016 (accessed on 16th July 2025).
9. Bell, L. C. K., & Noursadeghi, M. (2018). *Pathogenesis of HIV-1 and Mycobacterium tuberculosis co-infection.* https://core.ac.uk/download/151187028.pdf (accessed on 16th July 2025).
10. Friedman, A. J., Phan, J., Schairer, D. O., Champer, J., Qin, M., Pirouz, A., Blecher-Paz, K., Oren, A., Liu, P. T., Modlin, R. L., & Kim, J. (2013). Antimicrobial and anti-inflammatory activity of chitosan-alginate nanoparticles: a targeted therapy for cutaneous pathogens. *The Journal of investigative dermatology*, *133*(5), 1231–1239. https://doi.org/10.1038/jid.2012.399(accessed on 16th July 2025).
11. Brown, A. J. P., Brown, G. D., Chen, K., Drummond, R. A., et al. (2014). *Candida albicans* colonization and dissemination from the murine gastrointestinal tract: The influence of

morphology and Th17 immunity. https://core.ac.uk/download/29151197.pdf (accessed on 16th July 2025).

12. Catlett, J. L., Catazaro, J., Cashman, M., Carr, S., Powers, R., Cohen, M. B., & Buan, N. R. (2020). Metabolic Feedback Inhibition Influences Metabolite Secretion by the Human Gut Symbiont Bacteroides thetaiotaomicron. *mSystems*, *5*(5), e00252-20. https://doi.org/10.1128/mSystems.00252-20(accessed on 16th July 2025).
13. Cadwell, K., & Debnath, J. (2018). Beyond self-eating: The control of nonautophagic functions and signaling pathways by autophagy-related proteins. *The Journal of cell biology*, *217*(3), 813–822. https://doi.org/10.1083/jcb.201706157(accessed on 16th July 2025).
14. Cavalieri, D., Godaly, G., Hagberg, L., Hedges, S., Schappert, K., & Shahin, R. (2016). *Subversion of host innate immunity by uropathogenic Escherichia coli.* https://core.ac.uk/download/80494906.pdf (accessed on 16th July 2025).
15. Clark, J. J., Cumberworth, S., Donald, C. L., Kohl, A., et al. (2017). *Inhibition of type I interferon induction and signaling by mosquito-borne flaviviruses.* https://core.ac.uk/download/80697084.pdf (accessed on 16th July 2025).
16. Krachler, A. M., Sirisaengtaksin, N., Monteith, P., Paine, C. E. T., Coates, C. J., & Lim, J. (2021). Defective phagocyte association during infection of *Galleria mellonella* with *Yersinia pseudotuberculosis* is detrimental to both insect host and microbe. *Virulence*, *12*(1), 638–653. https://doi.org/10.1080/21505594.2021.1878672(accessed on 16th July 2025).
17. Crabbé, A., Liu, Y., Matthijs, N., Rigole, P., De La Fuente-Nùñez, C., Davis, R., Ledesma, M. A., Sarker, S., Van Houdt, R., Hancock, R. E., Coenye, T., & Nickerson, C. A. (2017). Antimicrobial efficacy against Pseudomonas aeruginosa biofilm formation in a three-dimensional lung epithelial model and the influence of fetal bovine serum. *Scientific reports*, *7*, 43321. https://doi.org/10.1038/srep43321(accessed on 16th July 2025).
18. Coenye, T., Crabbé, A., Tavernier, S., Vandeplassche, E., et al. (2019). *Influence of the lung microbiome on antibiotic susceptibility of cystic fibrosis pathogens.* https://core.ac.uk/download/227040537.pdf (accessed on 16th July 2025).
19. Coleman, F. T. (2016). *Influence of macrophage NF-kappaB activation on pneumococcal pneumonia.* https://open.bu.edu/bitstream/2144/14597/10/Coleman_bu_0017E_11688.pdf (accessed on 16th July 2025).
20. Paller, A. S., Kong, H. H., Seed, P., Naik, S., Scharschmidt, T. C., Gallo, R. L., Luger, T., & Irvine, A. D. (2019). The microbiome in patients with atopic dermatitis. *The Journal of allergy and clinical immunology*, *143*(1), 26–35. https://doi.org/10.1016/j.jaci.2018.11.015(accessed on 16th July 2025).
21. Soares, M. P., Gozzelino, R., & Weis, S. (2014). Tissue damage control in disease tolerance. *Trends in immunology*, *35*(10), 483–494. https://doi.org/10.1016/j.it.2014.08.001(accessed on 16th July 2025).
22. Huitema, E., Kulagina, N., Marques Monteiro Amaro, T. M., Motion, G., et al. (2015). *Nuclear processes associated with plant immunity and pathogen susceptibility.* https://core.ac.uk/download/30663567.pdf (accessed on 16th July 2025).
23. Polytarchou, Christos*; Koukos, Georgios*; Iliopoulos, Dimitrios. Systems biology in inflammatory bowel diseases: ready for prime time. Current Opinion in Gastroenterology 30(4):p 339-346, July 2014. | DOI: 10.1097/MOG.0000000000000081(accessed on 16th July 2025).

24. Jacobson, M. (2003). *Enteric diseases in pigs from weaning to slaughter.* https://core.ac.uk/download/11694636.pdf (accessed on 16th July 2025).

25. Jiang, H., & Wang, D. (2018). The Microbial Zoo in the C. elegans Intestine: Bacteria, Fungi and Viruses. *Viruses, 10*(2), 85. https://doi.org/10.3390/v10020085(accessed on 16th July 2025).

26. Martin, C. R., Osadchiy, V., Kalani, A., & Mayer, E. A. (2018). The Brain-Gut-Microbiome Axis. *Cellular and molecular gastroenterology and hepatology*, *6*(2), 133–148. https://doi.org/10.1016/j.jcmgh.2018.04.003(accessed on 16th July 2025).

27. Kirchner, S., Power, B. J., & Waters, A. P. (2016). *Recent Advances in Malaria Genomics and Epigenomics.* https://core.ac.uk/download/46580201.pdf (accessed on 16th July 2025).

28. Sharpton, S. R., Yong, G. J. M., Terrault, N. A., & Lynch, S. V. (2018). Gut Microbial Metabolism and Nonalcoholic Fatty Liver Disease. *Hepatology communications*, *3*(1), 29–43. https://doi.org/10.1002/hep4.1284(accessed on 16th July 2025).

29. McCullers, J. A. (2013). *Do specific virus–bacteria pairings drive clinical outcomes of pneumonia?* https://core.ac.uk/download/pdf/82071893.pdf (accessed on 16th July 2025).

30. Meeus, I., Smagghe, G., Swevers, L., Van Meulebroek, L., et al. (2020). *Metabolomic analysis of cricket paralysis virus infection in Drosophila S2 cells reveals divergent effects on central carbon metabolism as compared with silkworm Bm5 cells.* https://core.ac.uk/download/322827688.pdf (accessed on 16th July 2025).

31. Ngo, J. (2024). *An actin cross-linking effector of the Vibrio type six secretion system increases intestinal motility through macrophage redistribution.* https://core.ac.uk/download/613868205.pdf (accessed on 16th July 2025).

32. Patters, B. J. (2018). *The role of exosomal transport of viral agents in persistent HIV pathogenesis.* https://core.ac.uk/download/234018970.pdf (accessed on 16th July 2025).

33. Underwood, M. A., & Sohn, K. (2017). The Microbiota of the Extremely Preterm Infant. *Clinics in perinatology*, *44*(2), 407–427. https://doi.org/10.1016/j.clp.2017.01.005 (accessed on 16th July 2025).

34. Soni, J., & Pandey, R. (2024). *Single cell genomics based insights into the impact of cell-type specific microbial internalization on disease severity.* https://core.ac.uk/download/615303706.pdf (accessed on 16th July 2025).

35. Uehara, A., Ansari, A. A., Dang, A. T., Thurman, A. R., Dang, A. T., Dale, B. A., Shacklett, B. L., et al. (2013). *Transcription profiling reveals potential mechanisms of dysbiosis in the oral microbiome of rhesus macaques with chronic untreated SIV infection.* https://core.ac.uk/download/323071203.pdf (accessed on 16th July 2025).

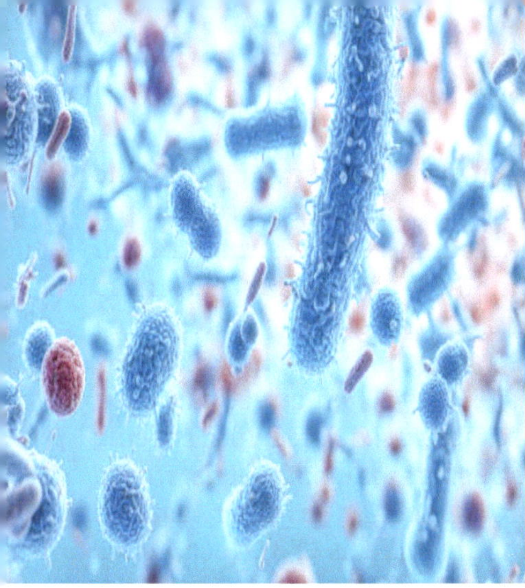

Chapter 5

MICROBIOLOGICAL OF INFECTIOUS DISEASES

Contents

Introduction

Identification in microbiology for patient treatment and care is crucial in managing infectious diseases. Precise pathogen detection through various diagnostic procedures can significantly influence outcomes, especially in severe cases requiring urgent intervention. Advances in laboratory testing have equipped clinicians with a broad spectrum of tools, including blood, urine, cerebrospinal fluid (CSF), and sputum cultures, along with serological assays. Each method possesses distinct advantages and limitations, underscoring the importance of understanding their specific roles in infection diagnosis. Proper utilisation of these microbiological techniques facilitates prompt treatment decisions, a factor of particular importance given the increasing prevalence of antibiotic resistance and the serious consequences of untreated infections. Culture techniques remain fundamental in clinical microbiology for isolating and identifying causative infectious agents, particularly in analysing specimens such as sputum and blood that can reveal critical diagnostic information. For example, sputum cultures are vital in diagnosing respiratory infections, while blood cultures are essential in identifying systemic infections. Emerging antigen detection methods have shown promise, especially in resource-limited regions where traditional culture techniques may be impractical. Research indicates that antigen detection can sometimes surpass conventional culture methods, notably in children who have received prior antimicrobial treatment (Lankinen, 2003). There is a clear trend toward integrating various diagnostic approaches to provide timely and accurate clinical information. Serological assays also serve as valuable adjuncts to culture and antigen detection, especially when direct pathogen identification is challenging. These tests can identify antibodies or antigens associated with specific infectious diseases and are extensively used in diagnosing infections such as viral pathogens, where cultures are often not feasible. Their significance is particularly pronounced in urgent situations requiring rapid diagnosis to prevent further transmission, such as in tuberculosis (TB). Techniques like the Microscopic Observation Drug Susceptibility Assay (MODS) have demonstrated superior sensitivity in high-prevalence settings compared to traditional methods, emphasising the need for innovative, resource-efficient diagnostics (Dang, 2012). Ultimately, an integrated approach combining multiple microbiological diagnostic tools is essential for optimising the detection and management of infectious diseases.

Definition of Microbiological Diagnosis

Microbiological diagnosis constitutes a vital pillar in the diagnosis and management of infectious diseases, utilising a comprehensive array of laboratory tests to identify pathogenic organisms. This process involves the integration of various methodologies capable of detecting microorganisms, including bacteria, viruses, fungi, and parasites. By analysing clinical specimens such as blood, urine, cerebrospinal fluid (CSF), and sputum, microbiological diagnostics support clinicians in determining the presence or absence of specific infections. A notable feature of this diagnostic approach is its reliance on both culture-dependent and non-culture-dependent techniques, each offering distinct advantages in terms of sensitivity and specificity. Traditional culture methods have historically been considered the gold standard, while advancements in molecular techniques such as PCR have enhanced pathogen detection, even in cases of low bacterial load. The effectiveness of microbiological diagnostics is exemplified in their application to clinical conditions such as tuberculosis (TB) and pneumonia. For TB, innovative culture methods like the MODS assay have demonstrated increased sensitivity compared to conventional smear microscopy, enabling the detection of cases that might otherwise remain undiagnosed. This development is particularly significant in resource-limited settings where TB is endemic and accurate diagnosis is crucial for disease control and treatment. Additionally, progress in antigen detection technologies has improved the identification of pathogens like pneumococci, which are traditionally difficult to culture through conventional techniques.

Furthermore, the expanded utilisation of diverse diagnostic methods enhances overall accuracy and provides a comprehensive overview of infectious disease prevalence within patient populations (Dang, 2012). Recognising the importance of standardisation in microbiological diagnostic procedures is essential to ensure accuracy and facilitate comparability among studies. In this context, adherence to standards such as those established by the World Health Organisation for pneumococcal disease is paramount, as harmonised methodologies improve the validity of diagnostic results. These standards are critical not only in clinical diagnostics but also in vaccine efficacy testing and epidemiological studies, where precise pathogen detection is fundamental for evaluating public health interventions. Moreover, ongoing innovations in immunoassays and molecular techniques continue to refine microbiological diagnostics towards greater sensitivity and specificity. As the field evolves, rigorous validation of novel methodologies remains vital to preserving the integrity of microbiological diagnosis, with the ultimate goal of enhancing patient outcomes in the prevention and treatment of infectious diseases (Lankinen, 2003) (Figure 5.1).

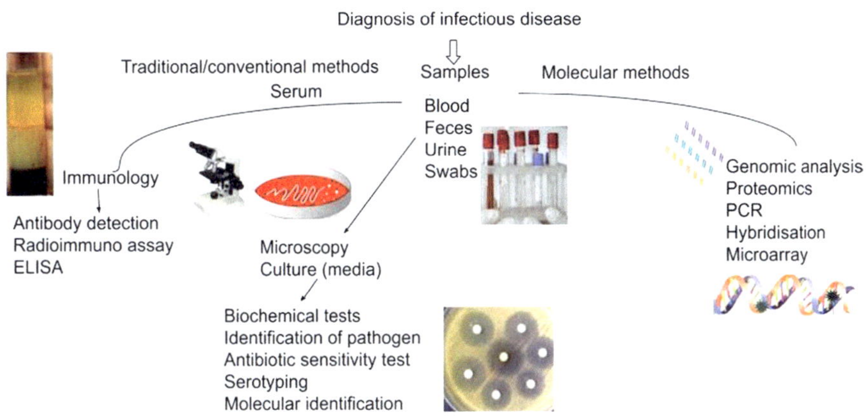

Figure 5.1. Sample processing for the diagnosis of infectious disease using conventional and molecular methods.

Source: https://www.researchgate.net/profile/Muazzam-Sheriff-Maqbul/publication/350878009/figure/fig1/AS:1012773744025604@1618475485473/Sample-processing-for-the-diagnosis-of-infectious-disease-using-conventional-and.jpg.

Importance in Clinical Settings

In clinical practice, microbiological diagnosis cannot be overstated, particularly regarding the detection and management of infectious diseases. Accurate and prompt identification of pathogens through blood, urine, and other body fluid cultures plays a vital role in influencing patient treatment outcomes. For example, blood cultures enable the detection of systemic infections such as septicemia, allowing healthcare professionals to prescribe suitable antimicrobial therapies promptly. Moreover, advanced techniques such as enzyme immunoassays and serological assays can identify specific antibodies or antigens, thereby enhancing the clinician's understanding of the patient's condition. The application of these diagnostic tools is integral to guiding therapy, optimising antibiotic use, and preventing antimicrobial resistance, ultimately leading to improved patient survival and public health outcomes. The importance of accurate diagnostic techniques is particularly evident in the management of diseases such as TB, where traditional methods are often inadequate. The use of the MODS, which demonstrates higher sensitivity compared to conventional smear microscopy — particularly in resource-limited settings where early diagnosis is vital — serves as an illustrative example. Comparative studies of MODS and other diagnostic techniques, such as the Mycobacteria Growth Indicator Tube (MGIT) test, unequivocally demonstrate their effectiveness in accurately identifying TB and drug-resistant TB strains. These advancements underscore the necessity for adopting innovative diagnostic technologies to enhance infection detection. Consequently, healthcare providers are better equipped to deliver timely and precise interventions, thereby improving patient outcomes and reducing the transmission of infectious agents within communities, as evidenced by research (Dang, 2012). Additionally, serological tests play a central role in clinical diagnosis by enabling the detection of pathogens that are difficult to culture.

For instance, antigen detection assays are valuable in diagnosing specific infections like pneumococcal disease, especially when standard culture methods are less effective — particularly following prior antimicrobial therapy, as seen in respiratory infections. The increased sensitivity of antigen detection with enrichment techniques allows for more accurate diagnosis in challenging cases. This capacity is particularly advantageous in epidemiological studies, where understanding incidence patterns is crucial for public health initiatives. The integration of various microbiological diagnostic tests into clinical practice not only enhances diagnostic accuracy but also informs healthcare policies aimed at improving patient outcomes and curbing the spread of infections (Lankinen, 2003).

5.1. Blood Cultures

Blood cultures are a vital component in the microbiological diagnosis of infectious diseases, especially when suspecting bacteremia or sepsis. The process involves collecting and incubating blood samples to identify pathogenic microorganisms present in the blood. Early and successful identification of these pathogens has a significant impact on patient treatment, as the timely administration of targeted antimicrobial therapy can greatly improve outcomes. The sensitivity of blood cultures is crucial because delayed detection can lead to increased morbidity and mortality in critically ill patients. Additionally, interpreting blood culture results can be complex, requiring a thorough understanding of local infection epidemiology and the patient's clinical context, highlighting the importance of microbiological data in clinical decision-making for effective treatment. Regarding the diagnosis of *Streptococcus pneumoniae* infection, newer methods such as antigen detection can improve blood culture sensitivity. Research has shown that antigen detection, particularly when combined with an enrichment step, may outperform traditional culture techniques in identifying pneumococcal pathogens in clinical samples. This is especially relevant for groups like children, who may have prior exposure to antimicrobials, where traditional culture methods can produce false negatives. The development of specific assays, such as enzyme immunoassays for pneumococcal capsular antigens, represents a significant advancement in diagnostics. These options can provide better results in settings lacking sophisticated laboratory facilities. Therefore, ongoing innovation in diagnostic methods is crucial in the fight against infection, underscoring the importance of collaboration between clinicians and researchers to improve and simplify testing techniques for wider application. Blood cultures are not without risks; careful attention must be paid during sample collection, storage, and processing. Contamination or mishandling can compromise the clinical integrity of blood cultures. Effective measures to prevent these issues include maintaining strict aseptic techniques during venipuncture and collecting adequate blood volumes to increase the likelihood of positive cultures. Moreover, the emergence of antibiotic-resistant organisms adds further challenges to managing infections identified through blood cultures, necessitating a focus on antibiotic stewardship. As sepsis continues to be a leading cause of morbidity and mortality in the intensive care unit, clinicians must be well-trained in interpreting blood culture results and understanding their implications for therapy, all while remaining vigilant to prevent contributing to antimicrobial resistance (Chan et al., 2017) (Figure 5.2.).

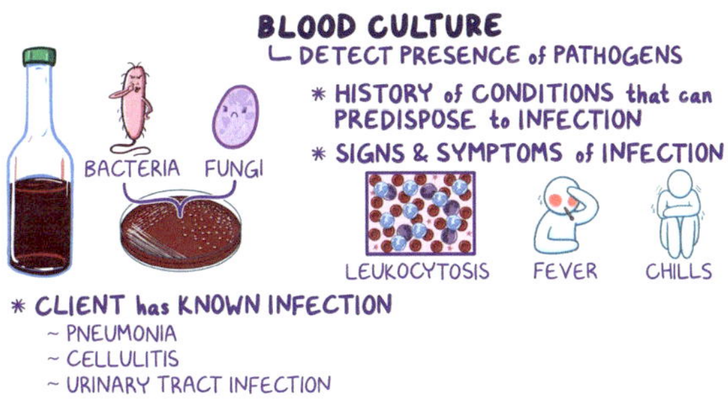

Figure 5.2. Blood culture.

Source: https://www.osmosis.org/_next/image?url=https%3A%2F%2Fd16qt3wv6xm098.cloudfront.net%2FGKnPOKI5TYCcBlYP5KdR3ORVQh2NSHNt%2F_.jpg&w=3840&q=75.

5.1.1. Purpose and Significance of Blood Cultures

The primary use of blood cultures is to confirm the presence of microbial infections in the blood, such as bacteremia or fungemia. These tests are vital for diagnosing, monitoring, and treating certain infectious diseases, like sepsis, which can develop into potentially fatal systemic complications if left untreated. By enabling clinicians to isolate and identify the pathogens causing an infection, blood cultures facilitate targeted antimicrobial therapy, thereby improving the chances of a successful cure. This diagnostic specificity is particularly crucial in life-threatening conditions where early intervention is key, underscoring the central role that blood cultures play in infectious disease management and microbiological diagnosis. Beyond identification, blood cultures provide vital information about the causative organisms and their susceptibility or resistance to various antibiotics. This data is essential for designing effective treatment plans and combating antibiotic resistance, a growing global concern.

Early detection of infections through blood culture results can significantly reduce the morbidity and mortality associated with sepsis by allowing healthcare professionals to initiate optimal treatment promptly. Moreover, advances in technologies like molecular diagnostics are making it easier and faster to obtain diagnostic results, supporting the continued relevance of blood cultures in modern practice and their contribution to antimicrobial stewardship programmes aimed at reducing resistance. Besides their clinical utility, blood cultures also assist in monitoring the epidemiology of infecting pathogens and informing public health initiatives. Data from these cultures can reveal trends in pathogen prevalence and resistance patterns within specific populations, aiding the development of targeted prevention strategies. Such epidemiological information has wide-ranging applications, especially in veterinary medicine, where understanding infectious disease dynamics in animal populations is essential for devising effective control measures. For example, research into enteric diseases affecting pigs has highlighted the importance of precise diagnostic methods, such as blood culture, in accurately identifying and managing health issues, ultimately benefiting both human and animal health interventions (Jacobson, 2003; Chiu et al., 2006) (Figure 5.3). Jacobson, 2003

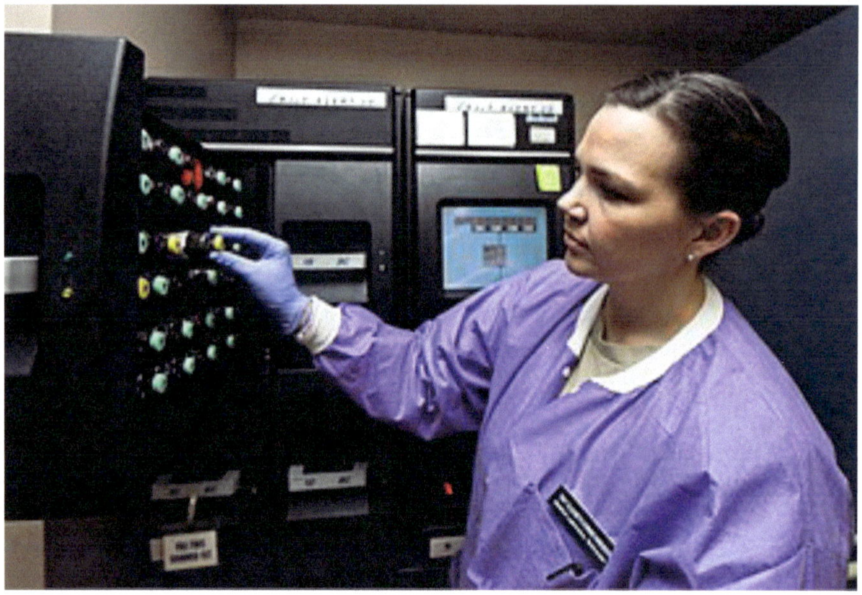

Figure 5.3. A laboratory worker unloads blood culture bottles from a BACT/Alert machine, an automated system used to incubate blood cultures and detect microbial growth.

Source: https://upload.wikimedia.org/wikipedia/commons/thumb/f/ff/National_Lab_Week_130410-F-TT327-090.jpg/330px-National_Lab_Week_130410-F-TT327-090.jpg.

5.1.2. Common Pathogens Detected in Blood Cultures

Blood cultures constitute an indispensable diagnostic tool for identifying pathogens responsible for bloodstream infections, which may escalate into sepsis and other severe conditions. Among the most identified pathogens, *Staphylococcus aureus*, particularly methicillin-resistant *Staphylococcus aureus* (MRSA), presents a significant clinical concern due to its increasing prevalence and resistance to standard antibiotic treatments. The detection of these bacteria in blood cultures is vital, as it informs the selection of effective antibiotic therapies and infection control measures. The identification of *Escherichia coli*, traditionally associated with urinary tract infections but increasingly linked to sepsis, further emphasises the necessity for comprehensive microbiological examination. Recognising the predominance of these bacteria in blood cultures is critical for achieving favourable outcomes in the management of life-threatening infections. Additionally, *Streptococcus pneumoniae*, a pathogen commonly recovered in blood cultures, is the etiological agent of various diseases, notably pneumonia and meningitis, with its presence in bloodstream infections correlating with elevated mortality and morbidity. Although blood culture remains the gold standard for diagnosis, advancements in antigen detection methods, such as enzyme immunoassays for pneumococcal polysaccharides, have shown promise in enhancing sensitivity, especially in patients who have previously received antibiotic treatment. These diagnostic innovations underscore the ongoing need for improved microbiological diagnostic techniques, particularly in the context of emerging infectious disease patterns. Given the evolving landscape of infectious diseases, maintaining robust surveillance and diagnostic capabilities is more crucial than ever for effective pathogen management (Lankinen, 2003). Furthermore, blood cultures frequently detect enteric pathogens such as *Klebsiella spp*. and *Enterobacter spp*., both of which are significant contributors to healthcare-associated infections.

These organisms, often exhibiting multidrug resistance, highlight the imperative for stringent antibiotic stewardship to counteract rising resistance rates. Prompt and accurate identification of these pathogens is essential for guiding effective therapeutic strategies. Moreover, blood culture results have implications beyond individual patient care, informing public health policies aimed at controlling the dissemination of multidrug-resistant pathogens within healthcare facilities. Continuous assessment of blood culture systems and the integration of novel diagnostic assays are necessary to mitigate the impact of these organisms on patient outcomes and the healthcare system at large (Chan et al., 2017) (Figure 5.4).

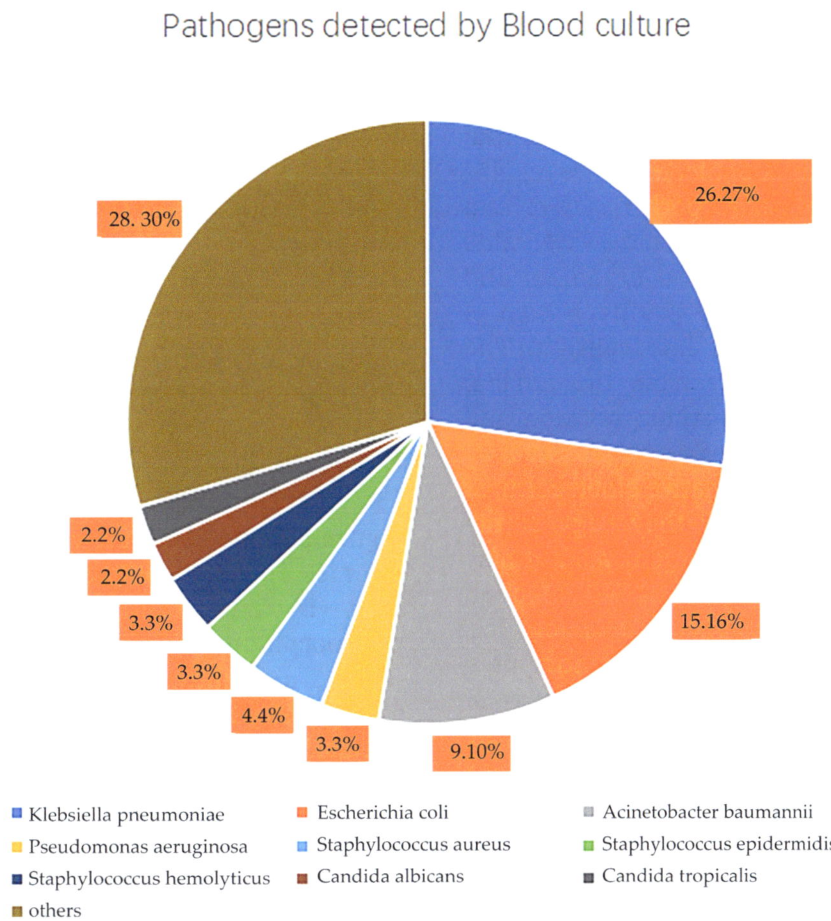

Figure 5.4. Pathogens detected by blood culture.

Source: https://www.researchgate.net/publication/368418187/figure/fig2/AS:11431281254264552@1719101784756/Pathogens-detected-by-blood-culture.tif.

5.1.3. Interpretation of Blood Culture Results

The interpretation of blood cultures is essential in the diagnosis of infectious diseases, especially those leading to sepsis. Blood cultures aim to detect pathogens within the bloodstream, and their results provide physicians with the foundation for devising customised antimicrobial therapies. The effectiveness of blood cultures depends on factors such as the timing of sample collection, the volume of blood obtained, and the method utilized for culturing. It necessitates a critical appraisal of these results, particularly in cases of suspected sepsis, as early identification of etiological agents may significantly influence patient outcomes. The study underscores that understanding the spectrum of pathogens is pivotal for guiding appropriate management and optimising antibiotic use to reduce morbidity and mortality related to infectious diseases (Lankinen, 2003). Therefore, a systematic evaluation of blood culture findings ensures that clinicians respond appropriately to potential infections. Upon receipt of blood culture results, it is imperative to assess both negative and positive outcomes. A positive culture warrants confirmation of the identified organism and its antibiotic susceptibility profile, which is vital for effective clinical intervention. The presence of contaminants from the normal skin biota may lead to misinterpretation and unnecessary concern unless corroborated by clinical data. Conversely, negative blood cultures can be highly informative; they suggest the absence of culturable microorganisms but may prompt consideration of alternative infection sources. Advances in diagnostic technologies, such as molecular techniques, are anticipated to enhance the sensitivity and specificity of pathogen detection, thereby increasing the overall diagnostic yield, especially in complex cases of blood culture interpretation (Lankinen, 2003). This integrative approach emphasises the importance of accurate result interpretation within the comprehensive diagnostic process. Moreover, understanding the epidemiological context is vital when interpreting blood culture data. The spectrum of potential pathogens varies according to geographic location, patient demographics, and regional disease prevalence, as demonstrated in various studies of community-acquired sepsis (Southeast Asia Infectious Disease Clinical Research Network, 2017). For example, clinicians must consider endemic pathogens specific to particular regions, such as the Dengue virus or *Leptospira spp.*, which may not be prevalent elsewhere. Diagnostic strategies should be adapted accordingly to account for these variations. Additionally, ongoing education for clinicians regarding emerging guidelines and interpretative methods can enhance diagnostic precision and treatment effectiveness. Feedback mechanisms linking laboratory results to clinical outcomes are crucial for refining diagnostic strategies and ultimately improving infectious disease management through evidence-based decisions (Figure 5.5).

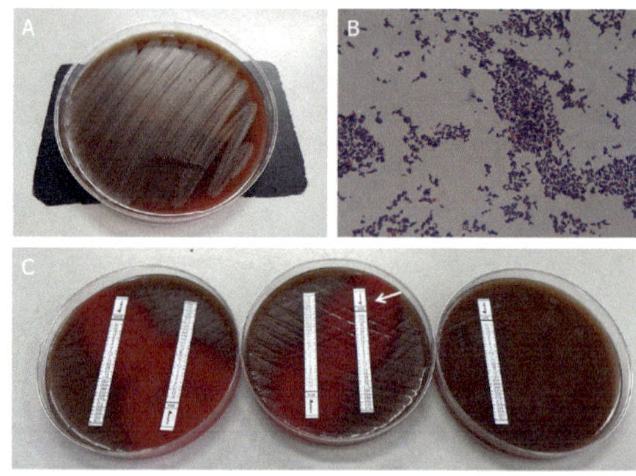

Figure 5.5. Blood culture results. (A) Growth of colonies of Abiotrophia defectiva in the blood agar. (B) Gram stain reveals Gram-positive pleomorphic coccobacilli, arranged in chains (original magnification, 1000×). (C) Antimicrobial susceptibility testing demonstrated susceptibility to vancomycin, imipenem, and meropenem, but resistance to penicillin and levofloxacin.

Source: https://www.researchgate.net/publication/359192467/figure/fig2/AS:1143128118792441 5@1694450724459/Blood-culture-results-A-Growth-of-colonies-of-Abiotrophia-defectiva-in-the-blood-agar.tif.

5.2. Urine Cultures

Urine culture is a fundamental diagnostic technique used to evaluate urinary tract infections (UTIS), one of the most common infectious diseases worldwide. The procedure involves the collection of urine samples and microbiological analysis to identify and quantify microbial organisms. Conventionally, urine cultures can isolate causative agents such as *Escherichia coli*, which accounts for the majority of UTIs, as well as other bacteria like *Klebsiella pneumoniae* and *Proteus mirabilis*. This examination not only confirms the presence of infection but also provides information regarding the antibiotic sensitivity of the identified pathogens, thereby guiding appropriate therapeutic strategies. Accurate detection of these organisms is particularly valuable in cases of complex or recurrent UTIa, as untreated infections may lead to severe complications, including pyelonephritis and renal failure, underscoring the critical role of urine cultures in clinical practice. Beyond bacterial identification, urine testing has expanded to include the detection of other biomarkers specific to certain infections. For example, microbial antigen detection and nucleic acid amplification tests can improve diagnostic accuracy, especially when standard cultures yield negative results. This is particularly relevant given the diverse etiological agents of UTIs, which can encompass viral and fungal pathogens, albeit less frequently. Furthermore, research on fever of unknown origin (FUO) has demonstrated that the prevalence of UTI as an underlying infection supports the inclusion of comprehensive urinary analysis within differential diagnosis protocols (Thangamathi et al., 2006). Such multidimensional approaches emphasise the significance of urine cultures in elucidating infectious disease etiology and informing targeted treatment interventions. Technological innovations have also enhanced the efficiency of urine cultures, including the development of automated systems that facilitate rapid sample processing and analysis. These advancements have considerably reduced the turnaround time for obtaining culture results, which is crucial in clinical settings where prompt intervention is required. The use of enriched media, as recent studies indicate, improves the detection of fastidious bacteria present in low numbers but associated with severe clinical manifestations (Lankinen, 2003). Ongoing research and improvements in test sensitivity and specificity promise to further refine diagnostic accuracy, thereby optimising the management of UTIs and other infections diagnosed through urine analysis. It is essential for healthcare practitioners to continually update their knowledge and adhere to evolving guidelines concerning urine cultures, in order to achieve optimal patient outcomes in the microbiological diagnosis of infectious diseases. *Escherichia coli*

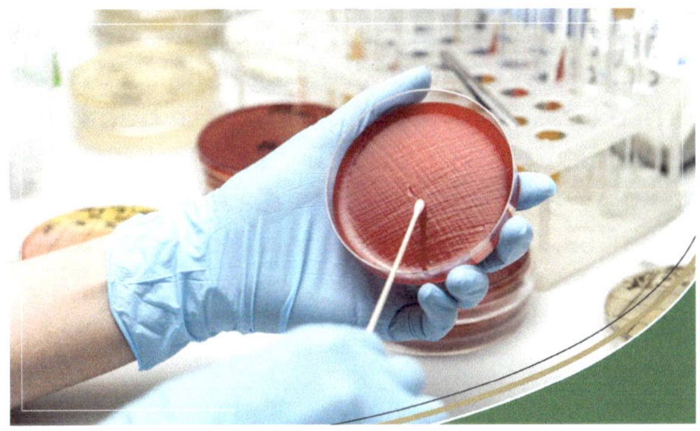

Figure 5.6. Urine culture test.

Source: https://www.sweetcures.co.uk/cdn/shop/articles/Urine-Culture-Test-Finding-the-Cause-of-UTI_2b3b778e-2fb8-46a7-9def-c08cf785d2ab.jpg?v=1633102104.

5.2.1. Indications for Performing Urine Cultures

The performance of urine cultures is a significant feature of microbiological diagnostics, especially in diagnosing urinary tract infections (UTIs). Urine cultures are mainly indicated when a patient exhibits signs or symptoms of infection, such as dysuria, frequent or urgent micturition, or flank pain. The presence of these symptoms warrants a thorough investigation to identify the pathogenic organisms causing the infection. In clinical practice, early diagnosis through urine culture is vital to guide effective antibiotic therapy and prevent infection-related complications. Additionally, the specificity and sensitivity of urine culture make it a reliable tool for diagnosing UTI, enabling targeted therapy against the causative microorganisms. Urine cultures are particularly valuable in specific patient groups, such as the elderly, pregnant women, and individuals with underlying conditions that increase their susceptibility to severe infections. These patients have an elevated risk of asymptomatic bacteriuria, which requires comprehensive assessment, as treatment may not be necessary and could lead to serious morbidity if overlooked. For example, in pregnant women, bacteriuria can predispose to pyelonephritis, resulting in maternal and fetal complications. Moreover, urine cultures are crucial in recurrent UTI cases to determine if persistent infection or complications like anatomical abnormalities or resistance are present, thus allowing for more precise prophylaxis or treatment. These points underscore the importance of urine cultures beyond mere diagnosis, impacting overall patient management. Apart from routine diagnosis, urine cultures are essential for guiding empirical antibiotic therapy, especially amid rising resistance patterns. In an era of increasing antibiotic resistance, urine cultures provide valuable insights into treatment options. While conventional culture methods often identify pathogens in most cases, chronic infections may necessitate advanced diagnostics, such as mNGS, to improve detection and tailor therapies for difficult cases. As mentioned earlier, traditional culture-based methods sometimes fail, particularly when dealing with complex or atypical infections (Chen et al., 2022). Therefore, urine cultures not only facilitate accurate diagnosis but also influence treatment decisions in complex clinical scenarios, making them a vital tool in microbiological infection diagnosis (Figure 5.7 7).

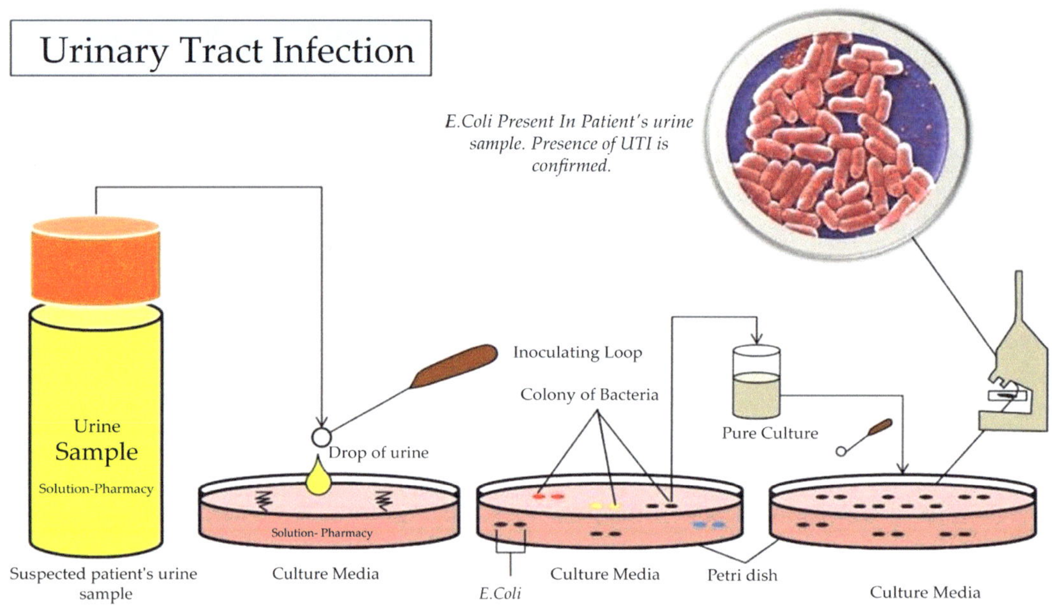

Figure 5.7. Example of laboratory workflow for Urinary tract infections (UTIs).

Source: https://bookmerilab.com/tests/wp-content/uploads/2022/04/maxresdefault-1024x576.jpg.

5.2.2. Common Urinary Pathogens and Their Implications

To understand the most common urinary pathogens and their significance, it is essential to identify the primary causative organism of urinary tract infection (UTI). Among these pathogens,

Escherichia coli is the most frequent, accounting for about 80% of infections. This organism resides in the gastrointestinal tract and typically accesses the urinary system through the urethra. Other noteworthy pathogens include *Klebsiella pneumoniae*, *Proteus mirabilis*, and *Enterococcus species*, all of which present unique diagnostic and treatment challenges. The importance of these pathogens extends beyond typical UTIs; for example, recurrent infections can lead to complications such as pyelonephritis and renal scarring. Additionally, the rise of antibiotic-resistant strains poses a significant public health concern, necessitating advanced microbiological diagnostic methods for effective and timely treatment. The classical diagnosis of UTIs involves urine culture, which identifies common pathogens. With advancements in serological testing and molecular identification, rapid and accurate detection has become promising, exemplified by the development of rapid antigen tests for specific pathogens. Such diagnostic tools not only enable targeted antimicrobial therapy but also aid in managing the broader epidemiological aspects of these infections. Early microbiological diagnosis is especially crucial in vulnerable groups such as the elderly and immunocompromised, where untreated infections can be fatal despite being initially treatable. A comprehensive understanding of the common urinary pathogens is therefore vital for effective disease management and public health surveillance. Beyond pathogen detection, understanding their resistance patterns is critical in addressing the growing challenge of antimicrobial resistance. Resistance often results from the misuse and overuse of antibiotics, forcing organisms like *E. coli* to develop mechanisms to evade conventional treatments. The increasing incidence of multidrug-resistant urinary pathogens greatly limits available therapeutic options, prompting healthcare providers to reassess antibiotic prescribing practices. Clinical guidelines advocate tailoring antibiotic therapy based on culture results and sensitivity profiles. Furthermore, combining microbiological diagnostics with targeted antimicrobial therapy can help mitigate the impact of resistant organisms on patient outcomes. Thus, a thorough knowledge of common urinary pathogens and their implications enhances clinical treatment and informs infection prevention and control strategies (Lankinen, 2003; Khanum et al., 2015) (Figure 5.8).*Escherichia coli*

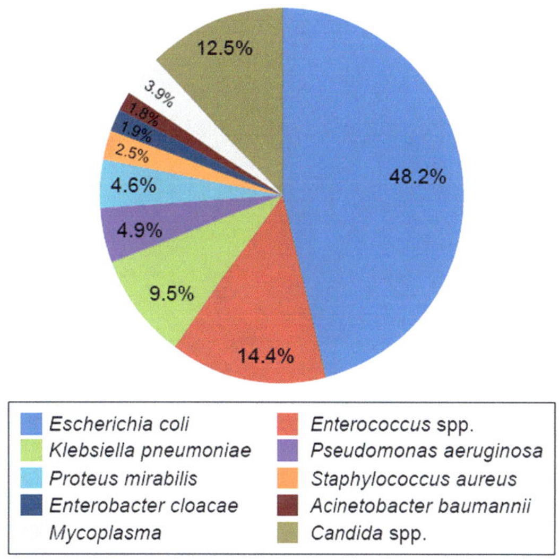

Figure 5.8. Most common pathogens detected in cUTI patients.

Source: https://www.researchgate.net/publication/320942080/figure/fig1/AS:11431281256676657@1719560982853/Most-common-pathogens-detected-in-cUTI-patients.jpg.

5.2.3. Techniques for Collecting and Processing Urine Samples

Sample urine collection is a vital step in microbiological diagnosis of infectious diseases, especially urinary tract infection (UTI). The accuracy of diagnosis largely depends on the technique used during sample collection. One effective technique is the clean catch midstream method, which reduces contamination from external genitalia and thus produces more reliable results. This involves the patient beginning to urinate, pausing, and then collecting midstream urine in a sterile container. In some cases, such as with young children or patients unable to provide midstream samples, catheterisation may be utilized. Each collection method has its own advantages and limitations, which influence the type of microorganisms detected and subsequently inform clinical decisions about treatment and management. After the urine samples are collected, prompt and proper processing is essential for microbiological diagnosis. The microbiology laboratory plays a crucial role here, where samples are filtered, centrifuged, and cultured on selective media to isolate potential pathogens. Traditional culture techniques enable the detection of urinary pathogens like *Escherichia coli*, a common cause of UTI. Rapid diagnostic tests, such as leukocyte esterase and nitrite dipsticks, can also provide preliminary indicators of urinary tract infection.

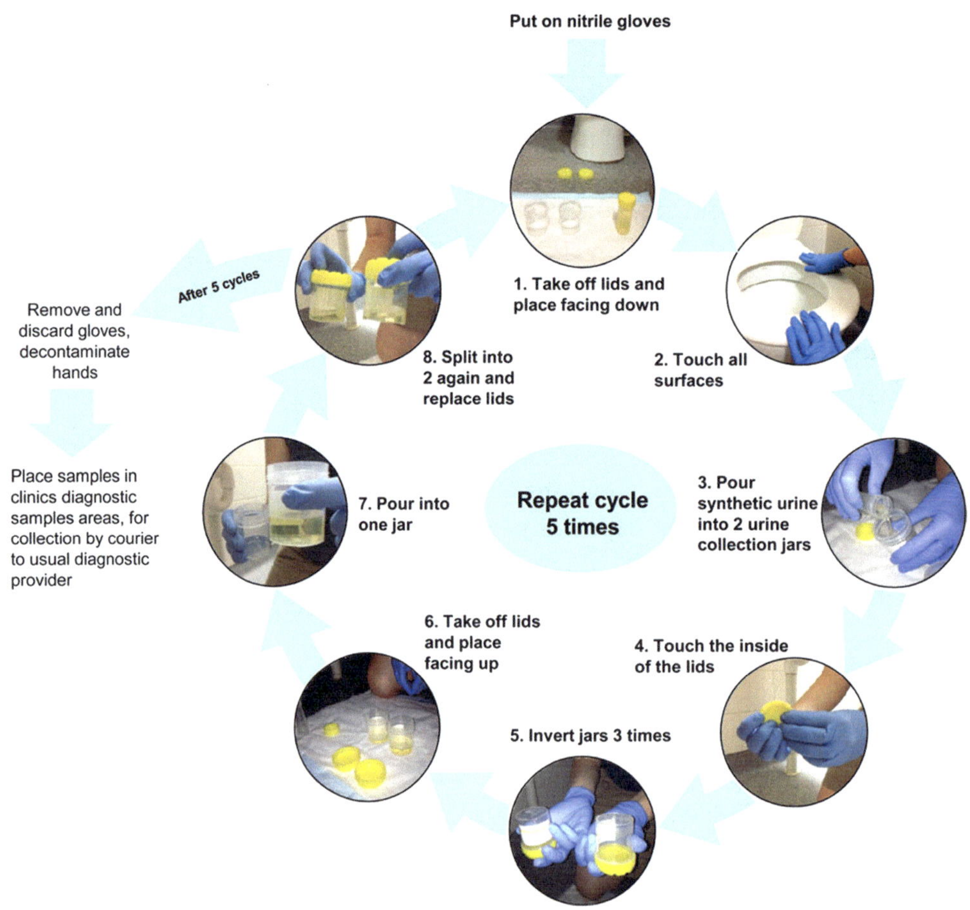

Figure 5.9. The method for simulation of collection of urine specimens using a urine surrogate solution.

Source: https://www.researchgate.net/profile/Patiyan-Andersson-2/publication/267742581/figure/fig1/AS:295741949005841@1447521783730/The-method-for-simulation-of-collection-of-urine-specimens-using-a-urine-surrogate.png.

Consistency of results is ensured by following standard protocols, giving clinicians confidence in diagnosing infections accurately and efficiently, supported by expert guidelines on testing procedures (Baron et al., 2013). Proper transport and storage of urine specimens are also critical, as they can affect microbial viability and test outcomes. To preserve samples effectively, they should be stored at appropriate temperatures, generally between 2° C and 8° C, to prevent bacterial overgrowth or deterioration. Delays in analysis may lead to false negatives or misinterpretation of microbial counts due to bacterial proliferation or death. Microbiology best practices recommend analysing specimens within two hours of collection; if immediate analysis is not feasible, precautions such as using preservatives should be employed to maintain sample integrity. These measures are essential to ensure reliable microbiological testing, thereby supporting more accurate clinical decisions in infectious disease management from urine samples (Morabe, 2022) (Figure 5.9).*Escherichia coli*

5.3. Cerebrospinal Fluid (CSF) Cultures

Culture analysis of cerebrospinal fluid (CSF) is a vital aspect of microbiological diagnosis of infectious diseases, particularly those affecting the central nervous system (CNS). CSF cultures are crucial in identifying pathogens responsible for infections such as meningitis and encephalitis, where rapid diagnosis impacts treatment outcomes. In clinical practice, collecting sterile CSF samples via lumbar puncture is essential. Once obtained, the samples can be subjected to various culturing techniques to detect fungi, viruses, and bacteria. The processing time of CSF samples significantly improves the chances of successfully isolating pathogens, with early initiation of appropriate therapy being vital for patient care. Understanding the microbiological growth requirements of different pathogens is key to developing effective CSF culture protocols in clinical laboratories. The pathogenesis of viral encephalitis can be better understood through detailed analysis of CSF cultures. A study on children found that enterovirus 71 was a leading cause of viral encephalitis, along with other viruses such as measles and herpes simplex virus (Beig et al., 2010). Using different isolation methods, including viral growth in specific cell lines and serological testing for IgM antibodies, can greatly enhance diagnostic accuracy. The study also demonstrated that patients presenting with generalised convulsions and altered sensorium are often associated with positive CSF culture results. Hence, combining clinical presentation with laboratory findings provides a clearer understanding of the infectious process, emphasising the importance of CSF cultures in effective patient management.

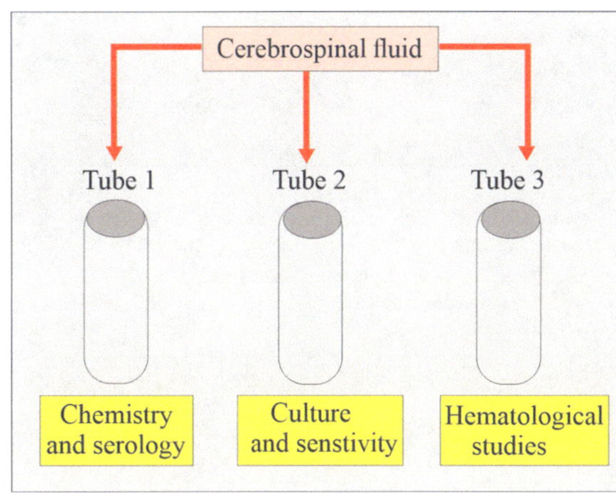

Figure 5.10. Cerebrospinal fluid.

Source: https://labpedia.net/wp-content/uploads/2020/01/CSF-tubes-collection.jpg.

Furthermore, CSF cultures are essential for detecting less common but clinically significant pathogens, especially fungi. *Cryptococcus neoformans*, a common fungal pathogen causing severe CNS infections, requires accurate diagnosis and treatment (Calandra et al., 2010). There is an ongoing need for novel antifungal agents, given the limitations of current therapies that often exhibit limited activity against specific fungi. CSF cultures are instrumental in identifying such pathogens to enable personalised treatment strategies and improve patient outcomes. The development of innovative diagnostic approaches, such as new antifungal peptides targeting specific fungal cell components, exemplifies ongoing progress in microbiology. Continued advancement in knowledge and treatment of infections involving CSF disturbances remains vital (Figure 5.10).

5.3.1. Role of CSF Cultures in Diagnosing Central Nervous System Infections

In the diagnosis of central nervous system infections, cerebrospinal fluid (CSF) cultures are essential. They play a vital role in identifying the causative agents of many infections, such as meningitis and encephalitis. By analysing CSF obtained through lumbar puncture, physicians can detect microbial agents since the fluid reflects the status of the central nervous system. Early CSF culture diagnosis is particularly important, as prompt administration of suitable antibiotics can significantly improve patient outcomes. Furthermore, the specificity of CSF cultures in distinguishing bacterial, viral, and fungal infections is valuable for selecting the correct treatment.

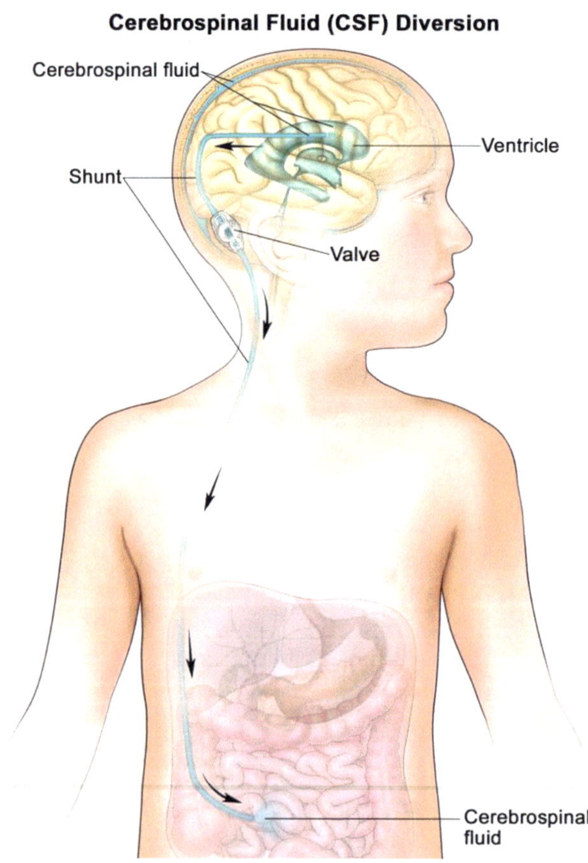

Figure 5.11. Cerebrospinal fluid (CSF) has an important function of protecting the central nervous system.

Source: https://storage.googleapis.com/prod-diagcorp/images/ckeditor/FZ3VknqPLDQpKYPIdDmrh TpzdhHe2rfO1awuZBhdy DUNOKBf9PpSmVMsdooc 4EKg4xEQXd9k9KWHRoHk_1612430552.jpg.

This specificity is especially critical, as inappropriate treatment can swiftly worsen the patient's condition or contribute to antibiotic resistance, thus complicating clinical management (Chan et al., 2017). Despite their high informativeness, CSF cultures have limitations. False negatives may occur due to various reasons, including suboptimal sampling techniques, prior antibiotic use, or contamination with fastidious organisms.

Therefore, clinicians often rely on a combination of diagnostic tests, such as imaging studies, evaluation of clinical symptoms, and CSF analysis. The accuracy of diagnosis improves when cultures are complemented by PCR techniques, which can detect pathogen nucleic acids in cases where conventional culture methods fail. This integrated approach ensures the most effective identification and treatment of central nervous system infections, thereby reducing the risk of long-term neurological sequelae. Additionally, identifying the causes of febrile illnesses, including those outlined in the context of fever of unknown origin (FUO), necessitates thorough investigations like CSF cultures for proper patient management (Thangamathi, 2006).

CSF cultures extend their value beyond diagnosis; they are crucial for informing public health responses during outbreaks of emerging infectious diseases. By detecting resistant strains or pathogens of public health significance, health authorities can implement interventions to contain outbreaks. Moreover, pooled CSF culture data provide valuable epidemiological insights into the incidence and spread of central nervous system infections, emphasising the importance of surveillance in public health policy. With increasing antibiotic resistance, the information gained from CSF cultures guides antimicrobial stewardship programmes to optimise drug use and prevent resistance development. Therefore, CSF cultures not only offer diagnostic clarity but also influence treatment strategies and public health policies (Chan et al., 2017) (Figure 5. 11).

5.3.2. Common Pathogens Associated with CSF Infections

Central nervous system (CNS) infection, especially cerebrospinal fluid (CSF) infection, is most often caused by a variety of pathogens with differing properties in virulence and clinical presentation. Acute bacterial meningitis is most commonly caused by the prevalent bacterial pathogens, namely *Neisseria meningitidis*, *Streptococcus pneumoniae*, and *Haemophilus influenzae*. Meningococcal infection, mainly affecting young adults, can lead to severe complications such as sepsis and enhanced morbidity if left untreated. Pneumococcal disease remains a major cause of death and illness despite vaccine availability, particularly in immunocompromised individuals and the elderly, where *S. pneumoniae* can cause meningitis, pneumonia, and bacteremia. Additionally, *H. influenzae* type b previously accounted for most cases in children before the advent of effective conjugate vaccines, but it remains relevant in unvaccinated populations. Besides bacterial pathogens, viral agents are also commonly involved in CSF infections. Herpes simplex virus (HSV) types 1 and 2 are well known to cause viral meningitis and occasional encephalitis, with significant neurological effects if untreated early. Other viruses, such as enteroviruses and cytomegalovirus, are responsible for a large proportion of viral meningitis cases, mainly in immunocompromised individuals. For example, enteroviruses are the most common cause of viral meningitis in children and tend to occur seasonally in warmer weather. Diagnosis often involves PCR techniques to improve sensitivity and specificity, as older methods like viral cultures may not quickly identify the diverse strains in circulation. Serological tests are also useful for differentiating viral from bacterial causes, allowing for more targeted treatment. Fungal and parasitic infections have become notable threats among certain groups, particularly immunocompromised hosts. *Cryptococcus neoformans* is one of the most common causes of CNS infections in AIDS patients, often leading to cryptococcal meningitis. Diagnosis typically involves organism identification in CSF through India ink preparation or cryptococcal antigen testing, highlighting the importance of awareness of opportunistic infections in at-risk populations.

Likewise, the protozoan *Toxoplasma gondii* can cause cerebral toxoplasmosis in immunocompromised individuals, adding further complexity to the CSF infection profile. Due to the diverse spectrum of pathogens, definitive microbiological diagnosis through proper CSF analysis—complemented by supportive serological testing—is essential for optimal treatment (Lankinen, 2003; Chan et al., 2017). Understanding the common pathogens responsible for CSF infections not only supports accurate diagnosis but also aids in guiding public health policies aimed at reducing infection rates among vulnerable populations (Figure 5.12).

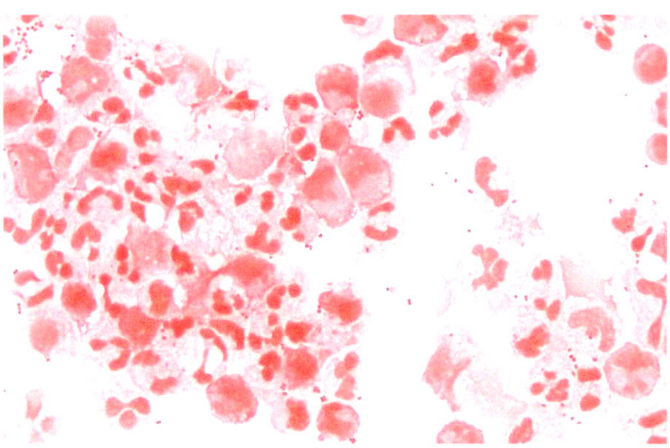

Figure 5.12. Neisseria meningitidis in cerebrospinal fluid (CSF) seen by gram stain at 1000× magnification.

Source: https://upload.wikimedia.org/wikipedia/commons/thumb/e/e6/Neisseria_meningitidis_CSF_Gram_1000.jpg/1024px-Neisseria_meningitidis_CSF_Gram_1000.jpg.

5.3.3. Procedures for CSF Collection and Analysis

The process of cerebrospinal fluid analysis and collection plays an essential role in the microbiological diagnosis of infections, particularly those affecting the central nervous system. Typically, the procedure is conducted via lumbar puncture, in which a needle is carefully inserted into the subarachnoid space to collect fluid for diagnostic purposes. It is imperative that the procedure be performed under strict aseptic conditions to prevent contamination and infection. Once collected, CSF undergoes various analyses, including cytological tests, biochemical investigations, and microbiological cultures, to detect potential pathogens and inflammatory markers. Handling and transportation of CSF specimens must be undertaken with utmost caution, as delays or harsh conditions can compromise sample integrity, thereby adversely affecting diagnostic accuracy. Strict adherence to established protocols is therefore indispensable for the successful collection and analysis of CSF.

Post-collection, CSF is examined for diagnostic markers indicative of infections such as meningitis or encephalitis. Key microscopy techniques, including Gram staining, along with culture methods, are employed to identify bacteria, fungi, or viruses. Additionally, Polymerase Chain Reaction (PCR) assays are now vital in rapidly and accurately identifying specific pathogens, especially when traditional culture methods require extended periods for results. Biochemical analyses assessing protein and glucose concentrations in CSF further provide insights into the inflammatory status of the meninges. In certain cases, serological testing may complement CSF analysis, particularly concerning conditions with evidence of immune activity (Ndege et al., 2020). Accurate interpretation of these results necessitates specialized expertise, as correlating various CSF parameters with clinical manifestations is crucial for accurate diagnosis. The clinical implications of CSF analysis extend beyond mere diagnosis; they significantly influence treatment decisions and prognosis assessments. For example, a CSF profile suggestive of bacterial meningitis typically warrants immediate administration of broad-spectrum antibiotics, whereas viral infections may be managed conservatively.

Furthermore, understanding the subtle distinctions in CSF findings aids in differentiating among various etiologies of central nervous system infections and minimizes the risk of ineffective therapeutic interventions. Recent studies have also demonstrated the benefits of combining traditional diagnostic methods with advanced technologies, such as urine Xpert and urine-lipoarabinomannan (LAM) tests, to enhance detection of concomitant systemic infections (Barr et al., 2017). Consequently, the meticulous procedure involved in CSF aspiration and analysis constitutes a vital component in the comprehensive microbiological assessment of infectious diseases.

5.4. Sputum Cultures

Sputum culture is a valuable microbiological test for diagnosing pulmonary infections and, once collected, can provide important information about the causative organism of pneumonia and other lung infections. Sputum collection and examination can be used to identify the pathogen, making it easier to implement targeted therapy. The test is particularly useful for diagnosing bacteria such as *Streptococcus pneumoniae*, which causes community-acquired pneumonia. Recent research indicates that certain antigen detection methods may be more sensitive than standard culture, especially in patients treated with antibiotics, suggesting that adding enrichment steps could improve diagnostic results. The findings highlight the importance of choosing appropriate methods based on patient background and local epidemiological data to achieve better clinical outcomes for respiratory infection patients (Lankinen, 2003). Additionally, sputum cultures support overall epidemiological surveillance of infectious diseases. For example, studies on microorganisms like pneumococci and atypical bacteria demonstrate the significance of conducting sputum tests to monitor the prevalence of these pathogens within specific groups. In Southeast Asia, where diverse pathogens can lead to sepsis and severe respiratory infections, detecting distinctive microbiological patterns can inform health interventions and antibiotic stewardship programmes.

Diagnosing pneumonia in low-resource settings remains challenging; however, standardized sputum culture techniques can improve diagnostic reliability and bolster responses to public health threats posed by emerging pathogens, strengthening healthcare systems (Southeast Asia Infectious Disease Clinical Research Network, 2017). Proper sample collection, processing, and interpretation are crucial for accurate sputum culture results. High-quality samples are essential, as contamination with oral flora may lead to misleading findings and hinder the identification of infection. Consequently, adhering to standardised methods is vital for obtaining precise results. Furthermore, additional diagnostic tests, such as enzyme immunoassays for specific antigen detection, are increasingly used alongside culture methods, thereby enhancing sensitivity and specificity. Combining these established and emerging techniques enables healthcare professionals to make better-informed treatment decisions without risking misdiagnosis. As diagnostic technology advances, continuous refinement of sputum culture methods is necessary to more effectively combat respiratory infections and improve patient care (Lankinen, 2003) (Figure 5.13).

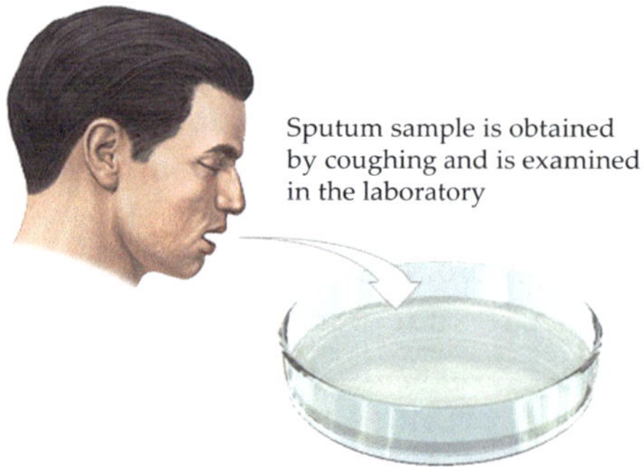

Figure 5.13. Sputum culture illustration.

Source: https://ssl.adam.com/graphics/images/en/9945.jpg.

5.4.1. Importance of Sputum Cultures in Respiratory Infections

Sputum cultures are critically important in understanding the microbiological causes of respiratory infections, especially in identifying the disease-causing agents of conditions such as pneumonia, chronic bronchitis, and tuberculosis. Sputum sampling and analysis provide immediate insights into bacterial pathogens of the respiratory tract. Isolating and identifying specific microorganisms enables healthcare professionals to tailor antibiotic treatments, which is crucial amid the increasing prevalence of drug-resistant strains. Moreover, the sensitivity of sputum cultures in detecting pathogens, particularly in cases of polymicrobial or atypical pneumonia, cannot be overstated. Research studies show that tests like antigen detection can boost the sensitivity of sputum cultures, supporting their use in diverse clinical settings, especially when standard microbiological facilities are unavailable (Lankinen, 2003). Beyond diagnosis, sputum cultures play a vital role in epidemiological research and public health monitoring. Cultivating pathogenic microorganisms from sputum can reveal trends in respiratory infections within specific populations, guiding vaccination and prevention strategies. Notably, studies highlight the significance of sputum testing in assessing the prevalence of *Streptococcus pneumoniae*, a leading cause of community-acquired pneumonia (Lankinen, 2003). As molecular diagnostic techniques advance, the accuracy and speed of sputum cultures are improving, enabling timely and correct diagnosis and treatment. Consequently, data obtained from sputum cultures influence not only individual patient care but also broader public health programmes aimed at controlling respiratory infections. In addition to guiding therapy and public health efforts, sputum cultures greatly impact clinical outcomes. Rapid identification of causative organisms allows clinicians to prescribe the most effective antimicrobial agents, potentially reducing complications and hospital stay durations for respiratory infections. Increasing evidence indicates that delays in administering appropriate antibiotics can raise morbidity and mortality, especially in high-risk groups. Sputum cultures also support the implementation of proper isolation protocols in infectious cases, which is essential for preventing the spread of highly contagious agents, such as those causing tuberculosis. Thus, they are a fundamental component of respiratory infection management and are integral to the microbiological diagnosis of infectious diseases (Figure 5.14).

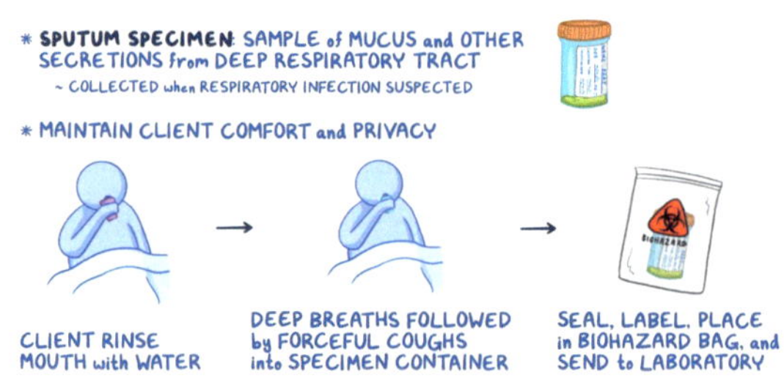

Figure 5.14. Sputum cultures for respiratory infections.

Source: https://www.osmosis.org/_next/image?url=https%3A%2F%2Fd16qt3wv6xm098.cloudfront.net%2F9PtTvA5oRN_0ChsyNEtD3JFwSNmD2EqC%2F_.jpg&w=3840&q=75.

5.4.2. Identification of Pathogens in Sputum Samples

Pathogen detection in sputum samples is essential for diagnosing respiratory infections, especially pneumonia, which poses a global public health challenge. Traditional methods, such as culture, have long been fundamental for microbial diagnosis. However, these conventional techniques are often insensitive and nonspecific, particularly in cases involving fastidious pathogens or polymicrobial infections. Accurate pathogen identification directly influences treatment decisions, underscoring the importance of reliable diagnostic methods. Advances in molecular diagnostics are effectively addressing these challenges, enabling clinicians to detect a broader spectrum of pathogens with enhanced precision. With the integration of new techniques, diagnostic approaches are evolving, making it vital for healthcare professionals to stay informed about innovations that improve patient care through rapid and accurate microbial identification. Molecular diagnostic tools like polymerase chain reaction (PCR) have transformed pathogen detection in sputum samples.

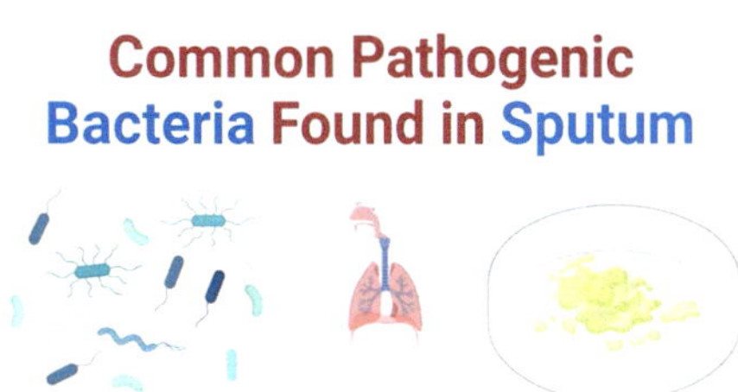

Figure 5.15. Common pathogenic bacteria found in sputum.

Source: https://microbenotes.com/wp-content/uploads/2022/05/Common-Pathogenic-Bacteria-Found-in-Sputum.jpeg.

These methods can amplify and identify specific microbial DNA or RNA at very high levels, allowing for the detection of numerous pathogens, including viruses, bacteria, and fungi. Such benefits are particularly significant when traditional culture methods produce inconclusive results, as these techniques can identify pathogens present in low quantities or with specific growth requirements. Additionally, multiplex PCR assays enable simultaneous detection of multiple pathogens, significantly speeding up the diagnostic process.

These technological advances enhance detection sensitivity and facilitate early initiation of effective antibiotic therapy, which is crucial for improving patient outcomes in severe respiratory infections, as evidenced by recent studies demonstrating increased clinical utility of molecular diagnostics in pneumonia treatment (Torres et al., 2019). Incorporating technologies like microarray analysis further advances sputum diagnosis. The Virochip, a high-throughput platform for detecting various viral pathogens, exemplifies such innovation.

A noteworthy case involved the detection of human parainfluenzavirus four via endotracheal aspirate, illustrating the value of microarray technology in identifying pathogens overlooked by conventional tests. This case not only confirmed the presence of a previously underestimated pathogen but also highlighted the significant clinical implications — enabling timely management in patients with potentially fatal diseases (Blackburn et al., 2006). As our understanding of the lung microbiome deepens, it becomes clear that the microbial environment is complex, emphasising the need for advanced diagnostic tools capable of unravelling the complexities of respiratory infections. This ongoing evolution in diagnostic technology heralds an exciting horizon for the effective management of infectious diseases (Figure 5.15).

5.4.3. Factors Affecting Sputum Culture Results

The validity of sputum culture findings depends on several key variables, including the quality of the received specimen on which testing is performed. Sample collection techniques are especially important; for example, excessive salivary contamination can suppress pathogen detection and result in false-negative outcomes. Collecting samples early in the morning, when patient secretions are at their highest, may increase the likelihood of recovering infectious agents. Both the patient population and their socioeconomic status also influence results; certain groups may have higher rates of specific infections, which affects the choice of microorganisms to be cultured and identified. Additionally, concurrent medical conditions, such as immunosuppressive diseases, impact both the quantity and diversity of recovered pathogens, complicating diagnosis and treatment plans (Thangamathi, 2006). Therefore, strict sample collection protocols are crucial for achieving optimal sputum culture yields. Sample transport and processing are also critical factors affecting culture outcomes. Once the specimen is collected, it must be processed promptly to preserve the viability of the organisms. Transport delays can lead to overgrowth of normal biota and reduce the viability of target organisms, especially in fastidious pathogens. Temperature fluctuations and environmental conditions during transit can also compromise microbial integrity. Appropriate culture media and techniques are necessary for isolating and identifying pathogens, allowing for the growth of those requiring special conditions or taking longer to grow. Recent advances, such as the GeneXpert assays described in other microbiological studies, suggest that rapid diagnostic methods could improve the sensitivity of pathogen detection from sputum cultures, thereby enhancing clinical outcomes (Morabe, 2022). The results of sputum cultures also depend on whether antibiotic therapy was initiated before specimen collection. Patients with a history of antibiotic use may have biased results, as such treatments can suppress the growth of certain pathogens, leading to underreporting in culture results. Consequently, obtaining a complete patient history of prior treatments is essential for accurate interpretation of results. Laboratory factors, including staff training and techniques, further influence the accuracy of sputum culture results. Regular implementation of quality assurance measures is vital, as these ensure proper identification and susceptibility testing of organisms from the isolates. Overall, the diverse factors affecting sputum culture results necessitate a comprehensive approach within clinical and laboratory settings to ensure accurate diagnosis and effective treatment of infectious diseases (Thangamathi et al., 2006).

5.5. Serological Tests

Serological tests are crucial in the microbiological diagnosis of infectious diseases by detecting specific antibodies or antigens in body fluids, mostly serum. They rely on the immune system's ability to produce antibodies when exposed to pathogens, thus enabling the detection of most infectious agents without the need for culturing. The advantages of serological tests include rapid results and the ability to identify infections that are difficult to detect with conventional culture methods. For example, serological testing has proven to be more sensitive in detecting pneumococcal infections, especially in patients who have already received antimicrobial treatment. The development of pneumococcal capsular polysaccharide antigen enzyme immunoassays exemplifies advancements in serological techniques, allowing for sensitive detection that can provide valuable epidemiological data (Lankinen, 2003). While they are essential for diagnosing individual pathogens like *Streptococcus pneumoniae*, serology also plays a vital role in understanding infection patterns overall, particularly in epidemiological studies. For instance, a study in Southeast Asia aimed to identify causative pathogens of community-acquired sepsis and highlighted the importance of various serological markers in informing treatment and management strategies. Notably, pathogens such as leptospirosis and dengue virus were found to be prevalent, illustrating the diverse microbial landscape across regions. Incorporating serological testing into diagnosis allows clinicians to target appropriate antimicrobial therapies, thereby improving clinical outcomes and potentially reducing mortality from serious infections (Southeast Asia Infectious Disease Clinical Research Network, 2017). This underscores the utility of serological testing as both a diagnostic and public health tool. Despite their benefits, serological tests have limitations. Interpretation can be challenging due to cross-reactivity between serotypes or related organisms, leading to false-positive or false-negative results. Additionally, the timing of testing is critical, as antibody levels vary significantly depending on the stage of infection. With ongoing technological advancements, there must be consensus on standardised methods for serological testing to improve reproducibility across laboratories. Increased research and standardisation are necessary to refine serological tests and establish optimal criteria for positivity, especially in regions with high prevalence of co-endemic infections. Addressing these challenges will help maintain serological tests as a key element in the diagnosis of infectious diseases, thereby supporting global health programmes (Lankinen, 2003) (Figure 5.16).

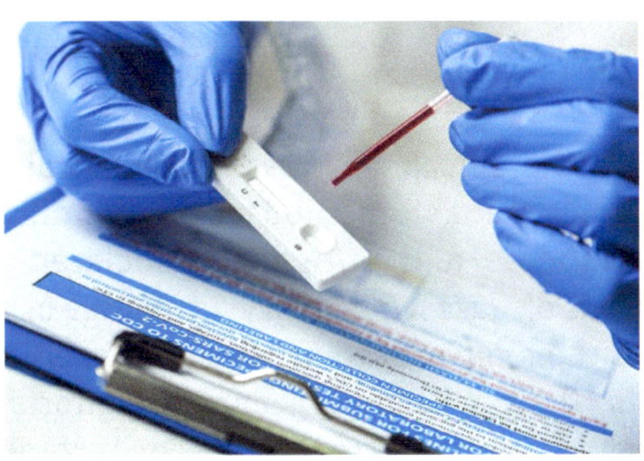

Figure 5.16. Performing serological test.

Source: https://www.news-medical.net/images/news/ImageForNews_705943_16462272081747550.jpg.

5.5.1. Overview of Serological Testing Methods

Serological test protocols are a vital component of microbiological diagnosis for infectious diseases, as they detect antibodies or antigens in various biological specimens. They are especially useful when standard culture techniques are time-consuming or less effective. For example, serological tests can deliver rapid diagnostic results for syphilis, HIV, and certain viral infections, enabling timely and effective clinical management. Techniques such as enzyme-linked immunosorbent assay (ELISA) and western blotting are commonly employed because of their high specificity and sensitivity, allowing for precise pathogen identification. Analysing the immune response to infection not only assists in diagnosis but also supports vaccination efforts and epidemiological research, exemplifying the importance of serological testing in public health. The accuracy of these tests relies heavily on several factors, including antigen selection, sample collection timing, and the inherent characteristics of the tests used. For instance, the sensitivity of antigen detection methods has been examined in various settings, with findings indicating that these methods can sometimes outperform traditional culture techniques, especially when patients have received prior antimicrobial treatment (Lankinen, 2003). Additionally, incorporating enrichment steps into serological assays enhances their sensitivity, making them more effective for diagnosis, particularly in resource-limited environments. However, issues such as cross-reactivity among related pathogens remain a challenge, complicating interpretation. Hence, ensuring these methods are robust against such factors is essential to improve their reliability for clinical diagnosis of infectious diseases. Beyond diagnosis, serological methods can also support other diagnostic approaches, forming a comprehensive infectious disease management system. For example, combining serological results with clinical presentation and other laboratory tests, such as polymerase chain reaction (PCR), can provide a more complete picture of the patient's condition. This multi-method approach is especially important for diseases like tuberculosis, where traditional diagnostic techniques often lack sufficient sensitivity (Dang, 2012). Furthermore, serological testing technology is continually advancing, with rapid and point-of-care tests now available that improve accessibility and practicality in clinical settings. These developments demonstrate the ongoing relevance of serological methods within microbiological diagnosis, paving the way for improved health outcomes.

5.5.2. Types of Infections Diagnosed Through Serological Tests

Serological tests are a vital diagnostic tool for identifying infections with diverse causes, enabling the detection of pathogens by identifying specific antibodies or antigens in a patient's serum. These tests are particularly valuable in diagnosing viral infections such as hepatitis B and C, where the presence of viral antigens or anti-HBV and anti-HCV antibodies indicates active infection or previous exposure. Additionally, serological tests play a crucial role in diagnosing infections like human immunodeficiency virus (HIV), allowing for early detection and treatment. Serological analysis can also be employed to diagnose autoimmune diseases that mimic infectious conditions, demonstrating its versatility and applicability in microbiological diagnosis. The rapid turnaround of serological test results makes them well-suited for acute clinical settings, where early intervention often results in better patient outcomes. Besides viral infections, serology is essential for diagnosing bacterial infections, especially when culture methods are too slow or less sensitive. For example, *Streptococcus pneumoniae* infections can be detected by identifying specific pneumococcal antigens in body fluids such as urine and nasopharyngeal secretions. Studies suggest that antigen detection may outperform culture techniques, particularly in children who are receiving antibiotics (Lankinen, 2003). Furthermore, serological testing aids in diagnosing conditions like systemic lupus erythematosus, where the presence of autoantibodies can clarify whether an infectious cause exists. Overall, incorporating serological tests into the diagnostic process enhances the ability to identify bacterial infections, leading to more targeted treatment decisions. Finally, serological tests are useful in parasitic infections when traditional diagnostic methods fall short. Conditions such as malaria, leishmaniasis, and typhus fever can be effectively diagnosed through serological testing, especially when rapid diagnostic tests are employed. For instance, detecting specific antibodies during malaria can confirm exposure even after recovery, supporting epidemiological studies and public health responses (Thangamathi, 2006). Similarly, serological techniques that identify antibodies against leptospires are crucial in suspected cases of leptospirosis in endemic areas. With ongoing advancements in serological methods, the capacity to detect a wide range of infections continues to grow, filling gaps that other laboratory techniques might overlook.

5.5.3. Limitations and Advantages of Serological Tests

In microbiological diagnosis, serological tests constitute a valuable method for the identification of antibodies and antigens associated with infectious diseases. A primary advantage of these tests is their capacity to produce relatively rapid results, thereby enabling early diagnosis and prompt initiation of treatment. For instance, in cases of suspected tuberculosis (TB), serological testing can identify individuals who may not yet exhibit clinical signs but are in the process of seroconversion, thus allowing early intervention to reduce disease transmission. Furthermore, serological tests are particularly beneficial in resource-limited settings where standard culture methods may lack specificity and sensitivity, thereby enhancing diagnostic accuracy in high-burden areas. As articulated by Dang (2012), the widespread availability and low cost of such tests further emphasise their role in expanding the diagnostic arsenal for infectious diseases. Nonetheless, serological tests are subject to certain limitations that can compromise their diagnostic utility. One such limitation is the potential for false-negative or false-positive results, which can significantly influence clinical decision-making. For example, the detection of antibodies can be delayed post-infection, resulting in late diagnosis during the early stages of disease. Additionally, cross-reactivity among different pathogens can generate misleading results, complicating clinical interpretation. In the case of candidemia, an emergent blood pathogen, serological tests are likely to yield unreliable outcomes due to the presence of non-albicans *Candida* species, which are occasionally undetectable with standard assays, as noted by Khanum et al. (2015). These limitations necessitate the integration of serological testing with other microbiological diagnostic methods to confirm results and enhance diagnostic accuracy. In conclusion, while serological tests offer significant advantages in the rapid and effective diagnosis of infectious diseases, their limitations must be carefully addressed. The reliability of these tests is particularly critical in managing diseases requiring immediate therapeutic intervention, such as TB and candidemia. As medicine advances, it is imperative to incorporate novel strategies and technologies to improve the validity of serological assessments. The development of more sensitive assays and innovative technologies, such as multiplex serology, will help overcome current limitations. Simultaneously, recognizing the importance of an integrated diagnostic system that combines serological procedures with culture methods will ultimately support improved clinical management and patient outcomes across various healthcare settings.

SUMMARY

Microbiological diagnosis of infections, especially through blood, urine, cerebrospinal fluid (CSF), sputum, and serology cultures, plays a vital role in modern medicine. Advances in diagnostic techniques such as enzyme immunoassays and antigen detection have significantly enhanced the sensitivity and specificity of pathogen identification, enabling more efficient and timely treatment options for patients. For instance, enhanced pneumococcal antigen development has yielded promising results, demonstrating that antigen detection can be more sensitive than traditional culture methods, particularly in cases where prior antimicrobial treatment was administered, as shown in the research by Lankinen (2003).

Such innovations highlight the potential for rapid pathogen identification and improved infectious disease management. However, it is also crucial to recognise the ongoing limitations within microbiological diagnosis. Despite advancements in tools like the Microscopic Observation Drug Susceptibility Assay (MODS) and LED fluorescence microscopy for tuberculosis diagnosis, challenges such as low sensitivity in detecting drug-resistant strains remain, as evidenced by the studies discussed (Dang, 2012). These constraints emphasise the need for continuous research and development in both diagnostic techniques and staff training. Achieving high diagnostic accuracy is essential for effective public health management, requiring collaborative efforts among researchers, clinicians, and public health officials to address current gaps. Moving forward, enhancing microbiological diagnosis involves establishing international standards and guidelines, which will facilitate better comparison of results across different settings and ensure standardised care quality. Combining traditional and novel diagnostic methods, supported by reliable epidemiological data, is vital for guiding clinical decisions and improving patient outcomes. As infectious disease diagnosis evolves, maintaining a commitment to advancing existing tools and approaches is paramount, drawing lessons from successes in pneumococcal diagnosis and tuberculosis evaluation, as highlighted by Lankinen (2003) and Dang (2012).

Microbiological diagnosis of infectious diseases from various biological samples, including blood, urine, cerebrospinal fluid (CSF), and sputum, constitutes a crucial aspect of clinical practice. Different specimen types provide diverse insights into the etiology of infections and the responsible pathogens. For instance, blood cultures are instrumental in diagnosing systemic infections such as bacteremia and septicemia, whereas urine cultures are essential for identifying urinary tract infections. Sputum cultures hold particular importance in detecting respiratory infections, including tuberculosis and pneumonia, where pathogens such as *Mycobacterium tuberculosis* can be isolated. The reliability of these diagnostic tests has direct implications for patient management, guiding treatment decisions and improving clinical outcomes, thereby underscoring the importance of rigorous microbiological techniques in clinical microbiology. Serological assays serve as an adjunct to culture methods by detecting specific antibodies or antigens in the patient's serum, adding another dimension to the diagnostic process.

These tests are especially valuable when cultures are cumbersome or impractical. In immunocompromised patients with opportunistic infections, for example, serological tests can rapidly determine the presence of infections caused by organisms such as *Candida spp.* or *Aspergillus spp.*, where prompt treatment is vital. The integration of serological diagnostics facilitates more efficient management of infectious diseases, notably fungal infections, as early detection significantly reduces morbidity and mortality among vulnerable populations (Akilamani et al., 2019). Advances in new diagnostic methods, including molecular techniques and rapid testing, have revolutionized microbiological diagnostics. These innovations enable faster and more accurate pathogen identification, particularly for organisms that are difficult to culture or in cases requiring immediate intervention. For example, recent studies have highlighted the efficacy of diagnostic tools such as the Microscopic Observation Drug Susceptibility Assay (MODS) in detecting tuberculosis with higher sensitivity than traditional methods (Dang, 2012). Concurrently, enhanced accuracy and consistency in modern serological testing for fungal infections considerably support patient treatment. Collectively, these technological advancements underscore the growing importance of integrated diagnostic approaches in effective infectious disease management, effectively bridging laboratory findings with clinical application.

CLOSER LOOK

QUALITY ASSURANCE IN DIAGNOSTIC MICROBIOLOGY

Quality assurance (QA) of diagnostic microbiology is a deliberate activity with the objective of providing reliable, accurate, and timely laboratory results. As most clinical choices are made on the basis of laboratory reports, good QA is essential to effective patient care, control of infections, and public health surveillance. QA consists of two primary components: Quality Control (QC) and Quality Improvement (QI). Quality control involves the regular surveillance of lab operations to ensure that test results are reproducible and reliable. This includes the use of internal controls (e.g., positive and negative controls) and external controls, such as proficiency testing, in which unknown samples from outside sources are tested in an attempt to assess performance (Figure 5.17).

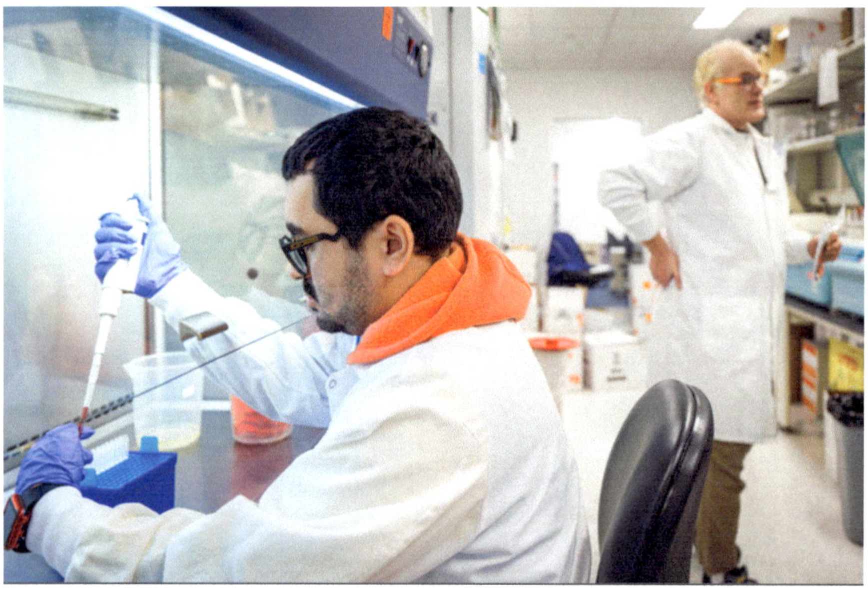

Figure 5.17. Researchers working in a clinical research laboratory, with one scientist preparing samples under a biosafety cabinet and another managing laboratory processes in the background.

Source: https://www.fredhutch.org/content/dam/www/shared-resources/crsp/Clinical%20 Research%20Specimen%20Processing-1.jpg.

Pre-analytical, analytical, and post-analytical processes of laboratory testing must be integrated into an overall QA program:

1. **Pre-Analytical Phase:** Proper specimen collection, labelling, transport, and storage are all included. Errors at this stage—such as the use of an incorrect container or delay in transport—can compromise sample integrity. QA procedures provide consistency in sample-handling procedures and training of staff.
2. **Analytical Phase:** In this phase, actual testing and processing of samples take place. QA ensures equipment gets properly calibrated, reagents get validated and testing processes adhere to standard operating procedures (SOPs). Participation in external quality assessment

(EQAS) joining schemes allows laboratories to compare their performance against national or international standards.

3. **Post-Analytical Phase:** The phase includes result interpretation, reporting, and clinician communication. QA ensures timely, unambiguous, and reliable reporting, including critical result information verification and patient confidentiality.

Staff competency is a significant feature of QA. Regular training, certification, and competency assessment allow the upkeep of superior standards. Laboratory accrediting agencies like NABL (India), CAP (USA), and ISO 15189 provide formal evidence of a lab's practice of QA.

Documentation is also important. Every activity, error, and corrective action must be documented and reviewed from time to time for ongoing improvement. Audit trail, incident log, and performance measures are the minimum QA tools.

REFERENCES

1. Beig, F. K., Malik, A., Rizvi, M., Acharya, D., & Khare, S. (2010). Etiology and clinico-epidemiological profile of acute viral encephalitis in children of western Uttar Pradesh, India. *International journal of infectious diseases : IJID : official publication of the International Society for Infectious Diseases*, *14*(2), e141–e146. https://doi.org/10.1016/j.ijid.2009.03.035(accessed on 16th July 2025).
2. Akilamani, M. (2019). *A study on the pattern of fungal infections and clinical profile in immunocompromised patients with special reference to characterization and molecular study of Candida species in a tertiary care hospital.* https://core.ac.uk/download/235670744.pdf (accessed on 16th July 2025).
3. Khanum, I., Mahmood, S., ali, f., Waqar, H., Awan, S. (2015). Clinical Characteristics and Risk Factors of Candidemia in Tertiary Care Hospital. Infectious Diseases Journal of Pakistan., 24(3), 859-864.(accessed on 16th July 2025).
4. Ndege, R., Ngome, O., Bani, F., Temba, Y., Wilson, H., Vanobberghen, F., Hella, J., Gingo, W., Sasamalo, M., Mnzava, D., Kimera, N., Hiza, H., Wigayi, J., Mapesi, H., Kato, I. B., Mhimbira, F., Reither, K., Battegay, M., Paris, D. H., Weisser, M., ... Rohacek, M. (2020). Ultrasound in managing extrapulmonary tuberculosis: a randomized controlled two-center study. *BMC infectious diseases*, *20*(1), 349. https://doi.org/10.1186/s12879-020-05073-**9**(accessed on 16th July 2025).
5. Baron, E. J., Bourbeau, P., Carroll, K. C., Chapin, K., et al. (2013). *A guide to utilization of the microbiology laboratory for diagnosis of infectious diseases: 2013 Recommendations by the Infectious Diseases Society of America (IDSA) and the American Society for Microbiology (ASM).* https://core.ac.uk/download/345206010.pdf (accessed on 16th July 2025).
6. Barr, D. A., Burton, R., Kerkhoff, A. D., Lawn, S. D., et al. (2017). *Disseminated tuberculosis among hospitalized HIV patients in South Africa: A common condition that can be rapidly diagnosed using urine-based assays.* https://core.ac.uk/download/96628002.pdf (accessed on 16th July 2025).
7. Chiu, C. Y., Rouskin, S., Koshy, A., Urisman, A., Fischer, K., Yagi, S., Schnurr, D., Eckburg, P. B., Tompkins, L. S., Blackburn, B. G., Merker, J. D., Patterson, B. K., Ganem, D., & DeRisi, J. L. (2006). Microarray detection of human parainfluenzavirus 4 infection associated with respiratory failure in an immunocompetent adult. *Clinical infectious diseases : an official publication of the Infectious Diseases Society of America*, *43*(8), e71–e76. https://doi.org/10.1086/507896 (accessed on 16th July 2025).
8. Calandra, T., Mikulska, M., Poulain, D., Sanguinetti, M., Third European Conference on Infections in Leukemia Group, & Viscoli, C. (2010). *The use of mannan antigen and anti-mannan antibodies in the diagnosis of invasive candidiasis: Recommendations from the Third European Conference on Infections in Leukemia.* https://core.ac.uk/download/pdf/8646118.pdf (accessed on 16th July 2025).
9. Carvalho, A. C. C., Matin, N., Mello, F. C. D. Q., Pontali, E., et al. (2017). *The cursed duet today: Tuberculosis and HIV-coinfection.* https://core.ac.uk/download/158171520.pdf (accessed on 16th July 2025).

10. Chan, L., Ibrahim, N. A., Mat Nor, M. B., Tai, C. C., et al. (2017). *Guide to Antimicrobial Therapy 2017.* Edition: 2017 Publisher: Malaysian Society Of Intensive care Editor: Louisa Chan ISBN: 978-967-11415-3-3 https://core.ac.uk/download/300453506.pdf (accessed on 16th July 2025).
11. Chen, J., Chen, Y., He, Q., Jalan, R., et al. (2022). *Rapid pathogen detection for infected ascites in cirrhosis using metagenome next-generation sequencing: A case series.* https://core.ac.uk/download/480394280.pdf (accessed on 16th July 2025).
12. Torres, A., Lee, N., Cilloniz, C., Vila, J., & Van der Eerden, M. (2016). Laboratory diagnosis of pneumonia in the molecular age. *The European respiratory journal*, *48*(6), 1764–1778. https://doi.org/10.1183/13993003.01144-2016(accessed on 16th July 2025).
13. Dang, T. M. H. (2012). *Diagnosis of Tuberculosis in a High Burden Resource-Limited Setting.* https://core.ac.uk/download/200153487.pdf (accessed on 16th July 2025).
14. Diederen, B. M. W. (2007). *New Approaches to the Laboratory Diagnosis of Legionnaires' Disease.* https://core.ac.uk/download/pdf/15452626.pdf (accessed on 16th July 2025).
15. Edelstein, P. H., Jørgensen, C. S., & Wolf, L. A. (2020). *Performance of the ImmuView and BinaxNOW assays for the detection of urine and cerebrospinal fluid Streptococcus pneumoniae and Legionella pneumophila serogroup 1 antigen in patients with Legionnaires' disease or pneumococcal pneumonia and meningitis.* https://core.ac.uk/download/328720978.pdf (accessed on 16th July 2025).
16. Jacobson, M. (2003). *Enteric Diseases in Pigs from Weaning to Slaughter.* https://core.ac.uk/download/11694636.pdf (accessed on 16th July 2025).
17. Lankinen, K. S. (2003). *Catching the pneumococcus: Studies focusing on carriage, epidemiology and microbiological methods.* https://core.ac.uk/download/628859937.pdf (accessed on 16th July 2025).
18. Morabe, N. G. (2022). *Validation of Genexpert machine using extrapulmonary samples at national tuberculosis referral laboratory in Lesotho.* https://core.ac.uk/download/616422470.pdf (accessed on 16th July 2025).
19. Southeast Asia Infectious Disease Clinical Research Network (2017). Causes and outcomes of sepsis in southeast Asia: a multinational multicentre cross-sectional study. *The Lancet. Global health*, *5*(2), e157–e167. https://doi.org/10.1016/S2214-109X(17)30007-4(accessed on 16th July 2025).
20. Thangamathi, G. (2006). *Etiological Profile of Infectious Fever – Bacterial and Parasitical.* https://core.ac.uk/download/235655444.pdf (accessed on 16th July 2025).
21. Zhang, W., Zhang, X., & Zhao, Y. (2024). *Application of metagenomic next-generation sequencing in the diagnosis of infectious diseases.* https://core.ac.uk/download/635409553.pdf (accessed on 16th July 2025).

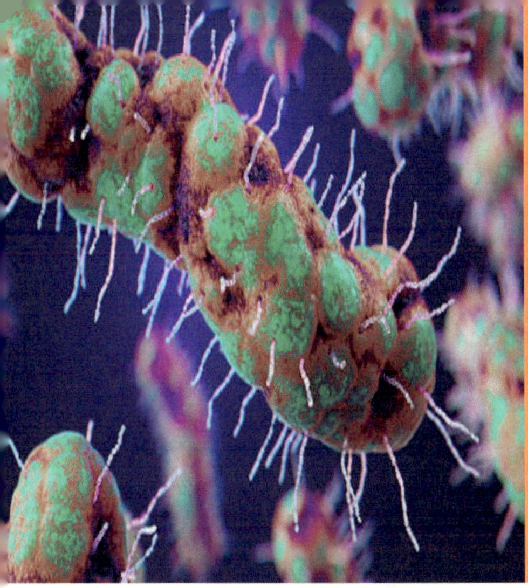

Chapter 6
BACTERIAL STRUCTURE AND GENETICS

Contents

Introduction

In microbiology, the study of bacterial structure and genetics forms the foundational basis for understanding life at the cellular level. Bacteria are unicellular organisms characterised by a wide array of structural features essential for survival and adaptation. The cell wall, a significant component of bacterial anatomy, varies among species and influences not only the bacterium's shape but also its interactions with the environment. For example, bacteria can be classified as Gram-negative or Gram-positive depending on their cell wall composition, which also determines their susceptibility to antibiotics and their overall pathogenic potential. The complexity inherent in bacterial architecture necessitates rigorous examination, given the critical roles of bacterial genetics in medicine, biotechnology, and ecology. Moreover, the bacterial genome demonstrates a remarkable capacity to withstand environmental pressures, underscoring the importance of its genetic study. Bacterial genomes can harbour a variety of traits, including antibiotic resistance and metabolic capabilities, which are often acquired through horizontal gene transfer mechanisms such as transformation, transduction, and conjugation. This genomic flexibility allows bacteria to evolve rapidly under selective pressures. A comprehensive understanding of bacterial genetics not only enhances insights into evolutionary biology but also facilitates practical applications, such as developing novel therapeutic strategies against resistant bacterial strains. For instance, plasmids — circular DNA molecules naturally found in bacteria—are utilized to demonstrate the application of genetic elements in producing recombinant proteins, exemplifying the intersection of bacterial design and genetic engineering. The examination of specific genetic elements, such as the nod-box in *Rhizobium* species, illustrates how regulatory mechanisms govern gene expression. The nod-box, a conserved cis-acting element, regulates nodulation genes in response to environmental stimuli. This specificity is significant because it exemplifies how bacteria adapt to their environment through sophisticated regulatory networks. Regulatory studies involving the nod-box, such as those conducted by Fallik and colleagues, reveal how these systems can lead to differential gene expression patterns essential for successful symbiosis with host plants. Analysing these genetic and structural paradigms enhances our understanding of bacterial life, opening new avenues for applications in agriculture and environmental management, and underscores the interconnectedness of bacterial genetics and structure within broader biological systems.

Importance of Studying Bacterial Structure and Genetics

Understanding the structure and genetics of bacteria is essential across numerous disciplines such as medicine, agriculture, and biotechnology. The structure of bacterial cells plays a pivotal role in determining how these microorganisms interact with their environment and host organisms. For example, the composition of the bacterial cell wall, whether Gram-positive or Gram-negative, critically influences susceptibility to antibiotics and mechanisms of infection. By comprehending these structural differences, researchers are able to develop targeted therapies that interfere with the survival processes of pathogens within host tissues. Insights gained from bacterial genetics also facilitate the genetic engineering of microorganisms for biotechnological purposes, including the production of biofuels and biodegradable plastics, thereby supporting sustainable industrial practices. An in-depth study of bacterial structure and genetics not only advances medical science but also addresses pressing environmental concerns. The evolutionary mechanisms and genetic adaptability of bacterial populations are fundamental to their ecological success. The rapid diversification observed within bacterial populations, exemplified by lineages such as the Wrinkly Spreader in *Pseudomonas fluorescens*, illustrates how genetic mutations can confer competitive advantages in diverse environments. This adaptability is crucial to understanding bacterial behaviour in ecosystems and during clinical infections. The capacity for biofilm formation exemplifies the influence of genetic factors on community behaviour and ecological dynamics, providing stability and resistance to treatments. Elucidating these genetic mechanisms enhances our understanding of pathways governing processes such as biofilm formation and antibiotic resistance, which are of considerable importance for managing bacterial infections and harnessing bacterial properties for industrial use (Jerdan et al., 2020). Beyond environmental and medical applications, the comprehension of bacterial structure and genetics is vital for the advancement of marine biotechnology and related sciences. As interest grows in marine environments as sources of novel bacterial species and biopharmaceuticals, understanding their genetic elements and structural capabilities allows for cost-effective access to their unique features. Research on bacterial strains can identify potential opportunities for academic-industry collaborations, increasing funding and cooperative research initiatives in biotechnology (Seaman & Whitehouse, 2001). Additionally, molecular tools derived from genetic research enhance our capacity to engineer bacteria for specific applications, such as bioremediation or nutrient cycling in marine ecosystems. Overall, comprehensive studies of bacterial structure and genetics provide innovative solutions to numerous scientific challenges, underscoring their significance in contemporary research (Figure 6.1).

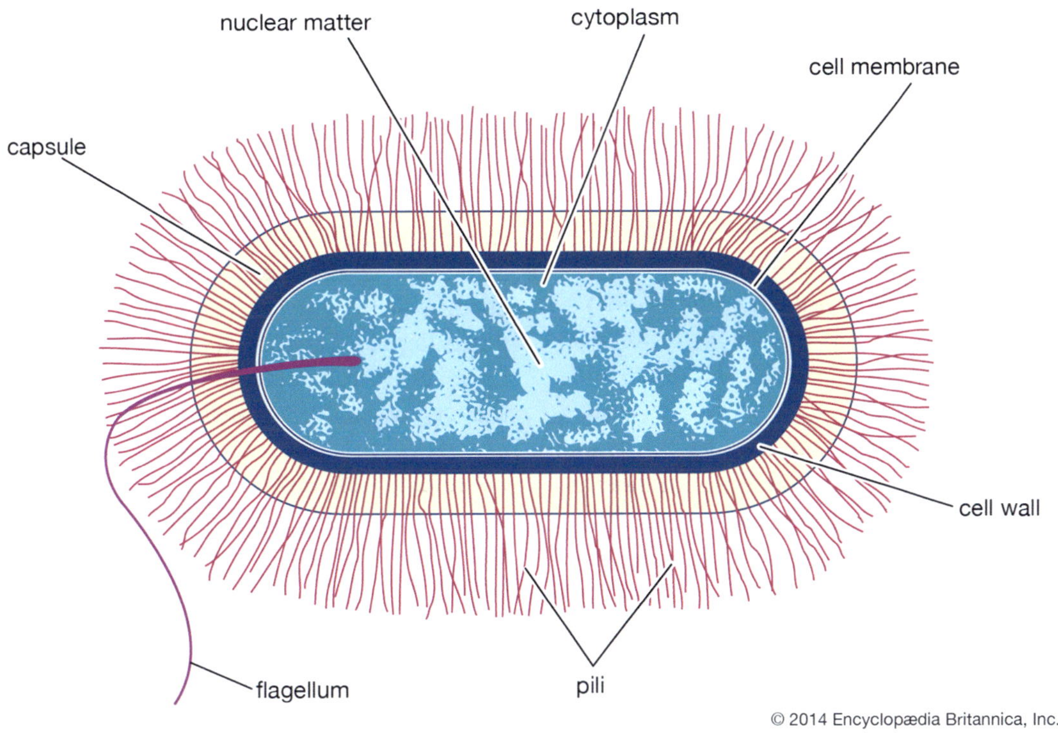

Figure 6.1. Bacterial structure.

Source: https://plantlet.org/wp-content/uploads/2020/10/drawing-structure-cell-bacillus-type.jpg.

6.1. Basic Structure of Bacteria

The overall organisation of bacteria is characterised by their typical cellular composition, which distinctly differentiates them from eukaryotic cells. At the core of bacterial organisation is the cell membrane that encases the cytoplasm and essential cellular components. This membrane functions not only as a boundary but also regulates nutrient absorption and waste elimination to maintain homeostasis within the cell. Some bacteria possess a rigid cell wall primarily composed of peptidoglycan, which provides structural support and contributes to resistance against osmotic pressure- an essential attribute for survival across various environments. The structural features of bacteria highlight their efficacy and versatility, enabling colonization across diverse ecological niches, ranging from soil to the human body, and underpinning their evolutionary role within the microbial kingdom. Bacteria contain essential genetic material in the cytoplasm, typically organised into a single circular chromosome devoid of a membrane envelope, unlike eukaryotic cells. This genomic organisation facilitates efficient replication and transcription, allowing rapid adaptation to environmental stresses.

Additionally, plasmids — small, extrachromosomal circular DNA molecules — are present in most bacteria. These plasmids often carry genes conferring advantageous traits such as antibiotic resistance, emphasising their significance in bacterial evolution and adaptability. The presence of ribosomes, crucial for protein synthesis, further exemplifies the complexity of bacterial genetics, as these organelles translate genetic information into functional proteins. The comprehensive genetic architecture of bacteria underscores their functional potential and capacity for adaptive evolution. External structures such as flagella and pili are vital for communication and environmental adaptation. Flagella, or whip-like appendages, facilitate motility by enabling bacteria to migrate between habitats in search of nutrients or favourable conditions. This motility is essential for survival, as it allows bacteria to escape unfavourable environments or locate resources. Pili are hair-like projections that support surface attachment and enable conjugation, an important mechanism of gene transfer. Conjugation plays a critical role in the dissemination of genetic traits, particularly antibiotic resistance, thereby contributing to bacterial evolution and genetic diversity. The integration of these external features with internal cellular structures results in highly adaptable organisms capable of resisting adverse conditions and thriving across a broad spectrum of ecological niches. This comprehensive understanding underscores the importance of studying bacterial structure within the wider context of bacterial genetics.

6.1.1. Cell Wall Composition and Function

The composition of bacterial cell walls is the primary determinant of their structural stability, with cell walls mainly comprising peptidoglycan, a polymer of sugars and amino acids. This structural feature imparts strength and shape to bacteria and protects against environmental stressors, such as osmotic pressure. In Gram-positive bacteria, the thick peptidoglycan layer retains crystal violet stain during Gram staining, resulting in a purple colouration. Conversely, Gram-negative bacteria have a thin peptidoglycan layer located between an inner and an outer membrane, leading to a pink appearance upon staining. The structural variations in the cell wall influence not only the physical properties of these organisms but also their susceptibility to antibiotics; certain antibiotics inhibit the synthesis of the peptidoglycan layer, thereby underscoring its importance for bacterial viability. Furthermore, the cell wall contributes to the pathogenicity of specific bacteria, with some pathogens exploiting its composition to evade immune responses or facilitate infection. For example, the presence of surface proteins such as lipopolysaccharides in Gram-negative bacteria triggers vigorous inflammatory responses in the host and enhances adhesion to host tissues. Structural modifications of the cell wall can also confer antibiotic resistance; mutations or acquisition of resistance genes enable bacteria to alter their peptidoglycan layer, rendering standard treatments ineffective. This adaptive capacity highlights the evolutionary significance of cell wall composition in bacteria and raises urgent concerns for public health, especially amid increasing antibiotic resistance worldwide. Additionally, the relationship between bacterial cell walls and their functions within microbiomes underscores the importance of a comprehensive understanding of bacterial structure. For instance, the role of the cell wall in maintaining homeostasis and mediating interactions with eukaryotic cells is a key focus of microbiome research. Recent workshops have explored the characteristics of healthy gut microbiomes and their influence on human health, providing insights into how bacterial morphology, such as cell wall structure, impacts host interactions and health outcomes. The complexity of these interactions emphasises the necessity of understanding cell wall composition in addressing broader issues related to microbial health and disease. Ongoing research aims to elucidate the functional implications of cell wall differences among bacterial populations, which may inform the development of novel treatment strategies for managing dysbiosis and promoting microbial balance in human health (Bandurski & Singh, 1983; McBurney et al., 2019) (Figure 6.2.).

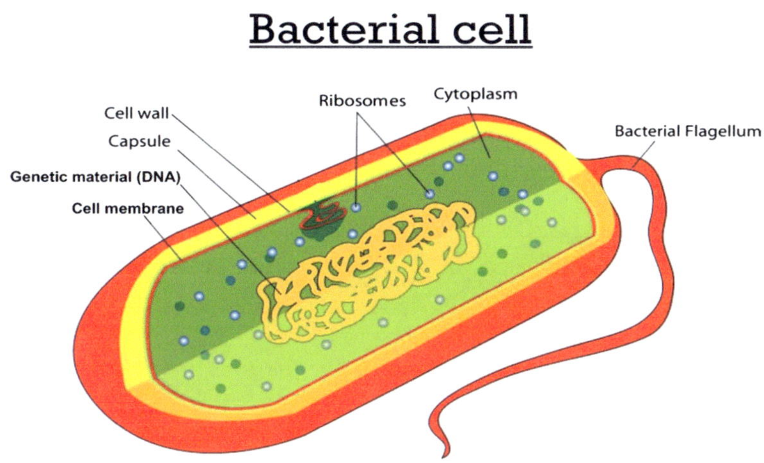

Figure 6.2. Bacteria cell structure.

Source: https://i.ytimg.com/vi/4DYgGA9jdlE/hq720.jpg?sqp=-oaymwEhCK4FEIIDSFryq4qpAxMIA RUAAAAAGAElAADIQj0AgKJD&rs=AOn4CLDia-7NpwGUfPENvIBkoxVXx-9Szw.

6.1.2. Plasma Membrane Characteristics

The plasma membrane constitutes a fundamental component of bacterial architecture, essential for maintaining cellular integrity and mediating interactions with the environment. Primarily composed of a phospholipid bilayer, its selective permeability permits the ingress of vital nutrients while excluding detrimental agents. This selective permeability is indispensable for bacterial survival and functionality, especially given their typical habitation within dynamic environments. Furthermore, the presence of various proteins embedded within the membrane enhances its functionality, such as transport proteins facilitating molecular movement across the bilayer. This dynamic structure not only sustains cellular homeostasis but also enables bacteria to respond to environmental signals, which is vital for their capacity to adapt and evolve, as highlighted in current studies on microbial resilience. Beyond its fundamental role in substance transport and environmental exposure, the plasma membrane is integral to signaling processes and energy generation within bacterial cells. Most bacteria utilize proton gradients across the membrane to synthesize ATP, a process heavily dependent on membrane integrity. This is particularly relevant for respiring or fermenting bacterial species, where the membrane's capacity to support multiple electron transport chains directly influences energy production. Recent research into membrane composition, including the identification of specific lipid types affecting membrane fluidity, may have significant implications for understanding bacterial growth and survival mechanisms. Such research broadens the functional complexity of the plasma membrane beyond its physical barrier role, illustrating its capacity as a responsive organism adapting to metabolic needs and external stresses. Additionally, the plasma membrane plays a critical role in determining bacterial cell shape and division, linking its properties to both structural and genetic attributes. The membrane's structural regulation is vital for maintaining cell shape, thereby affecting overall functionality and gene expression. For example, during cell division, the plasma membrane facilitates the segregation of genetic material, ensuring each daughter cell inherits a complete complement of genetic information. This connection between genetic stability and membrane integrity underscores an evolutionary trend where structural adaptations enhance reproductive success and survival among bacterial populations. The implications of these findings are global; as evidenced by existing research, understanding the characteristics of the plasma membrane could lead to advancements in combating bacterial infections and developing agricultural resistance to pathogens, such as root-knot nematodes discussed in agricultural studies with broad impacts on crop yield (Kaloshian & Teixeira, 2019). Consequently, the plasma membrane is a key organizer of bacterial structure, function, and genetics, warranting ongoing investigation and discovery in microbial biology (Horowitz & Owen, 1954) (Figure 6.3).

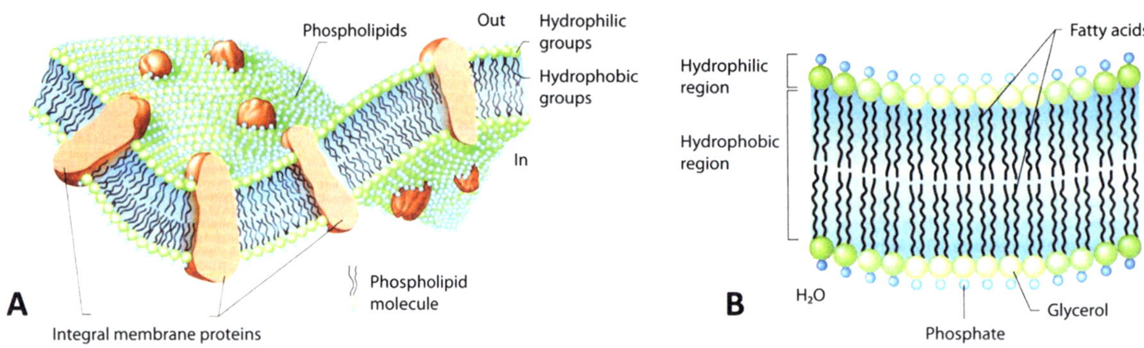

Figure 6.3. Schematic structure of a bacterial phospholipid bilayer membrane. (A) Cytoplasmic membrane showing the lipid molecules and transmembrane proteins. The inner surface faces the cytoplasm, and the outer part faces the environment. (B) Detailed view of the lipid bilayer.

Source: https://www.researchgate.net/profile/Julius-Lipp/publication/27336292/figure/fig7/AS:669391620427785@1536606807787/Schematic-structure-of-a-bacterial-phospholipid-bilayer-membrane-A-Cytoplasmic.png.

6.1.3. Cytoplasm and Its Components

The cytoplasm functions as an essential medium within bacterial cells, facilitating necessary biochemical activities. Composed of a gel-like substance known as cytosol, the cytoplasm is characterised by the presence of numerous macromolecules, dissolved ions, and metabolic enzymes that perform vital functions within the cell. Embedded within this environment, ribosomes — integral to protein synthesis — move freely and are central to translating genetic information into functional proteins. This dynamic environment not only supports metabolic processes but also coordinates various cellular functions, underscoring the central role of cytoplasmic composition in maintaining bacterial viability. Furthermore, the cytoplasm plays a significant role in cell division and environmental adaptation, reflecting its multifaceted nature within the overarching structure and genetics of bacteria. Aside from ribosomes, the cytoplasm contains heterogeneous structures such as inclusions and granules that serve as storage sites for nutrients, energy reserves, and structural compounds. For instance, polyhydroxybutyrate granules facilitate carbon and energy storage, while magnetosomes- composed of magnetic iron oxides- enable geomagnetic orientation. These inclusions enhance bacteria's ability to adapt to diverse environmental conditions, thereby promoting stability and viability. Additionally, the presence of nucleoid regions — containing the bacterial chromosome — highlights the importance of cytoplasmic organisation in genetic replication and regulation. The spatial arrangement of genetic material within the cytoplasm is critical for efficient transcription and translation, as it allows the rapid movement of genetic components and associated proteins, supporting fundamental bacterial functions. Current research on engineered bacteria indicates that the cytoplasm actively contributes to enzyme expression, further advancing biotechnological applications. For example, studies have demonstrated that certain strains of *Escherichia coli*, subjected to oxidative cytoplasmic conditions, can significantly enhance glycosyltransferase production- key enzymes in glycoprotein synthesis (Skretas et al., 2009). This showcases the functional potential of the cytoplasm and its optimisation prospects in microbial engineering. Moreover, understanding how DNA is compacted within bacterial cells provides insight into the structural stability of genetic information in the cytoplasm, as evidenced by the pressures and forces exerted on DNA during phage infection (Panja & Molineux, 2010). Analysing these intricacies enables researchers to manipulate bacterial processes, thereby fostering advancements in genetic engineering and synthetic biology (Figure 6.4).*Escherichia coli*

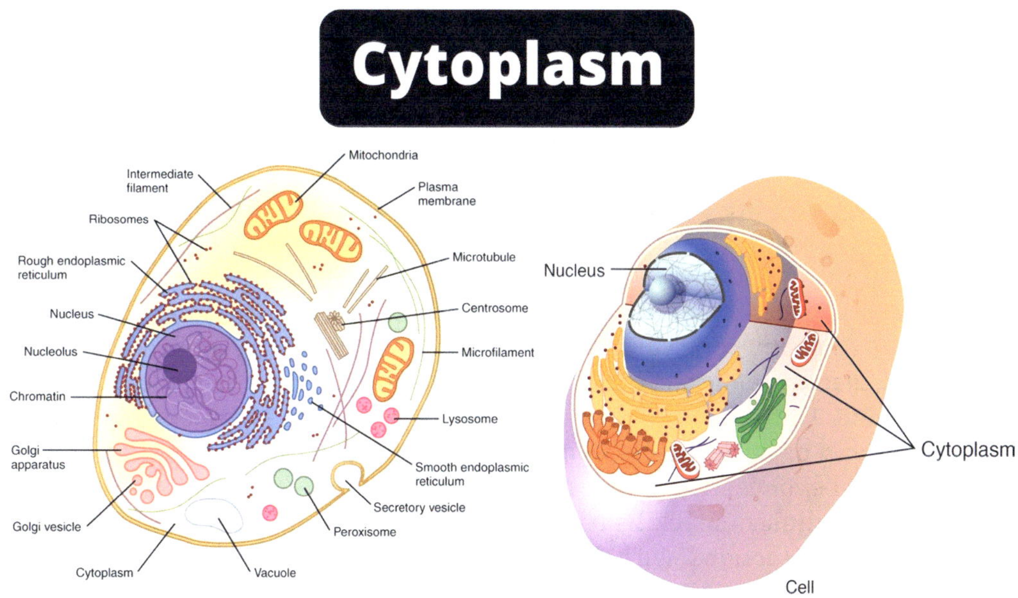

Figure 6.4. Cytoplasm.

Source: https://biologynotesonline.com/wp-content/uploads/2021/11/Cytoplasm.jpg.

6.2. Bacterial Cell Types

The variability among bacterial cell types forms the foundation for their genetic and structural composition. Bacteria can be broadly classified into two main categories: Gram-positive and Gram-negative, which differ primarily in cell wall structure. Gram-positive bacteria feature a thick peptidoglycan layer that retains the crystal violet dye used in Gram staining, resulting in a purple colouration under microscopy. Conversely, Gram-negative bacteria are characterised by a thinner peptidoglycan layer and an outer lipid-rich membrane containing lipopolysaccharides, which stain pink. These structural distinctions not only influence their interactions with antibiotics but also affect their environmental adaptability and pathogenic potential. The structural differences underscore the evolutionary significance of bacterial cell types and illustrate how these organisms have adapted to occupy diverse ecological niches while preserving cellular integrity and function. In addition to variations in cell wall architecture, bacterial cells exhibit substantial diversity in genetic organisation and replication mechanisms. Typically, bacterial chromosomal DNA exists as a single circular molecule, unlike the linear chromosomes observed in eukaryotes. Furthermore, most bacteria contain plasmids — smaller, circular DNA fragments — that may carry genes critical for survival, such as those conferring antibiotic resistance. Prior research has elucidated essential bacterial DNA repair mechanisms analogous to those in eukaryotes, including non-homologous end-joining pathways. This indicates a sophisticated level of genetic regulation aimed at maintaining genomic integrity and facilitating adaptation under environmental stresses, including pathogenic pressures and antibiotic challenges, thereby rendering bacteria evolutionarily resilient (Bowater & Doherty, 2006). The implications of bacterial cell-type heterogeneity extend beyond structural and genetic differences; cellular specialisation plays a vital role in interactions with host environments, particularly in immune responses. For example, studies have demonstrated that bacterial populations residing in the healthy murine middle ear display notable cellular heterogeneity and functional specialisation when confronted with pathogenic challenges. In such contexts, innate immune responses are paramount, with each cell type — such as monocytes and epithelial cells — exhibiting distinct patterns of immune gene expression. This cellular heterogeneity provides immediate and effective protection against infection, highlighting the importance of understanding how bacterial cell types interact with host immune systems- a key area of ongoing research (Ryan et al., 2020). These dynamics are essential for advancing our comprehension of bacterial behaviour in both disease and health conditions.

6.2.1. Differences Between Gram-positive and Gram-negative Bacteria

The distinction between Gram-positive and Gram-negative bacteria is a fundamental concept in microbiology, primarily concerning their cell wall structure and composition. Gram-positive cells are characterised by a thick peptidoglycan layer that retains the crystal violet stain used in Gram staining procedures, resulting in a purple colouration under microscopy. This substantial peptidoglycan layer constitutes up to 90% of the cell wall, contributing significantly to the rigidity and resilience of the bacteria against environmental stresses. Conversely, Gram-negative bacteria possess a thinner peptidoglycan layer, accounting for approximately 10–20% of their cell wall, which is external to an outer membrane and the plasma membrane. The outer membrane contains lipopolysaccharides (LPS), which are known to elicit strong immune responses in host organisms and are often implicated in the virulence of these bacteria. This fundamental structural difference critically influences their susceptibility to antibiotics and their pathogenic mechanisms. Furthermore, these structural variations extend beyond mere identification, affecting the interactions of the bacteria with their environments. For instance, the robustness of Gram-positive bacteria allows them to withstand harsher conditions compared to Gram-negative bacteria, which are more prone to physical injury and dehydration. Additionally, the outer membrane in Gram-negative bacteria provides a protective barrier against many antibiotics, necessitating targeted therapeutic strategies for infections caused by such pathogens. For example, treating infections involving bacteria like *E. coli*, *Salmonella enterica,* and *Campylobacter jejuni* is particularly challenging due to their Gram-negative nature, as determined by differential testing methods such as ozonation, which effectively deactivate these pathogens (Goudie et al., 2003). A comprehensive understanding of these differences is essential for developing effective antimicrobial strategies. Moreover, the genetic and metabolic profiles of Gram-positive and Gram-negative bacteria differ markedly. Gram-positive bacteria, such as *Staphylococcus* and *Streptococcus* species, tend to possess simpler genetic compositions and readily acquire advantageous genes, including those conferring antibiotic resistance, through horizontal gene transfer mechanisms like transformation and transduction. In contrast, Gram-negative bacteria often exhibit complex regulatory networks and metabolic pathways, allowing them flexibility in nutrient utilisation and adaptation to various environmental conditions, including those shaped by ecological interactions (Baldwin et al., 2019). This adaptability enables them to colonise diverse ecosystems, including plant-microbe systems, where interactions can promote survival and growth while providing protection against environmental stressors. Consequently, a thorough understanding of the differences between these bacteria is vital for research and applications in medicine and environmental management (Figure 6 .5).

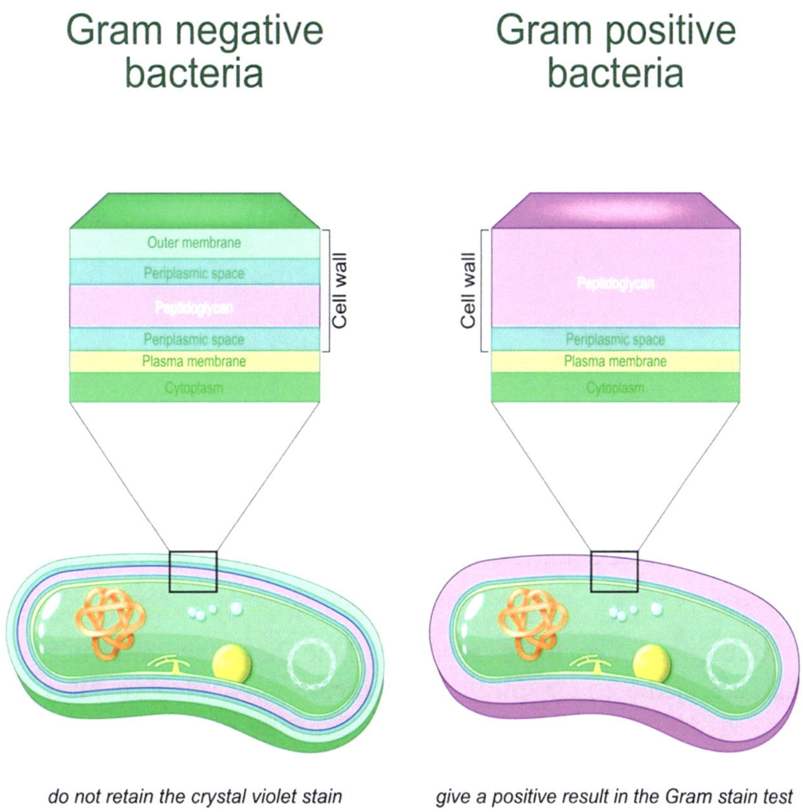

Figure 6.5. Gram-positive versus Gram-negative bacteria.

Source: https://blogger.googleusercontent.com/img/b/R29vZ2xl/AVvXsEi4fKbB4e7SjWWIkHh8VeAl4934sFxiF2bSpgxq6PICwkb2IQKMnlKCWwgAm-aXdPwQxcjLBhRwV45uQLaIhp_huIqMJXsHwAhXmzpry7piPcHw1JHFgEpcUzgY25odA_A4tANrpwWdgC90FR8tm9VCC1OQk56cxEgP5T3wOOVZoeXw9LmqcQYRNeCfBRU/s1000/Differences%20Between%20Gram%20Positive%20And%20Gram%20Negative%20Bacteria.jpg.

6.2.2. Shapes of Bacteria: Cocci, Bacilli, and Spirilla

Bacterial morphology, classified into three primary groups—cocci, bacilli, and spirilla—constitutes fundamental structural units with substantial influence on their environmental functions and interactions. Cocci are spherical bacteria that occur either as single cells or in various arrangements, such as pairs (diplococci), chains (streptococci), or clusters (staphylococci). This adaptability allows cocci to thrive in diverse environments, thereby contributing to their prevalence and significance in both pathogenic and symbiotic contexts. Conversely, bacilli are rod-shaped bacteria that tend to form chains due to their binary fission process.

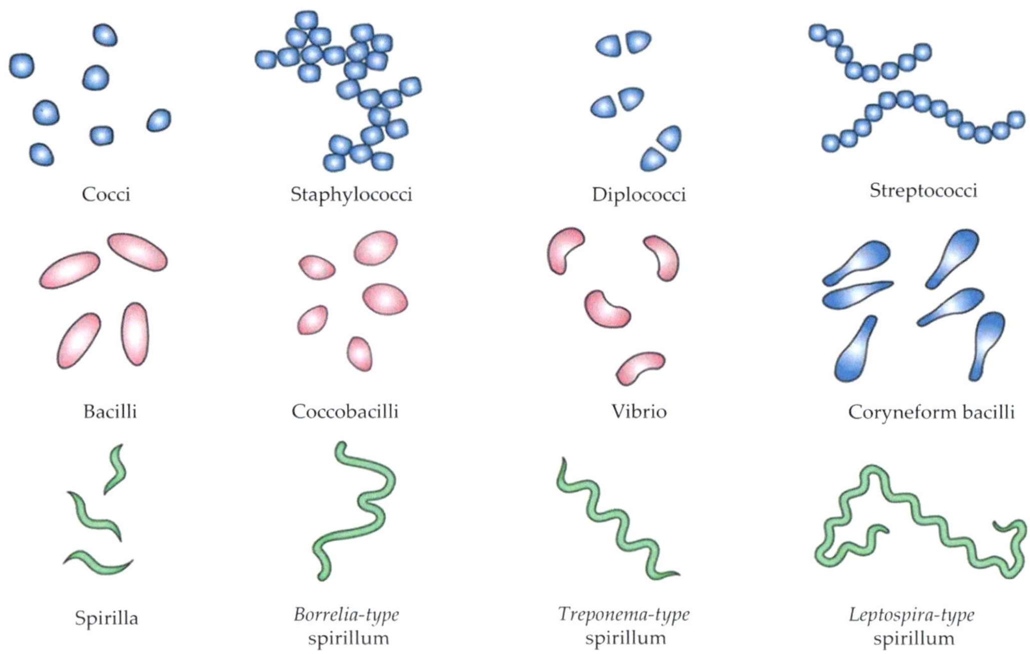

Figure 6.6. Shapes of bacteria.

Source: https://i0.wp.com/microbeonline.com/wp-content/uploads/2021/05/Basic-morphologies-of-various-bacteria.png?ssl=1.

The structural robustness of bacilli is crucial, as their shape facilitates nutrient absorption and motility. Spirilla, characterised by their spiral or corkscrew morphology, exhibit a unique adaptation for movement within viscous environments such as mucous membranes, where they often play critical roles in infection and nutrient recycling. Bacterial shape is influenced not solely by taxonomic classification but also by genetic mechanisms underlying specific morphologies. Environmental and genetic factors influence the general structure and function of various bacterial forms. For example, research has explored how particular genes are associated with the development of the characteristic shapes of cocci, bacilli, and spirilla. Regulation of peptidoglycan synthesis, essential for maintaining cell wall integrity, is a significant aspect of this relationship. Certain shapes confer advantages in specific ecological niches, affecting bacterial survival, which underscores the importance of genetic studies in understanding bacterial adaptability and evolution. Recent research indicates that environmental conditions — such as nutrient availability, temperature, and soil depth

— may significantly impact the morphological diversity of bacteria in natural habitats, thereby further emphasising the intricate linkages between structure and genetics (Wheeler, 2017). Detecting morphological variations among bacteria is particularly effective in laboratory settings, facilitating the identification and study of distinct species. Practical exercises, such as those conducted in microbiology courses, integrate hands-on experiments with morphological analysis, enhancing understanding of bacterial physiology and behaviour (Ahern & Habashi, 2020). Through interactive laboratory techniques, students gain insights into how bacterial shape relates to their ecological roles, including host interactions and participation in biogeochemical cycles. Ultimately, bacterial morphology is not merely descriptive but also integral to their genetic and functional organisation, opening avenues for exploration across various scientific disciplines. The integration of morphological and genetic perspectives underscores the importance of employing both concepts to comprehensively understand the complexity and significance of bacterial life (Figure 6.6).

6.2.3. Specialized Structures: Flagella and Pili

The composition and function of specialized structures such as flagella and pili are central to bacterial motility and adaptability research. Flagella are whip-like, elongated appendages that enable bacteria to swim in liquid environments, a vital trait for survival and colonization. These structures are powered by a motor system within the bacterial cell envelope, allowing high-vvelocity rotation to propel the organism forwars. In spirochetes, with their characteristic periplasmic flagella, the flagellar hook- primarily composed of the FlgE protein — plays a crucial role in connecting the motor to the filament. These hooks are distinguished by their resilience to harsh conditions, highlighting the role of these proteins in enabling motility across various environments. This advanced structural design demonstrates the complexity of bacterial motility mechanisms, which allow bacteria to adapt to diverse ecological niches (Miller et al., 2014). Although pili, in contrast to flagella, perform other functions apart from motility, such as biofilm formation and adherence, these hair-like, short structures are vital for surface attachment, including host tissue adherence, thereby increasing the bacterium's potential to cause infection.

Fimbriae, also known as micro- pili, exemplify such adherence capabilities. They enable bacteria to attach to specific receptors, facilitating colony formation. The diversity in form and function among pili illustrates the adaptability of microbes to environmental challenges. Recent genomic studies confirm that new types of pili can evolve according to ecological and evolutionary requirements. Through these mechanisms, pili contribute not only to bacterial survival but also influence their mechanisms of genetic exchange, promoting genetic diversity and evolution (Taoka et al., 2020). The coordinated action of flagella and pili provides an intriguing aspect of bacterial locomotion and environmental interaction. Since flagella primarily enhance mobility, pili mediate surface interactions, which are equally crucial for survival. This dual functionality allows bacteria to respond to environmental challenges-whether swimming towards nutrients or firmly adhering to surfaces. Moreover, the molecular composition of these structures, specifically the proteins forming flagella and pili, remains an active area of research. Understanding the stability and interactions of these proteins, such as the covalent cross-linking of FlgE within the flagellar hook, offers insights into the general mechanisms underpinning bacterial motility and fitness. The distinctive structures of flagella and pili are fundamental to the broader concepts of bacterial architecture and genetics, integrating physical and genetic systems that enable these microorganisms to thrive (Miller et al., 2014) (Figure 6.7)

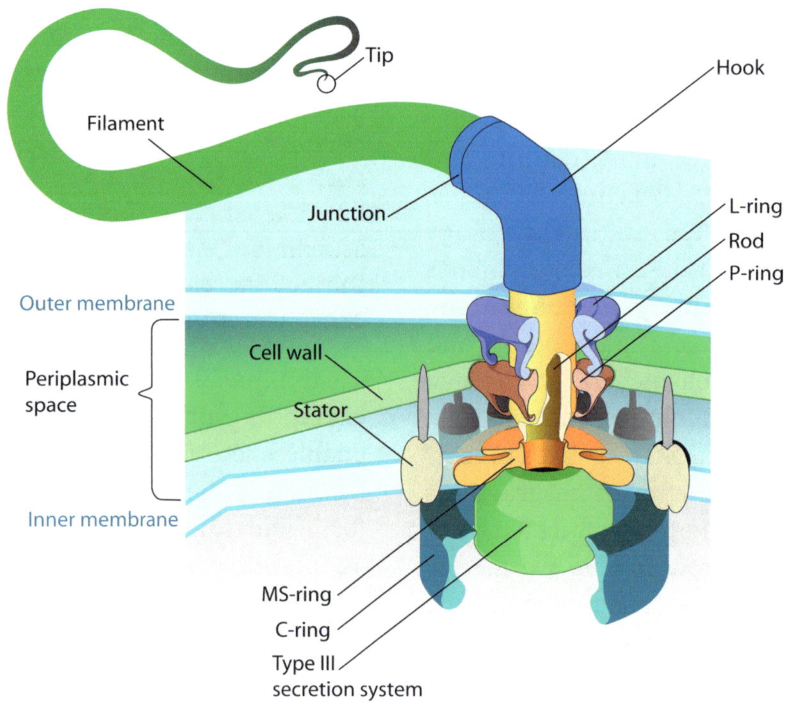

Figure 6.7. Structure of bacterial flagellum.

Source: https://upload.wikimedia.org/wikipedia/commons/thumb/4/40/Flagellum_base_diagram-en.svg/1024px-Flagellum_base_diagram-en.svg.png.

6.3. Genetic Material in Bacteria

The bacterial genetic material mainly consists of deoxyribonucleic acid (DNA), which differs from that of eukaryotic organisms. In prokaryotic cells, DNA exists as a single ring-shaped chromosome located in a region called the nucleoid. This structural organisation enables efficient regulation and replication necessary for the rapid proliferation typical of bacteria. Watson and Crick's DNA model describes the double helix with an emphasis on base pairing complementarity, ensuring the fidelity of genetic material during replication. One strand of DNA acts as a template for synthesising its complement, facilitating accurate duplication and transmission of genetic information. This inherent characteristic of DNA not only aids in trait transmission but also forms the basis of genetic diversity through mutations and horizontal gene transfer, playing a crucial role in bacterial adaptation and evolution (Horowitz & Owen, 1954).

Besides chromosomal DNA, most bacteria possess extrachromosomal DNA elements known as plasmids. These doughnut-shaped DNA molecules vary in size and can carry genes that confer advantages to their bacterial host, such as antibiotic resistance or virulence factors. The presence of plasmids is also vital for bacterial versatility since they can be transferred between cells via mechanisms like conjugation, transformation, or transduction. This horizontal gene transfer is essential for spreading rapidly evolving traits throughout bacterial populations and highlights the dynamic nature of bacterial genetics. Furthermore, some plasmids can integrate into chromosomal DNA, leading to the development of new functionalities and metabolic capacities, thereby enhancing bacterial survival in diverse environments (Boutry et al., 2008). Bacterial DNA includes not only chromosomal and plasmid DNA but also mobile genetic elements like transposons and insertion sequences. These elements increase genetic variability and plasticity within bacterial populations. Transposons can move within the genome and influence gene expression while generating antibiotic-resistant mutations. Their ability to catalyse genomic rearrangements demonstrates the plasticity of bacterial genetics and the evolutionary pressures exerted by environmental selection and medical interventions. Because bacteria are continually evolving in response to selective pressures, understanding these genetic mechanisms is vital for developing effective therapies and managing antibiotic resistance. Overall, the complex interactions among various forms of genetic material in bacteria showcase the sophistication of their gene structures and the dynamic nature of their genetic architecture (Horowitz & Owen, 1954).

6.3.1. Structure of Bacterial DNA

The bacterial DNA is mainly characterised by its unique double-stranded structure, which contrasts unfavourably with the linear eukaryotic DNA. In bacteria, DNA exists as a single circular chromosome folded within the nucleoid region of the cell. This arrangement enables efficient use of genetic material space and ensures essential genes are easily accessible during replication and transcription. Additionally, this compact topology allows bacteria to adapt quickly and survive in dynamic environments. Understanding this organisation is important because it sheds light on gene expression and regulation mechanisms in prokaryotes, which can differ significantly from those in eukaryotic systems and offer new insights for genetic engineering and synthetic biology. Besides the single large circular chromosome, most bacteria also possess plasmids — small, circular DNA molecules capable of autonomous replication. Plasmids often carry genes that provide advantageous traits, such as antibiotic resistance, which poses a major public health concern. The presence of plasmids introduces a second layer of genetic diversity, enabling bacterial populations to adapt to selective pressures like antibiotic use rapidly. This feature is a key factor in pathogen management, as pathogenic bacteria frequently mobilise plasmids to acquire and spread resistance genes through lateral gene transfer mechanisms. The interaction between chromosomal and plasmid DNA highlights the complexity of bacterial genetics and the strategies involved in adapting to diverse environments.

Furthermore, the topological structure of bacterial DNA plays a vital role in its functional capacity. Supercoiling of DNA permits tighter packing, facilitating efficient storage of genetic information within the limited cellular space available in bacteria. This structural configuration not only supports physical containment of DNA but also influences gene expression regulation. Changes in supercoiling can affect the accessibility of specific genes and, consequently, the ability of transcriptional machinery to initiate gene expression. As evidenced by research on pathogenic microorganisms, the dynamics of supercoiling are crucial for understanding how bacteria respond to environmental stresses and adapt accordingly, providing insights into broader trends in microbial evolution (Hofvander, 2004; Emmett & Rabadan, 2014) (Figure 6.8).

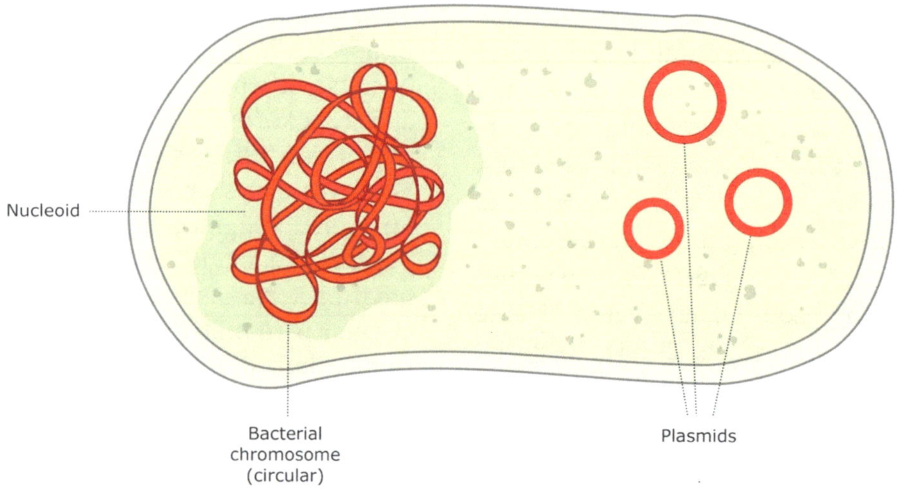

Figure 6.8. Bacterial DNA.

Source: https://www.sciencelearn.org.nz/_next/image?url=https%3A%2F%2Fwww.datocms-assets.com%2F117510%2F1722387675-enzymes_bacterialdna.jpg%3Fw%3D1840%26h%3D920&w=1920&q=85&dpl=dpl_3rhusQfrbXYfrm8BSLwuTDgVSr8n.

6.3.2. Plasmids and Their Role in Genetic Diversity

Plasmids play a significant role as contributors to bacterial genetic variation, acting as vectors for the transfer of genetic information between species and strains. They are extrachromosomal DNA molecules responsible for conferring a diverse array of genes upon an organism, ranging from antibiotic resistance to virulence factors and metabolic capabilities. The independence of plasmid replication from the bacterial chromosome permits the rapid dissemination of advantageous traits, particularly in environments subjected to selective pressures, such as the presence of antibiotics. Plasmid transfer occurs via mechanisms such as conjugation and transduction, thereby facilitating horizontal gene transfer (HGT) and promoting genetic diversity within bacterial populations. The study of plasmids underscores their importance not only in bacterial adaptation but also in the formation of pathogenic strains that resist treatment and control measures (Haaber et al., 2017). The structural variability of plasmids significantly influences the evolutionary dynamics of bacterial populations.

These elements can vary considerably in size, origin, and function, and may carry genes essential for survival in specific environments, such as plasmids that promote nitrogen fixation in rhizobia. For example, *Sinorhizobium meliloti* possesses a substantial amount of plasmid DNA, accounting for up to 45% of its genome. The presence of multiple plasmids enables bacteria to adapt to changing conditions during symbiotic interactions with legumes. Importantly, the conjugative nature of most plasmids facilitates the horizontal transfer of desirable traits across species, further enhancing genetic diversity. This complexity is especially relevant considering the rapid evolution of bacterial populations in response to environmental changes; thus, plasmids are integral to ecological and evolutionary studies (Lagares et al., 2014). Furthermore, the role of plasmids in increasing bacterial genetic diversity holds significant implications for public health. The acquisition of plasmids carrying antibiotic resistance determinants by pathogenic bacteria often leads to treatment failures. In organisms such as *Staphylococcus aureus*, the ability to develop resistance rapidly through plasmid acquisition renders existing antibiotics ineffective. Research indicates that mechanisms such as conjugation and transduction can facilitate extensive gene exchange, complicating infection management.

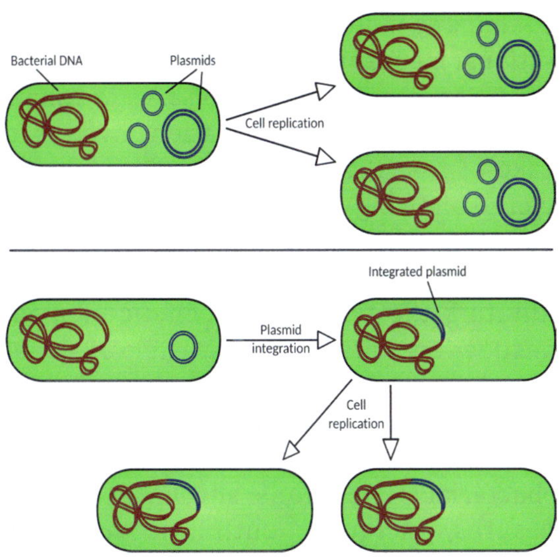

Figure 6.9. There are two types of plasmid integration into a host bacterium: Non-integrating plasmids replicate as shown in the top instance, whereas episomes, the lower example, can integrate into the host chromosome.

Source: https://upload.wikimedia.org/wikipedia/commons/thumb/4/42/Plasmid_replication_%28english%29.svg/1024px-Plasmid_replication_%28english%29.svg.png.

As these mobile genetic elements disseminate within bacterial populations, they generate rapidly evolving genetic landscapes that challenge conventional therapeutic approaches. A comprehensive understanding of plasmid-mediated gene transfer mechanisms and their impact on bacterial genetics is essential for developing new strategies to combat antibiotic-resistant pathogens (Haaber et al., 2017) (Figure 6. 6.9).

6.3.3. Comparison with Eukaryotic Genetic Material

The distinction between bacterial and eukaryotic DNA elucidates widespread differences in structure, organisation, and function, which reflect the evolutionary divergence of the two domains of life. Bacterial genomes are generally composed of a single circular chromosome, often supplemented with small plasmids that can carry additional genetic information, such as traits conferring antibiotic resistance. Conversely, eukaryotic DNA is arranged into multiple linear chromosomes within a membrane-enclosed nucleus. This segregation allows for increased regulatory complexity in eukaryotic gene expression and interaction, facilitating a broad range of cellular functions that are frequently absent in prokaryotes. Due to the absence of this nuclear organisation, bacterial transcription and translation are coupled processes, enabling bacteria to respond swiftly to environmental stimuli — a stark contrast to the separated transcription and translation observed in eukaryotic cells. Furthermore, the genetic material of eukaryotes exhibits greater complexity, partly attributable to the presence of introns within genes. Eukaryotic genes often contain non-coding introns that interrupt coding sequences, necessitating intricate splicing mechanisms during RNA maturation to produce functional messenger RNA (mRNA). In contrast, bacterial genes are predominantly devoid of introns, with coding sequences directly translated into proteins without splicing. This efficient genomic organisation enables bacteria to express genes more rapidly, thus allowing prompt responses to environmental changes. In eukaryotes, the elaborate organisation of regulatory elements and introns provides enhanced genetic control, which is essential for the development of complex multicellular organisms, permitting specialisation of functions across different tissue types. These structural differences have profound implications beyond mere variability; they influence evolutionary dynamics and adaptability. For example, bacteria can acquire genetic material through horizontal gene transfer, thereby increasing genetic diversity and versatility under selective pressures such as antibiotic exposure — a process differing significantly from the predominantly vertical inheritance in eukaryotes, where genetic changes occur via mutation and recombination during sexual reproduction. These inherent differences are embedded within their genomic architectures. Recent research has uncovered long-range fluctuations in the guanine-cytosine (GC% %) content of eukaryotic genomes, which may underscore evolutionary forces shaping genetic variability and stability, as discussed by Li and Holste (2004). Understanding these genetic distinctions enhances our comprehension of bacterial diversity and informs the development of targeted therapeutics that exploit these differences, thereby advancing strategies for treating bacterial infections rather than eukaryotic diseases.

6.4. Bacterial Reproduction

Bacterial growth is primarily characterised by the process of binary fission, whereby a single bacterial cell divides into two identical daughter cells. This process is highly effective in facilitating rapid population increases, allowing bacteria to thrive in various environments. Under favourable conditions, binary fission occurs approximately every 20 minutes, leading to exponential population growth that can quickly deplete available resources. During this process, genetic material is meticulously replicated so that each new cell inherits a complete copy of the parent cell's genome. Furthermore, the simplicity of binary fission underscores the straightforward nature of bacterial structure, where the efficient replication and segregation of genetic information offset the absence of a complex mitotic apparatus. This rapid reproduction mechanism is central to bacterial evolution and adaptation, enabling swift responses to environmental changes and promoting genetic diversity through horizontal gene transfer and mutation. Horizontal gene transfer among bacterial populations significantly contributes to their evolutionary processes. Although binary fission is the predominant mode of bacterial reproduction, additional mechanisms such as transformation, conjugation, and transduction serve to enhance genetic diversity. Transformation involves the uptake of free DNA from the environment by bacteria, allowing them to acquire novel traits from lysed cells. Conjugation, often mediated by plasmids, involves direct cell-to-cell contact, facilitating the transfer of genetic elements. Transduction entails the transfer of genetic material via bacteriophages. These mechanisms complement the genetic toolkit necessary for adaptation, which gains increasing relevance as bacterial populations encounter selective pressures, including antibiotic resistance. The interaction of these genetic exchange mechanisms enables bacteria to evolve strategies that enhance survival and proliferation, both structurally and within their ecological niches. The interdependence between bacterial life cycles and environmental adaptability underscores the evolutionary significance of genetic regulation and mutation rates. Studies have demonstrated that gene content scaling in prokaryotic genomes correlates with lifestyle differences, spontaneous mutation rates, and evolutionary pressures. The RAevol model suggests that scaling laws are driven by selective robustness pressures, which influence bacterial genome size and organisation (Beslon et al., 2010). Additionally, viral satellites, such as staphylococcal pathogenicity islands (SaPIs), exemplify the complexity of host-virus interactions during bacterial reproduction. These satellites can impose selective pressures on helper viruses, fostering coevolution and increasing genetic diversity within bacterial populations (Buckling et al., 2015). Such evolutionary processes not only reflect bacterial adaptability but also provide insights into bacterial genetics and structure in rapidly changing environments.

6.4.1. Asexual Reproduction Through Binary Fission

Asexual reproduction through binary fission is a straightforward process by which bacteria replicate their genetic material and multiply efficiently. This method enables a single bacterial cell to divide into two genetically identical daughter cells. Before division, the bacterium's DNA replicates, ensuring that each daughter cell inherits a complete set of genetic material. This mechanism is particularly advantageous in unstable environments where rapid population growth confers a survival benefit. The swift transfer of genetic material via binary fission reflects the streamlined structure of the bacterial genome, which typically consists of a singular, circular chromosome devoid of significant non-coding regions. This simplicity underscores how bacterial organisation directly correlates with reproductive strategies, facilitating rapid adaptation and evolutionary responses to ecological stresses. The efficiency of binary fission significantly contributes to the swift proliferation of bacterial populations, with bacteria capable of doubling in numbers within approximately 20 minutes under optimal conditions. Such exponential growth can lead to the swift colonization of available niches and dominance over other biological entities. However, this reproductive method is not without limitations. Mutations can occur during DNA replication, introducing genetic variation even among seemingly identical offspring. Notably, research has demonstrated that, under controlled conditions, nearly 10% of *E. coli* cultures exhibit variability in size and volume following binary fission, indicative of random developmental discrepancies despite identical replication circumstances (Bois et al., 2019). Consequently, while binary fission facilitates rapid bacterial proliferation, it also fosters genetic diversity essential for adaptation. The importance of binary fission and the resulting genetic variability becomes especially salient when examining patterns of evolution and population dynamics. This asexual reproductive process influences broader ecological and evolutionary phenomena, particularly in response to environmental pressures.

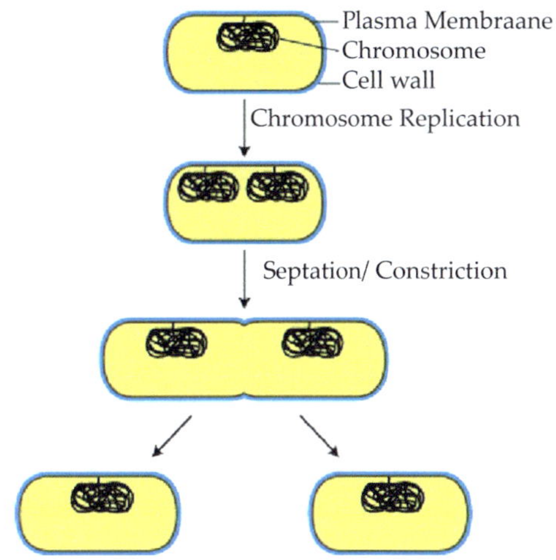

Figure 6.10. Binary fission in bacteria.

Source: https://www.researchgate.net/profile/Andrew-Watkinson-2/publication/43492619/figure/fig3/AS:527493390372864@1502775632813/Binary-Fission-in-Bacteria-Parent-cell-divides-into-two-identical-daughter-cells-through.png.

For example, in rapidly changing environments or dynamic communities, the swift multiplication via binary fission can induce significant shifts in ecosystem organisation and community structure, as bacteria preempt resource competition. Such insights are increasingly relevant in the context of the Anthropocene Epoch, where human activity markedly alters environmental conditions. Recent research in physical and evolutionary biology highlights potential pathways through which bacteria respond to extinction and recovery, emphasising the complex interplay among bacterial structure, genetics, and their role in maintaining ecological equilibrium (King et al., 2015) (Figure 6. 10).

6.4.2. Genetic Exchange Mechanisms: Transformation, Transduction, and Conjugation

There are three principal mechanisms of genetic transfer in bacterial genetics: transformation, transduction, and conjugation. All three processes are crucial for maintaining genetic diversity within bacterial populations to facilitate adaptation to changing environments. Transformation involves the uptake of extracellular DNA by a competent cell, potentially resulting in phenotypic alteration. This process exemplifies how bacteria can acquire advantageous traits, such as antibiotic resistance, from their environment rather than solely through vertical gene transfer. By promoting greater genetic variability, transformation serves as a fundamental factor in bacterial evolution and adaptation to pathogenic conditions. Transduction is another vital gene transfer mechanism that involves bacteriophages, viruses that infect bacteria. During this process, a bacteriophage may inadvertently transfer genetic material from one bacterial host to another during replication. Consequently, this mechanism enables horizontal gene transfer, facilitating the dissemination of genes related to virulence or antibiotic resistance. Recent studies have increasingly emphasised the importance of transduction in gene transfer, particularly in pathogenic bacteria such as *Staphylococcus aureus*. This bacterium demonstrates remarkable adaptability, notably through the acquisition of antibiotic resistance genes, highlighting the efficiency of transduction as a genetic transfer method — especially in medical settings where rapid adaptability is essential (Haaber et al., 2017). Conjugation, the third mechanism, is distinguished primarily by cell-to-cell contact and the transfer of plasmids — circular DNA molecules typically encoding antibiotic resistance genes. This process involves the formation of a pilus by one bacterium to establish a connection with another, thereby facilitating genetic exchange. Conjugation is especially significant under conditions of high selective pressure, where it promotes the effective spread of resistance traits. The dynamic nature of conjugation underscores the selective advantages conferred upon bacteria capable of effectively transferring beneficial genes. As microbial populations evolve, understanding these resistance-transfer mechanisms is imperative for developing strategies to prevent antibiotic resistance development and safeguard public health (Milka, 2018).

6.4.3. Impact of Reproduction on Bacterial Evolution

The reproductive processes employed by bacteria are fundamental to their evolutionary history and play a pivotal role in the adaptation and survival of these microorganisms. Binary fission stands as the primary mechanism of prokaryotic reproduction, involving rapid cell division that results in two genetically identical daughter cells. This asexual process facilitates swift population expansion and serves as an efficient means of transmitting advantageous traits within a population. Nonetheless, the absence of genetic recombination inherent to this mode of reproduction may constrain genetic diversity. To mitigate this limitation, most bacteria utilize horizontal gene transfer (HGT), which permits the acquisition of novel genetic material from other organisms. This multifaceted reproductive strategy not only enables the inheritance of adaptive traits but also fosters the development of new functions, thereby influencing the evolutionary trajectory of bacterial populations. Furthermore, the relationship between reproductive mechanisms and environmental stresses bears significant implications for bacterial evolution. In fluctuating environments, the capacity of bacteria to reproduce asexually in conjunction with HGT facilitates rapid adaptation to selective pressures. For instance, evidence indicates that in the context of staphylococcal pathogenicity islands (SaPIs), helper viruses adapt swiftly to gain resistance against satellite counterparts, exemplifying a co-evolutionary arms race that propels genetic innovation and adaptability (Buckling et al., 2015). These mechanisms illustrate that bacterial reproduction transcends mere survival; it is intricately intertwined with ecological interactions and evolutionary selection, capable of inducing abrupt genetic modifications. Consequently, the impact of reproductive strategies on evolution must be understood as a dynamic interplay between inherent biological processes and external environmental influences.

The evolutionary history of bacterial reproduction also underscores a transition from collective genetic sharing to individual vertical inheritance. Primitive life forms likely depended heavily on HGT, fostering a communal genetic environment where traits were exchanged freely. Over time, selective pressures may have favoured the emergence of more individualised reproductive strategies to promote greater stability and specialisation within bacterial lineages (Arnoldt et al., 2015). This transformation marks a significant milestone in microbial evolution, laying the groundwork for the extensive diversity observed in modern bacteria. As prokaryotes adapt to ever-changing environments, their reproductive strategies determine not only short-term survival but also long-term evolutionary trends. An in-depth understanding of bacterial reproductive complexity will ultimately enhance our knowledge of microbial persistence and the ongoing, dynamic adjustments these organisms make in response to changing conditions in an ever-evolving world (Figure 6. 11).

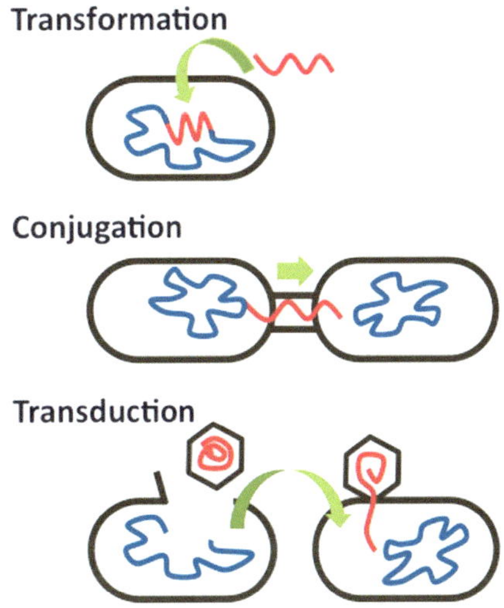

Figure 6.11. Mechanisms of bacterial horizontal gene transfer (HGT).

Source: https://www.researchgate.net/publication/280584808/figure/fig1/AS:324966294802456@1454489410517/Mechanisms-of-bacterial-horizontal-gene-transfer.png.

6.5. Gene Regulation in Bacteria

Gene regulation in bacteria is a significant process that allows bacteria to respond to fluctuating environmental conditions in an effective way. Bacterial genes are regulated by various systems including transcription factors, operons, and promoter regions that allow sets of genes to be co-expressed coordinately. An example is the lac operon, which regulates lactose metabolism in *Escherichia coli*. In the presence of lactose, it will bind to the repressor protein, enabling the transcription of genes that are required for lactose use. This adaptability serves to illustrate how gene regulation is not simply an exercise in biological control but also a reaction to altered nutrient availability, illustrating the evolutionary benefits provided by such mechanisms. Furthermore, the comprehension of such regulatory mechanisms is able to provide insight into universal principles of genetic adaptation, correlating this fundamental concept in the context of bacterial genetics and structure. At a molecular level, gene regulation in bacteria is influenced by various intrinsic and extrinsic factors that contribute to gene expression diversity. Gene expression has been revealed to be prone to random fluctuations, causing variation in the synthesis of proteins among genetically related organisms. This "phenotypic noise," as it has come to be known, emphasizes the importance of regulatory mechanisms in maintaining the stability of gene expression. Noise can interestingly originate in transcriptional and translational stages, and specific promoter sites are essential in establishing the level of noise. *E. coli* has demonstrated that evolutionarily highly conserved key genes retain promoters that confer lower phenotypic noise, thus maintaining essential cellular functions in a progressively resilient manner. Such findings have been identified to suggest that natural selection dictates the expression noise of genes, thus lending support to the activity of regulatory elements in bacterial population evolutionary progress (Silander et al., 2012). One of the most intriguing aspects of regulation in bacterial genes is how flexibility and stability coexist in each other in scaling properties within their genomes. The newer models, for instance, such as the RAevol model, have begun to uncover the mechanisms of genome scaling and regulatory network complexity factors. Such work shows that scaling laws that are seen in bacterial gene content are not so many characteristics of variation in lifestyle, but could be more deeply connected to spontaneous mutation rates and selective pressures for genomic stability. As bacteria traverse their universe, these scaling features tell us about how genome size and shape variation influence gene regulation. Hence, an understanding of gene regulation and genome organization can reveal how bacteria evolved to foster their survival in different ecological niches and further reinforce the connection between their structural genetics and regulatory plans (Beslon et al., 2010).

6.5.1. Operons and Their Function

The concept of operons is fundamental to gene expression and regulation in prokaryotes, representing a defining characteristic of their genetic organisation. An operon comprises multiple genes transcribed collectively under the control of a single promoter, thereby enabling the regulated expression of genes with similar functions. This structural arrangement is notably economical for bacteria, as it permits the concurrent synthesis of proteins involved in specific metabolic pathways or environmental responses. An illustrative example is the lac operon of *Escherichia coli*, in which genes involved in lactose metabolism are coordinated as a single unit, thus optimising resource utilisation based on lactose §availability. These systems exemplify how bacterial cells adapt rapidly to new environmental conditions without the need for elaborate regulatory mechanisms, thereby modelling effective evolutionary strategies. Operon regulation occurs through various mechanisms, ensuring that genes are expressed solely when required. For instance, in the lac operon, the presence of lactose inactivates a repressor protein, allowing RNA polymerase to bind and initiate transcription. Conversely, the absence of lactose results in the repressor binding to the operator region, inhibiting transcription. The bistable, toggle-like behaviour of this system underscores the flexibility and efficiency of operons in resource allocation. Furthermore, studies on operons have significant implications for understanding bacterial adaptation and survival, as demonstrated through experimental evolution research. For example, in *Pseudomonas fluorescens*, the phenotype of the Wrinkly Spreader mutant illustrates how mutational disturbances in regulatory networks can enhance fitness by functioning as operon-like clusters, enabling bacterial communities to access novel ecological niches and resources (Spiers, 2014). Additionally, the origins and evolution of operons extend beyond transcriptional control, reflecting the phylogenetic relationships among bacteria. Operons often display conserved features indicative of common ancestry and functional homology across diverse bacterial taxa. Magnetotactic bacteria (MTB) provide a particularly intriguing context for studying operon dynamics, especially regarding biomineralisation processes. These bacteria possess specialized operons responsible for magnetosome formation, organelles central to their magnetic orientation (McCausland & Komeili, 2020). By examining the genetic architectures underlying operon function in MTB, researchers gain profound insights into biochemical pathways and their evolutionary adaptations, illuminating the intricate networks linking bacterial structure, genetics, and ecological success. Consequently, the study of operons not only enhances understanding of bacterial functions but also serves as a window into the mechanisms of evolutionary adaptation (Figure 6.12).

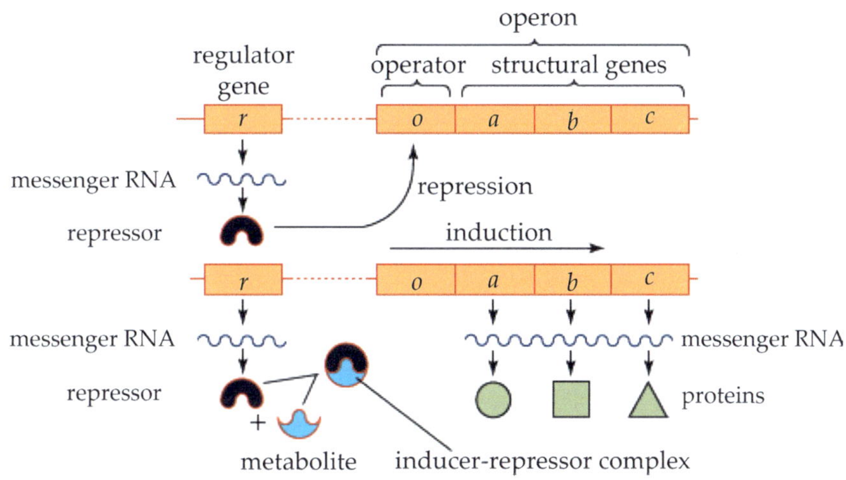

Figure 6.12. Model of the operon and its relation to the regulator gene.

Source: https://cdn.britannica.com/81/781-004-CA10795E/Model-operon-relation-regulator-gene.jpg?w=400&h=300&c=crop.

6.5.2. Environmental Factors Influencing Gene Expression

Environmental signals exert a significant influence on gene expression in bacteria, forming the foundation of their adaptability and survival. Multiple environmental cues, such as temperature, pH, and nutrient levels, can modulate the processes of transcription and translation, resulting in a variety of phenotypes in genetically identical organisms. This adaptability is vital for bacteria, as they frequently encounter changing environments. For example, alterations in the promoter regions of individual genes can lead to variations in protein production, contributing to what is known as' phenotypic noise." Experimental investigations with *Escherichia coli* have demonstrated that genes essential for survival possess promoter distributions that minimise noise levels; in other words, natural selection appears to counteract variability in critical gene expression under environmental stressors (Arkin et al., 2012). Understanding how bacteria regulate their genetic responses to environmental stimuli enhances our comprehension of their evolutionary strategies. The interaction between environmental cues and gene expression is also observable in the context of multifactorial diseases, such as inflammatory bowel disease (IBD). While IBD has a strong genetic component, environmental factors — including diet and microbial exposure — interact with host genetics to influence disease susceptibility and progression. Recent research highlights the roles of specific genes, such as NOD2/CARD15, which not only predispose individuals to IBD but also mediate responses to environmental stimuli that can trigger disease outbreaks. Given that bacteria are integral components of the gut microbiome, investigating how these microorganisms adjust their gene expression based on both genetic and environmental signals may shed light on disease pathogenesis and potential therapeutic targets (Lakatos et al., 2006). This dual regulatory mechanism underscores the importance of incorporating environmental factors into genetic research, particularly with regard to microbial pathogenicity. Furthermore, the regulation of gene expression by environmental forces directly relates to principles of evolutionary biology. Bacterial adaptation driven by environmental pressures, through modifications in gene expression, exemplifies the dynamic nature of genetic responses to external stimuli. Under environmental stress, bacteria can undergo epigenetic modifications that enable rapid adaptation without altering the underlying genetic code. The ability to regulate gene expression not only enhances survival under stress but also facilitates immune evasion and ecological diversification. This phenotypic versatility is evidenced by the diversity within bacterial populations, which can thrive and persist in various habitats by modulating their genetic responses accordingly. Consequently, understanding the mechanisms by which environmental factors influence gene expression is essential for elucidating the complex interactions among bacterial structure, genetics, and adaptation (Figure 6. 13).*Escherichia coli*

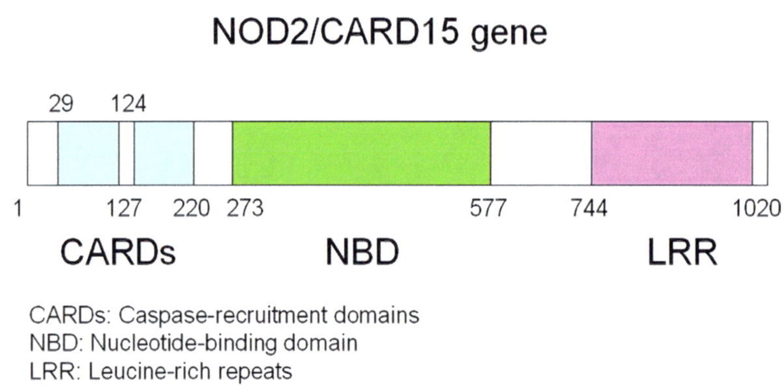

Figure 6.13. *NOD2/CARD15* gene.

Source: https://upload.wikimedia.org/wikipedia/en/3/33/NOD2_CARD15.jpg.

6.5.3. Role of Regulatory Proteins in Gene Control

The complexities of gene regulation in bacteria are primarily orchestrated through the actions of regulatory proteins, which play a significant role in overseeing the expression of genes necessary for various physiological functions. These proteins, including transcription factors and repressors, facilitate the detection of environmental stimuli, enabling bacteria to respond swiftly to changing conditions. Effective modulation of gene expression is crucial for survival, particularly in fluctuating environments characterised by nutrient scarcity or stress. Regulatory proteins influence promoter activity or interact with RNA polymerase to enhance or inhibit transcription, thus permitting precise regulation of protein synthesis essential for growth and metabolic processes. This sophisticated regulatory mechanism exemplifies the adaptability of bacterial systems, allowing them to flourish in diverse ecological niches. Within this regulatory framework, post-transcriptional control is highlighted as a primary determinant of gene expression. Regulatory proteins operate not only at the transcriptional level but also interact with mechanisms governing mRNA stability and translation. For example, small non-coding RNAs (sRNAs) may bind messenger RNA to modulate its degradation or translation efficiency, playing a vital role in post-transcriptional gene regulation. Such interactions enable organisms to respond rapidly to environmental changes without necessitating new transcription. Regulatory networks incorporating sRNAs introduce an additional layer of complexity to bacterial gene regulation, reflecting the multidimensional strategies bacteria employ to control their gene expression machinery. An illustrative example of regulatory protein control involves the regulation of genes within *Salmonella enterica* pathogenicity island I (SPI-1), which is essential for the bacterium's ability to invade epithelial cells. SPI-1 gene expression is stringently regulated and activated under specific conditions, representing a strategic adaptation. Experimental evidence indicates that the CRP-camp complex is a key factor repressing SPI-1 gene expression under non-permissive conditions. The regulatory protein HilD, known as the invasion master regulator in Salmonella, is unexpectedly controlled by CRP-camp, underscoring the central role of regulatory networks in bacteria. This interplay highlights the critical function of regulatory proteins in tightly regulating gene expression, influencing bacterial behaviour and pathogenicity, and reaffirming their pivotal role in bacterial structure and genetics (Beslon et al., 2010; Balsalobre et al., 2018).

6.6. Applications of Bacterial Genetics

Bacterial genetics plays a pivotal role in numerous applications extending beyond initial scientific inquiry, exerting a significant influence on disciplines such as medicine, biotechnology, and environmental science. Bacterial genes can be genetically engineered to enable the creation of GMOs capable of producing vital pharmaceuticals such as insulin and vaccines.

These advancements are particularly pertinent amid escalating global health challenges, where conventional drug development processes may prove economically burdensome. Leveraging techniques such as gene cloning and gene expression vectors, bacteria can synthesize complex biological molecules more efficiently than traditional methods. Consequently, understanding bacterial genetics not only advances medical capabilities but also underscores the importance of these microorganisms as vehicles for biotechnological innovation (Seaman & Whitehouse, 2001). Moreover, the development of high-resolution genomic tools has expanded the horizons of bacterial genetics. Platforms such as CRISPR/Cas 9 have transformed gene editing by enabling unprecedented precision, facilitating applications in disease modelling and gene therapy. Bacterial systems have been instrumental in the design and validation of such genome editing technologies, serving as platforms for studying genetic function and interaction.

As these methodologies continue to evolve, the potential for employing genetically modified bacteria to enhance agricultural sustainability and ensure food security becomes increasingly promising. Progress in bacterial genetics is crucial for developing crops with improved resistance to environmental stresses and pests, thereby supporting global food security amidst a growing population (Gartland et al., 2017). Beyond medicine and agriculture, bacterial genetics also finds applications in environmental decontamination and biotechnology. Bacteria can be engineered to degrade toxins, making them valuable agents in bioremediation processes.

Through genetic modification for specific metabolic capacities, bacteria can be employed in the remediation of oil spills, heavy metal contamination, and other hazardous wastes.

Additionally, such microorganisms can contribute to sustainability by converting waste into biofuels or other useful substrates. Continuous advancements in bacterial genetic methods and knowledge benefit ecological sustainability and highlight the interconnectedness of scientific disciplines. Therefore, the applications of bacterial genetics underscore its vital role in addressing some of the most urgent issues facing humanity today (Seaman & Whitehouse, 2001).Seaman & Whitehouse, 2001Seaman & Whitehouse, 2001

6.6.1. Use of Bacteria in Biotechnology

The application of bacteria within the field of biotechnology exemplifies a quintessential integration of microbiology and genetic engineering, leveraging the inherent capabilities of these microorganisms to develop products and processes. Bacteria constitute the primary contributors to this innovative domain due to their simplicity, rapid growth, and adaptability across diverse environments. Genetic manipulation techniques empower researchers to modify bacterial genomes, thereby enhancing their utility for biotechnological applications. For example, methods such as CRISPR/Cas9 have revolutionised genetic editing by enabling precise insertion or deletion of genetic material, resulting in the creation of genetically modified bacteria capable of synthesising essential substances such as insulin, growth hormones, and biofuels.

This remarkable capability positions bacteria at the forefront of efforts to address global health and energy sustainability challenges. Furthermore, bacterial applications extend beyond the medical and energy sectors, notably impacting agricultural biotechnology. Genetic modification of bacteria has facilitated the production of biofertilizers and biopesticides, promoting environmentally sustainable farming practices that mitigate ecological harm while increasing crop yields. The utilisation of bacteria capable of nitrogen fixation or pesticide degradation renders agricultural practices more environmentally friendly and efficient. Additionally, biotechnology employs bacteria to synthesize vital nutrients, including vitamins and amino acids, directly contributing to food security. These advancements underscore the importance of understanding bacterial genetics, especially as the world faces escalating demands for food production amidst rapid population growth. Research into marine bacteria further exemplifies the diverse potential of microorganisms in biotechnology. Recent investigations have identified novel genetic traits among marine bacteria, whose potential for discovering new compounds and enzymes of therapeutic relevance remains largely unexplored.

These organisms are significant not only within their marine ecosystems but are increasingly recognised as valuable sources of bioactive molecules with pharmaceutical applications. Recent studies in marine biotechnology highlight the importance of fostering collaboration between academic institutions and industry to facilitate the translation of research findings into practical applications, thus harnessing the full potential of marine biodiversity for healthcare and industrial purposes (Gary et al., 2001; Seaman & Whitehouse, 2001). Continuing research into bacterial structure and genetics will undoubtedly promote these developments, fostering a future where bacteria play a central role in addressing various technological and sustainability challenges.Seaman & Whitehouse, 2001

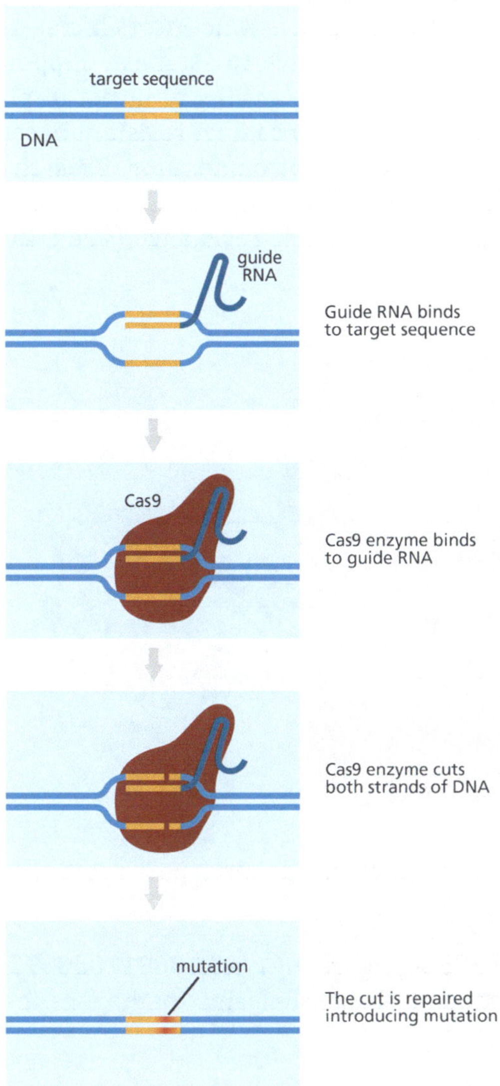

Figure 6.14. Diagram showing how the CRISPR-Cas9 editing tool works.

Source: https://www.yourgenome.org/wp-content/uploads/2023/12/1301-CRISPR-in-action-372x768.png.

6.6.2. Role of Bacteria in Medicine and Antibiotic Resistance

The expanding understanding of the medical functions of bacteria has increasingly become a subject of scholarly interest as researchers examine their roles beyond mere pathology, notably in areas such as antibiotic resistance. Traditionally, antibiotics have served as a fundamental component of contemporary medicine, effectively treating numerous bacterial infections. However, the emergence of antibiotic-resistant strains poses a significant challenge, necessitating a reassessment of how these microorganisms are perceived and utilized. The rising prevalence of resistance has driven the development of novel therapeutic strategies that target not only the bacteria themselves but also the mechanisms responsible for resistance. Consequently, investigating the structural and genetic aspects of bacteria has become essential, offering insights into how DNA modifications can confer resistance and potentially guiding the development of new treatments. In light of the antibiotic resistance crisis, researchers are increasingly considering bacteriophages — viruses that specifically infect and eradicate bacteria — as promising therapeutic agents. Bacteriophages offer the advantage of specificity, which may help to mitigate collateral damage to commensal microbiota, a notable concern associated with broad-spectrum antibiotics. This approach relies on the complex genetics and structural interactions between phages and bacterial hosts and suggests an ongoing co-evolutionary arms race. The demand for phage therapy has also been driven by the limitations of traditional antibiotics, as many existing drugs exhibit reduced efficacy due to widespread resistance mechanisms. Enhancing our understanding of bacteriophage interactions with bacterial genetics is therefore crucial for optimising phage application, emphasising the importance of bacteria not only as agents of disease but also as target entities in the development of novel pharmaceuticals. Within the context of emerging bacterial therapeutics, the legal and economic frameworks that underpin drug development are undergoing reevaluation. The substantial investments required for pharmaceutical research and development often depend on robust patent protections; however, recent Supreme Court rulings have cast uncertainty on the patentability of phage therapies, which could hinder innovation within this domain. As scientific efforts increasingly advocate for the replacement of antibiotics with phages, it is imperative to establish supportive structures that provide the necessary funding to industry stakeholders willing to invest in phage therapy. Absent adequate protections, the potential of bacteriophages to combat resistant bacterial diseases may remain unrealised. Consequently, creating a conducive environment for research and development — potentially through alternative regulatory mechanisms or incentives — is vital for the advancement of medicine in the ongoing battle against antibiotic resistance (Todd, 2014) (Figure 6. 15).

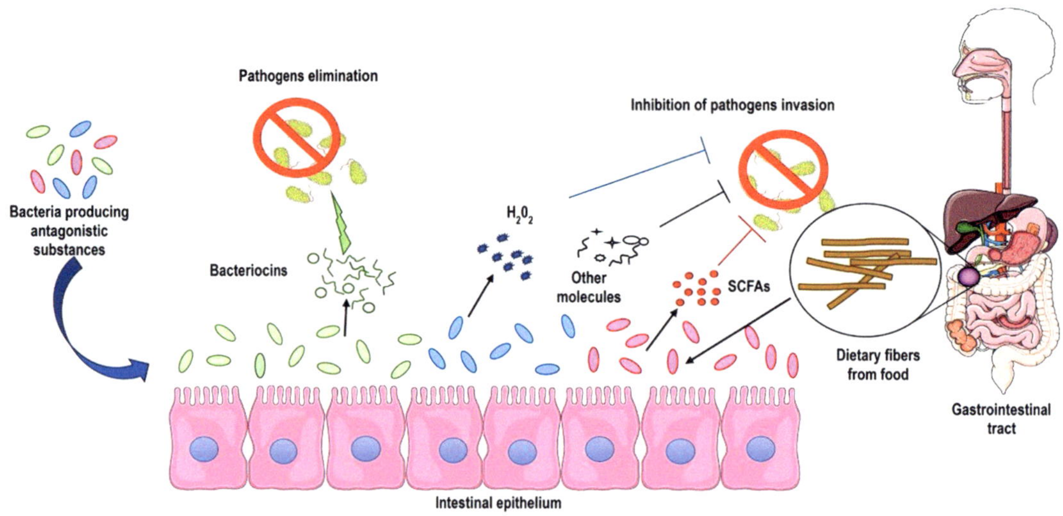

Figure 6.15. Protective effects and inhibitory actions of bacteria against pathogens in the gastrointestinal tract.

Source: https://www.researchgate.net/publication/354587584/figure/fig1/AS:1068170588721165@1631683122969/Protective-effects-and-inhibitory-actions-of-bacteria-against-pathogens-in-the.png.

6.6.3. Bacterial Genetics in Environmental Science

The intersection of environmental science and bacterial genetics is pivotal in elucidating ecological processes and biogeochemical cycling. Bacteria are involved in fundamental nutrient cycling processes, such as the cycling of carbon and nitrogen, and their genetic diversity enables adaptation to various environmental stresses. Advanced genetic techniques, including metagenomics and CRISPR-based technologies, allow researchers to investigate the metabolic capacities of bacterial communities across ecosystems. By analysing the genetic composition of environmental bacteria, scientists can determine their roles in bioremediation and thus harness their potential for pollutant degradation and ecological restoration. This genetic information holds both theoretical significance and practical applications, underscoring the importance of bacterial genetics within the interdisciplinary scope of environmental science in addressing critical issues such as climate change and pollution. Certain bacterial groups have garnered special attention due to their unique genetic adaptations. For example, magnetotactic bacteria (MTB) have developed organelles called magnetosomes that enable orientation within magnetic fields in marine environments. The molecular processes involved in magnetosome biogenesis are complex, involving multiple genes that regulate biomineralisation. This research not only deepens our understanding of bacterial functions but also presents opportunities in biotechnology and environmental remediation. Since these bacteria inhabit diverse environments from freshwater to marine habitats, understanding their genetics can shed light on microbial environmental sensing and adaptation mechanisms, thereby emphasising the necessity for continued research into bacterial genetics, ecological function, and sustainability (McCausland & Komeili, 2020). Moreover, the genetic diversity within bacterial populations serves as a reservoir of valuable adaptive traits. Horizontal gene transfer (HGT) plays a vital role by enabling bacteria to acquire advantageous genes from nearby organisms, facilitating rapid adaptation to environmental pressures. HGT is particularly significant in stressed environments, such as contaminated or extreme habitats, where it enhances bacterial efficiency in bioremediation, accelerating the breakdown of toxic compounds. Furthermore, bacterial genetics is crucial for understanding and monitoring antimicrobial resistance, which poses an increasing concern for public safety and environmental health. Consequently, understanding bacterial genetic processes is essential for advancing research and developing strategies to combat environmental degradation and protect human health (Seaman & Whitehouse, 2001).Seaman & Whitehouse, 2001

SUMMARY

In elucidating the complex relationship between bacterial structure and genetics, it becomes evident that these aspects are interconnected and fundamentally essential to bacterial survival. Structural features of bacteria, such as their rigid cell walls and distinctive membrane compositions, facilitate various physiological functions that are governed by their genetic information. For example, the genetic instructions encoded within bacterial DNA regulate cellular activities, including the synthesis of essential structures such as flagella and pili. These structures enable motility and adhesion, respectively, thereby exemplifying the intrinsic link between bacterial genetics and their structural capabilities. An understanding of this relationship not only enhances our fundamental comprehension of microbiology but also suggests potential strategies in biotechnology, whereby the regulation of these structures could lead to novel applications in medicine and environmental management. The genetic diversity among bacterial species is extensive, illustrating the evolutionary capacity that allows these organisms to adapt to diverse environments. Mechanisms such as horizontal gene transfer, mutation, and recombination contribute to this diversity and underscore the significant influence of genetics on bacterial adaptability and survival. Notably, DNA repair mechanisms, including the recently described prokaryotic non-homologous end-joining pathways, provide insights into bacterial resilience under environmental stresses and contribute to genomic stability. This emerging knowledge highlights the dynamic nature of bacterial genetics and its impact on structural integrity, emphasising the importance of genetic research in understanding bacterial life cycles and phage-bacterial interactions. Such information is vital, as it opens avenues for future research aimed at identifying novel genetic tools for regulating bacterial behaviour. Overall, this investigation into bacterial structure and genetics reveals the complexities and interconnections that define life at the microscopic level. Studies on specialized bacterial structures, such as magnetosomes, reveal the sophisticated adaptations microorganisms have evolved, reflecting their evolutionary history and environmental interactions. As documented in the literature, processes such as biomineralisation and organelle biogenesis are heavily influenced by genetic factors, offering promising directions for future studies (McCausland & Komeili, 2020). Concurrently, the complexity of DNA repair mechanisms underscores the necessity to protect bacterial genomes from environmental challenges and mutations (Bowater & Doherty, 2006). Collectively, these findings deepen our understanding of bacterial biology and provide critical insights into the relevance of bacterial genetics in biotechnology, ecology, and medicine, thereby affirming the enduring importance of this research to the global scientific community.

Bacterial genetics and structure studies offer valuable insights into processes that control cell division and growth. A key topic in this area is the adder principle, which states that bacteria maintain a fixed volume from birth to division but show variation even among genetically identical individuals. This principle challenges traditional models of growth because stochastic processes are thought to regulate the timing of cell division. This regulation might involve a time-keeper protein expressed proportionally to volume, highlighting the role of intrinsic cellular factors in size homeostasis. The experimental data support this model, showing that the additional volume added between division events remains constant regardless of fluctuations in newborn cell size, thereby indicating a simple mechanism for controlling bacterial growth dynamics (Ghusinga et al., 2015). The discussion of bacterial genetics also covers the stability and heritability of genetic information in these microorganisms. The structural composition of bacterial cells plays a crucial role in genetic transfer, especially processes such as horizontal gene transfer. Bacteria employ various mechanisms — transformation, transduction, and conjugation — to acquire gene diversity, which significantly enhances their adaptability and survival. These mechanisms have implications for agriculture, particularly in the use of genetically modified organisms (GMOs) and related issues concerning their role in organic farming practices. These considerations underscore the importance of understanding DNA's fate under different environmental conditions, including its survival in soil and its horizontal transfer via livestock feed (Clarke et al., 2001). Furthermore, the relationship between bacterial structure and gene regulation is central to understanding pathogenesis and antibiotic resistance. Bacteria have characteristic structural features, such as peptidoglycan cell walls and diverse membrane compositions, which not only serve as physical barriers but are also involved in signalling and gene expression. The bacterial structure influences how bacteria respond to environmental stresses, including antibiotics. It is essential to comprehend these relationships when developing new strategies to combat bacterial infections and improve treatment outcomes. The study of genomic organisation and regulatory networks offers additional perspectives on bacterial genetics, paving the way for further research aimed at translating these findings into biotechnological and therapeutic applications (Ghusinga et al., 2015).

CLOSER LOOK

BACTERIAL TRANSFORMATION

Bacterial transformation is a natural or induced process in which bacteria take up free DNA from their environment and incorporate it into their genome. It is one of the principal modes of horizontal gene transfer, the others being transduction and conjugation, and makes an important contribution to bacterial evolution, gene diversity, and horizontal transmission of antibiotic resistance (Figure 6.16).

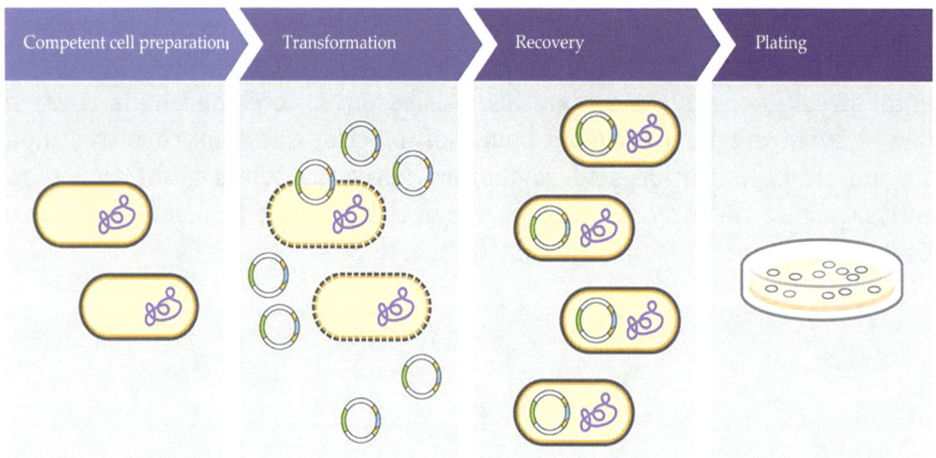

Figure 6.16. Diagram illustrating the process of bacterial transformation, including competent cell preparation, introduction of plasmid DNA, recovery, and plating to select transformed colonies.

Source: https://external-content.duckduckgo.com/iu/?u=https%3A%2F%2Fmicrobenotes.com%2Fwp-content%2Fuploads%2F2020%2F05%2FBacterial-Transformation.jpg&f=1&nofb=1&ipt=bea9bc48ddc2839e7953ae4614ec678bb744369a97fca1748028a2dede3b815d.

Transformation can occur spontaneously in certain "competent" bacteria such as *Streptococcus pneumoniae*, *Bacillus subtilis*, *Neisseria gonorrhoeae*, and *Haemophilus influenzae*. The competence is generally regulated and induced under specific conditions, such as starvation or cell density (quorum sensing). These bacteria release specialized proteins that are used in foreign DNA binding, uptake, and integration.

During natural transformation, extracellular DNA—usually from lysed bacterial cells—is bound to the surface of the recipient cell. The DNA is then transferred across the cell membrane, usually in the form of a single strand, with degradation of the complementary strand. Once inside, the DNA may be integrated into the host genome through homologous recombination if sequence homology exists, or it may be retained as a plasmid if it has an independent replication origin.

Artificial conversion is widely applied in molecular biology and biotechnology. Bacteria such as *Escherichia coli* may be made competent in the laboratory using chemical treatment (e.g., calcium chloride) or electroporation (through the use of electric pulses to temporarily permeabilize the cell membrane) to enable them to take up plasmid DNA. The process serves as a basis for cloning, genetic engineering, and the synthesis of recombinant proteins. Bacterial transformation has significant implications in clinical microbiology. It is a major mechanism behind the spread of antibiotic resistance genes and virulence factors. For example, transformation allows *Streptococcus pneumoniae* to acquire new capsule genes, changing its serotype and evading host immunity.

The discovery of transformation was key to history in proving that DNA is genetic material. Frederick Griffith's work with *S. pneumoniae* in 1928 revealed the "transforming principle," and Avery, MacLeod, and McCarty discovered it to be DNA in 1944.

REFERENCES

1. Beslon, G., Parsons, D. P., Sanchez-Dehesa, Y., Peña, J. M., & Knibbe, C. (2010). Scaling laws in bacterial genomes: a side-effect of selection of mutational robustness?. *Bio Systems, 102*(1), 32–40. https://doi.org/10.1016/j.biosystems.2010.07.009(accessed on 16th July 2025).
2. Ahern, H., & Habashi, J. (2020). *Cereus Fun: An Introduction to Microbiological Techniques.* https://core.ac.uk/download/395019283.pdf (accessed on 16th July 2025).
3. Goudie, A. C., Olateju, F., Anderson, J. G., Rowan, N., & MacGregor, S. J. (2003). Inactivation of pathogens on food and contact surfaces using ozone as a biocidal agent. Poster session presented at Society for General Microbiology – 152nd Meeting – –, University of Edinburgh. (accessed on 16th July 2025).
4. McBurney, M. I., Davis, C., Fraser, C. M., Schneeman, B. O., Huttenhower, C., Verbeke, K., Walter, J., & Latulippe, M. E. (2019). Establishing What Constitutes a Healthy Human Gut Microbiome: State of the Science, Regulatory Considerations, and Future Directions. *The Journal of nutrition, 149*(11), 1882–1895. https://doi.org/10.1093/jn/nxz154(accessed on 16th July 2025).
5. Silander, O. K., Nikolic, N., Zaslaver, A., Bren, A., Kikoin, I., Alon, U., & Ackermann, M. (2012). A genome-wide analysis of promoter-mediated phenotypic noise in Escherichia coli. *PLoS genetics, 8*(1), e1002443. https://doi.org/10.1371/journal.pgen.1002443(accessed on 16th July 2025).
6. Arnoldt, H., Strogatz, S. H., & Timme, M. (2015). *Simple model for the Darwinian transition in early evolution.* http://arxiv.org/abs/1501.05073 (accessed on 16th July 2025).
7. Azuma Taoka, Kaito, C., Nakane, D., Wada, H., Mori, H., Tulum, I., Shimabukuro, K., et al. (2020). *Tree of motility – A proposed history of motility systems in the tree of life.* https://core.ac.uk/download/327172571.pdf (accessed on 16th July 2025).
8. Baldwin, I. T., Dorcheh, E. K., Li, R., Rameshkumar, A., et al. (2019). *Antimicrobial peptide expression in a wild tobacco plant reveals the limits of host-microbe-manipulations in the field.* https://core.ac.uk/download/225124661.pdf (accessed on 16th July 2025).
9. Balsalobre, C., El Mouali, Y., Gaviria-Cantin, T., Gilbert, S. F., et al. (2018). *CRP-cAMP mediates silencing of Salmonella virulence at the post-transcriptional level.* https://core.ac.uk/download/161254135.pdf (accessed on 16th July 2025).
10. Bandurski, Robert S, Neelam Singh, issuing body Michigan State University. Department of Botany and Plant Pathology, and sponsoring body United States. National Aeronautics and Space Administration. 1983. *The Alpha-Helix Concept : Innovative Utilization of the Space Station Program : A Report to the National Aeronautic and Space Administration Requesting Establishment of a Sensory Physiology Laboratory on the Space Station.* East Lansing, MI: [Michigan State Univ., Dept. of Botany and Plant Pathology].(accessed on 16th July 2025).
11. Bankevich, A., Darling, A. E., Page, A. J., Kislyuk, A. O., Charlesworth, B., Buckee, C., et al. (2020). *Bacterial Microevolution and the Pangenome.* https://core.ac.uk/download/323058045.pdf (accessed on 16th July 2025).
12. Baumdicker, F., Hess, W. R., & Pfaffelhuber, P. (2010). *The diversity of a distributed genome in bacterial populations.* http://arxiv.org/abs/0907.2572 (accessed on 16th July 2025).

13. Gartland, Kevan M.A., et al. "Advances in biotechnology: Genomics and genome editing" The EuroBiotech Journal, vol. 1, no. 1, European Biotechnology Thematic Network Association, 2017, pp. 2-9. https://doi.org/10.24190/ISSN2564-615X/2017/01.02f (accessed on 16th July 2025).

14. WENTIAN LI and DIRK HOLSTE

15. (2004)*Spectral analysis of guanine and cytosine fluctuations of mouse genomic DNA.* Fluctuation and Noise Letters 2004 04:03, L453-L464 http://arxiv.org/abs/q-bio/0411017 (accessed on 16th July 2025).

16. King, K. C., Stelkens, R. B., Webster, J. P., Smith, D. F., & Brockhurst, M. A. (2015). Hybridization in Parasites: Consequences for Adaptive Evolution, Pathogenesis, and Public Health in a Changing World. *PLoS pathogens*, *11*(9), e1005098. https://doi.org/10.1371/journal.ppat.1005098(accessed on 16th July 2025).

17. Bois, A., Garcia-Roger, E. M., Hong, E., Hutzler, S., et al. (2019). *Congenital anomalies from a physics perspective: The key role of "manufacturing" volatility.* http://arxiv.org/abs/1905.04357 (accessed on 16th July 2025).

18. Boutry, S., Brisse, S., Bui Thi Ngoc, L., Gagnevin, L., et al. (2008). *From local surveys to global surveillance: Three high-throughput genotyping methods for epidemiological monitoring of Xanthomonas citri pv. citri pathotypes.* http://agritrop.cirad.fr/548014/1/document_548014.pdf (accessed on 16th July 2025).

19. Bowater, R., & Doherty, A. J. (2006). *Making ends meet: Repairing breaks in bacterial DNA by non-homologous end-joining.* https://core.ac.uk/download/2728184.pdf (accessed on 16th July 2025).

20. Buckling, A., Donderis, J., Elena, S. F., Frígols, B., et al. (2015). *Virus satellites drive viral evolution and ecology.* https://core.ac.uk/download/42366344.pdf (accessed on 16th July 2025).

21. Skretas, G., Carroll, S., DeFrees, S., Schwartz, M. F., Johnson, K. F., & Georgiou, G. (2009). Expression of active human sialyltransferase ST6GalNAcI in Escherichia coli. *Microbial cell factories*, *8*, 50. https://doi.org/10.1186/1475-2859-8-50(accessed on 16th July 2025).

22. Clarke, B., Dale, P., Fontes, E., Martin, D. R., et al. (2001). *A review of knowledge of the potential impacts of GMOs on organic agriculture.* https://core.ac.uk/download/10923231.pdf (accessed on 16th July 2025).

23. Miller, K. A., Motaleb, M. A., Liu, J., Hu, B., Caimano, M. J., Miller, M. R., & Charon, N. W. (2014). Initial characterization of the FlgE hook high molecular weight complex of Borrelia burgdorferi. *PloS one*, *9*(5), e98338. https://doi.org/10.1371/journal.pone.0098338(accessed on 16th July 2025).

24. Ryan, A. F., Nasamran, C. A., Pak, K., Draf, C., Fisch, K. M., Webster, N., & Kurabi, A. (2020). Single-Cell Transcriptomes Reveal a Complex Cellular Landscape in the Middle Ear and Differential Capacities for Acute Response to Infection. *Frontiers in genetics*, *11*, 358. https://doi.org/10.3389/fgene.2020.00358(accessed on 16th July 2025).

25. Lakatos PL, Fischer S, Lakatos L, Gal I, Papp J. Current concept on the pathogenesis of inflammatory bowel disease-crosstalk between genetic and microbial factors: Pathogenic bacteria and altered bacterial sensing or changes in mucosal integrity take "toll". World J Gastroenterol 2006; 12(12): 1829-1841 (accessed on 16th July 2025).

26. Ghusinga, K. R., Singh, A., & Vargas-Garcia, C. A. (2015). *A mechanistic first-passage time framework for bacterial cell-division timing.* http://arxiv.org/abs/1512.07864 (accessed on 16th July 2025).

27. Haaber, J., Ingmer, H., & Penadés, J. R. (2017). *Transfer of antibiotic resistance in Staphylococcus aureus.* https://core.ac.uk/download/84148494.pdf (accessed on 16th July 2025).

28. Hofvander, P. (2004). *Production of amylopectin and high-amylose starch in separate potato genotypes.* https://core.ac.uk/download/11694800.pdf (accessed on 16th July 2025).

29. Emmett, K. J. and Rabadan, R., "Characterizing Scales of Genetic Recombination and Antibiotic Resistance in Pathogenic Bacteria Using Topological Data Analysis", <i>arXiv e-prints</i>, Art. no. arXiv:1406.1219, 2014. doi:10.48550/arXiv.1406.1219. (accessed on 16th July 2025).

30. Horowitz, N. H., & Owen, R. D. (1954). *Physiological Aspects of Genetics.* https://core.ac.uk/download/4869317.pdf (accessed on 16th July 2025).

31. Jerdan, R., Iungin, O., V. Moshynets, O., Potters, G., & J. Spiers, A. (2020). Extending an Eco-Evolutionary Understanding of Biofilm-Formation at the Air-Liquid Interface to Community Biofilms. IntechOpen. doi: 10.5772/intechopen.90955(accessed on 16th July 2025).

32. Kaloshian, I., & Teixeira, M. (2019). *Advances in plant-nematode interactions with emphasis on the notorious nematode genus Meloidogyne.* https://core.ac.uk/download/305123985.pdf (accessed on 16th July 2025).

33. King, D. M. (2015). *Evolutionary Dynamics of Speciation and Extinction.* https://core.ac.uk/download/217321608.pdf (accessed on 16th July 2025).

34. McCausland, H. C., & Komeili, A. (2020). Magnetic genes: Studying the genetics of biomineralization in magnetotactic bacteria. *PLoS genetics*, *16*(2), e1008499. https://doi.org/10.1371/journal.pgen.1008499(accessed on 16th July 2025).

35. Lagares, A., Pistorio, M., & Sanjuán Pinilla, J. (2014). *The plasmid mobilome of the model plant-symbiont Sinorhizobium meliloti: Coming up with new questions and answers.* https://core.ac.uk/download/159287717.pdf (accessed on 16th July 2025).

36. McGowan, T. L. (1996). Construction of a novel fungal *gus* expression plasmid, and its evaluation in *Aspergillus nidulans*: A thesis presented in partial fulfilment of the requirements for the degree of Master of Science in Genetics at Massey University. https://core.ac.uk/download/148645080.pdf (accessed on 16th July 2025).

37. Milka, M. (2018). *Role of Horizontal Gene Transfer in Bacteria.* https://core.ac.uk/download/234687733.pdf (accessed on 16th July 2025).

38. Panja, D., & Molineux, I. J. (2010). Dynamics of bacteriophage genome ejection in vitro and in vivo. *Physical biology*, *7*(4), 045006. https://doi.org/10.1088/1478-3975/7/4/045006(accessed on 16th July 2025).

39. Parry, S. K. (1993). Construction and utilization of a bidirectional reporter vector in the analysis of two nod-boxes in *Rhizobium loti*: A thesis presented in partial fulfilment of the requirements for the degree of Master of Science in Molecular Genetics at Massey University. https://core.ac.uk/download/222793743.pdf (accessed on 16th July 2025).

40. Seaman, W., & Whitehouse, J. H. (2001). *Florida marine biotechnology: Research, development and training capabilities to advance science and commerce.* Sea Grant Technical Paper Number 110 https://core.ac.uk/download/11016354.pdf (accessed on 16th July 2025).

41. Spiers, A. J. (2014). *A mechanistic explanation linking adaptive mutation, niche change, and fitness advantage for the Wrinkly Spreader*. https://core.ac.uk/download/228177282.pdf (accessed on 16th July 2025).

42. Todd, K. (2014). *The promising viral threat to bacterial resistance: The uncertain patentability of phage therapeutics and the necessity of alternative incentives.* https://core.ac.uk/download/213020895.pdf (accessed on 16th July 2025).

43. Toenniessen, G. H., O'Toole, J. C., Harris, R. R., Herdt, R. W., & Murashige, T. (2001). *The Rockefeller Foundation's International Program on Rice Biotechnology.* https://core.ac.uk/download/71354545.pdf (accessed on 16th July 2025).

44. Wheeler, V. (2017). *Preliminary analyses of the diversity of soil microbes on the campus of the University of the Incarnate Word*. https://core.ac.uk/download/217400695.pdf (accessed on 16th July 2025).

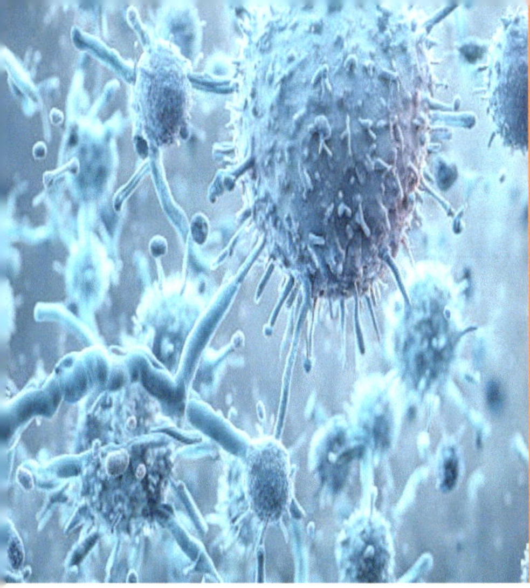

Chapter 7

GRAM-NEGATIVE BACTERIAL INFECTIONS

Contents

Introduction

Barnard, 2019The field of infectious diseases is increasingly dominated by Gram-negative bacteria, which are renowned for their resilience and antibiotic resistance. Characterised by their lipopolysaccharide outer membrane, these microorganisms pose unique challenges in both treatment and diagnosis. Infections caused by Gram-negative bacteria can result in significant morbidity and mortality, with diseases such as sepsis, pneumonia, and urinary tract infections frequently linked to them. The importance of detecting Gram-negative infections extends beyond immediate clinical implications to encompass broader public health concerns associated with their rising prevalence. As evidenced by the literature, a substantial proportion of pathogens responsible for cervico-facial sepsis are gram-negative, although their presence may not always be detected through culturing techniques (Barnard, 2019). This discrepancy reflects ongoing challenges faced by clinicians in accurately diagnosing and effectively treating these infections. The emergence of antimicrobial resistance (AMR) further complicates the management of Gram-negative bacterial infections. The widespread overuse and misuse of antibiotics in human and animal populations have led to the rise of multidrug-resistant

(MDR) strains, which diminish the efficacy of many current treatment options. This situation underscores the urgent necessity for innovative approaches in the diagnosis, vaccination, and treatment of resistant microorganisms (Jenner et al., 2017). The critical role of effective governance in strategising global and local responses to AMR cannot be overstated, as failures in one region can have far-reaching implications worldwide. To address the complex nature of AMR, cross-sector collaboration must be harnessed to promote research and development (R&D) efforts that not only provide new pharmaceutical options but also ensure stewardship of existing therapies. In mitigating the polymorphic challenges posed by Gram-negative bacterial infections, a comprehensive approach becomes imperative. Healthcare professionals and scientists must consider not only the development of novel treatments but also the implementation of prudent stewardship practices to curb the emergence of resistance. Additionally, the establishment of a timely global framework is essential to facilitate the development and distribution of new diagnostics and therapeutics, particularly in resource-limited settings (Jenner et al., 2017). The integration of intellectual property mechanisms can incentivise R&D investments and promote equitable access to innovations. This overarching strategy is vital for improving health outcomes and mitigating the public health risks associated with Gram-negative bacterial infections.

Definition of Gram-negative Bacteria

Understanding the Gram-negative definition of bacteria is crucial in grasping their unique features and significance in medical microbiology. These bacteria are characterised by their cell wall, which features a thin peptidoglycan layer between two membranes. This structure prevents them from retaining the crystal violet stain in the Gram staining process, categorising them as Gram-negative. Their outer membrane contains lipopolysaccharides that trigger strong immune responses, making them important in infection and inflammation. Their complex cell wall contributes to antibiotic resistance, complicating treatment and necessitating ongoing research for new therapies. Recognizing their clinical relevance involves more than just structure; it includes their prevalence in various environments and their ability to cause disease. Common genera like *Escherichia*, *Salmonella*, and *Pseudomonas* cause a broad spectrum of infections, from gastrointestinal illnesses to hospital-acquired infections. Many Gram-negative pathogens are opportunistic, exploiting weakened immune systems, especially in individuals with underlying health issues. Additionally, biofilm formation on medical devices like catheters and prosthetic joints makes infections harder to treat and clean, as these biofilms resist antibiotics and immune defences, leading to chronic conditions with increased morbidity (Zabielska et al., 2016) (Figure 7.1).

Advancements in diagnostic technologies are crucial for the prompt identification of Gram-negative bacteria, especially within hospital environments where swift intervention is imperative. Traditional bacteriological identification methods can be slow and laborious, often resulting in delayed therapeutic responses. Conversely, emerging technologies such as terahertz time-domain spectroscopy are under investigation for their potential to accelerate microbial detection. These methods offer rapid, non-invasive, and non-destructive identification of microbial populations, facilitating early detection of infections and accurate determination of bacterial Gram types (Berrier et al., 2012). As understanding of the clinical significance of Gram-negative bacteria deepens, continued innovation in detection and treatment strategies will be essential in addressing the escalating threat posed by Gram-negative bacterial infections.

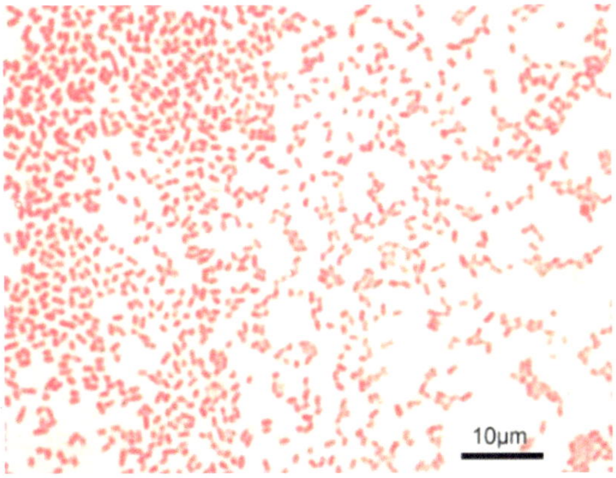

Figure 7.1. Microscopic image of Gram-negative *Pseudomonas aeruginosa* bacteria (pink-red rods).

Source: https://en.wikipedia.org/wiki/Gram-negative_bacteria#/media/File:Pseudomonas_aeruginosa_Gram.jpg.

Importance of Studying Gram-negative Infections

Gram-negative infections warrant thorough investigation due to the complexity of Gram-negative bacteria and their inherent resistance to most antibiotics. These bacteria possess a double membrane that functions as a natural barrier against therapeutic agents, rendering them difficult to treat. Understanding the mechanisms by which these pathogens resist antibiotics and evade immune responses is crucial for the development of effective therapeutic interventions. Furthermore, with the increasing incidence of multidrug-resistant Gram-negative bacterial infections, such as *Klebsiella pneumoniae* and *Escherichia coli*, which place a substantial burden on healthcare systems and result in higher morbidity and mortality, there is an escalating imperative to conduct comprehensive studies on the behaviour and characteristics of Gram-negative bacteria. Such research is essential for informing clinical practices and guiding public health interventions. Additionally, the epidemiological trends of Gram-negative infections underscore the importance of studying these organisms. Hospital infections, predominantly associated with Gram-negative bacteria, remain a significant concern within healthcare settings, particularly in intensive care units.

These infections can lead to severe complications, prolonged hospital stays, and increased healthcare costs. Moreover, research indicates that these bacteria are prevalent not only in clinical environments but also in agriculture, where antibiotic-resistant strains have been identified in livestock farms, as demonstrated in recent studies (Chapin et al., 2004). This interconnectedness between agricultural and human health highlights the need for multidisciplinary approaches in studying Gram-negative infections, as combating these pathogens necessitates integrated strategies encompassing environmental, clinical, and public health dimensions. Equally concerning is the stagnation in antibiotic development for Gram-negative bacterial infections. Despite a significant decline in the rate of novel antibiotic discovery since the mid-20th century, the emergence and proliferation of resistant strains pose a direct threat to human health (PEW Charitable Trust Report, 2016). As bacteria continue to develop new resistance mechanisms, the remaining effective antibiotics may soon become obsolete, turning previously manageable infections into potentially lethal conditions. This emphasises the critical need for ongoing research into novel therapeutic agents and treatments. By analysing the genetic makeup and resistance patterns of Gram-negative bacteria, researchers can identify new targets for drug development and inform policies regarding antibiotic use in both clinical and agricultural settings. Studying Gram-negative infections is thus not only a laboratory pursuit but also an essential component of ensuring global health security and protecting public health.*Escherichia coli*

7.1. Characteristics of Gram-negative Bacteria

The distinguishing characteristics of Gram-negative bacteria are crucial in determining their pathogenicity and their roles in various infections. Gram-negative bacteria possess a cell wall composed of a thin layer of peptidoglycan covered by an outer membrane. This outer membrane consists of lipopolysaccharides, which serve as characteristic antigenic determinants capable of eliciting robust immune responses in the host. The composition of this outer membrane contributes to the resistance to certain antibiotics and detergents, thereby rendering conventional treatments ineffective. This additional protective layer is particularly significant in the case of multidrug-resistant organisms (MDROs), as it allows bacteria to evade both immune defences and pharmacological interventions. Furthermore, Gram-negative bacteria tend to naturally form biofilms, which enhance their survival in adverse conditions and complicate clinical eradication (Di Domenico et al., 2017).

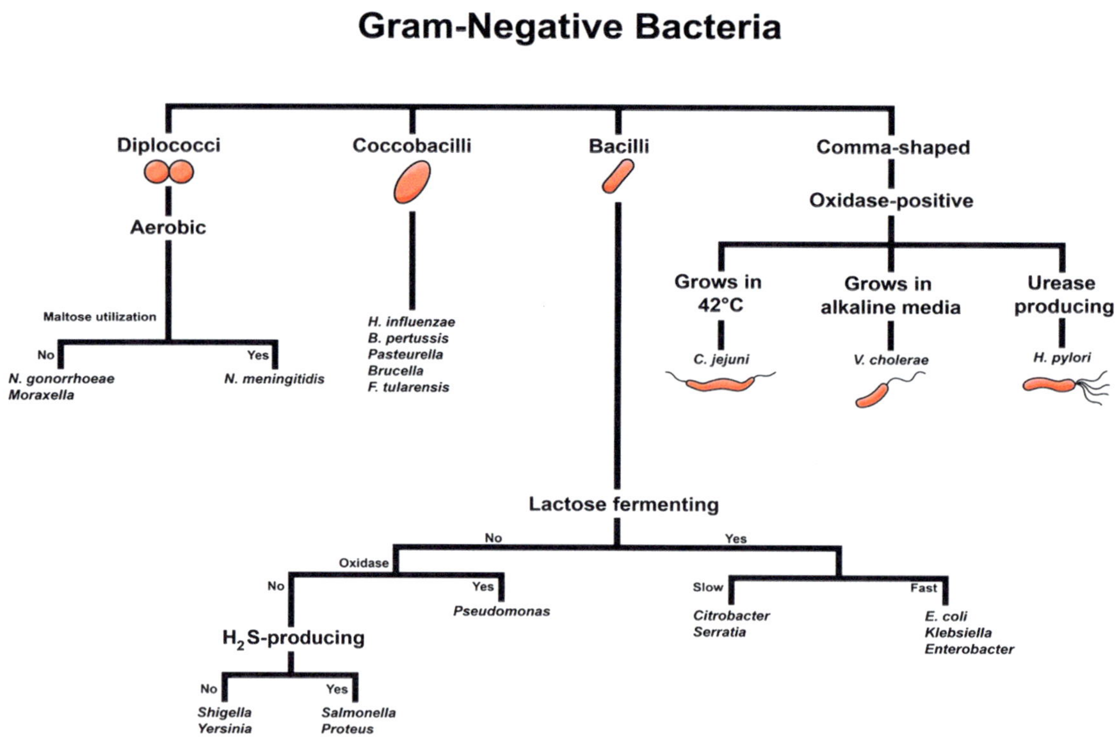

Figure 7.2. Overview of Gram-negative bacteria.

Source: https://step1.medbullets.com/microbiology/104193/gram-negative-bacteria.

Biofilm formation is prevalent among most Gram-negative species, increasing their virulence and resistance to antimicrobial therapies. Studies demonstrate that a substantial proportion of these bacteria can develop biofilms, notably in recurrent infections such as wounds or catheter-associated infections. Specifically, a study indicates that 80% of clinical isolates from patients exhibited biofilm production, underscoring its prevalence among Gram-negative pathogens. The formation of biofilms significantly impairs treatment efficacy, as cells within the biofilm matrix undergo altered metabolic activity, conferring resistance to antibiotics. This phenomenon is particularly concerning in the context of MDROs, which are becoming increasingly prevalent in healthcare environments. Consequently, understanding and interfering with biofilm development has become a vital area of research aimed at managing persistent Gram-negative infections (Di Domenico et al., 2017). Moreover, the pattern of antibiotic resistance in Gram-negative pathogens has been exacerbated by the overuse and misuse of broad-spectrum antibiotics, such as tetracyclines. Since the advent of penicillin in 1928, the widespread use of antimicrobial therapy has precipitated a dramatic increase in resistant bacterial strains. As resistance mechanisms are progressively elucidated, it becomes evident that these bacteria can alter their genetic makeup to survive despite antimicrobial agents. In the United States alone, thousands of lives are lost annually due to infections caused by resistant Gram-negative bacteria, underscoring the urgent need for novel treatments. In less developed countries, the challenge is even more pronounced, given limited access to effective antibiotics, thereby amplifying the threat posed by such microorganisms. The ongoing battle against antimicrobial resistance underscores the necessity for continuous research and funding to develop strategies capable of mitigating the impact of Gram-negative bacterial infections on global health (Figure 7.2).

7.1.1. Cell Wall Structure and Composition

The structure and composition of the Gram-negative bacterial cell wall are pivotal to their antimicrobial resistance and pathogenicity. Unlike Gram-positive bacteria, which feature a thick peptidoglycan layer, Gram-negative bacteria possess a slender peptidoglycan layer situated between two membranes: a cytoplasmic inner membrane and an outer membrane containing lipopolysaccharides (LPS).

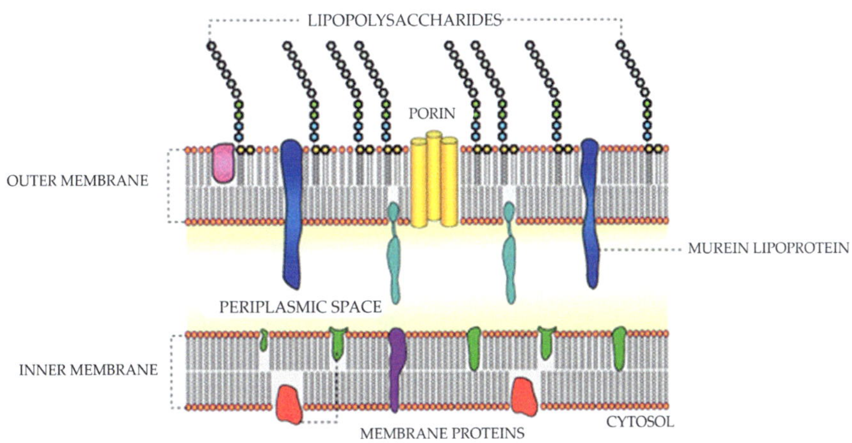

Figure 7.3. Gram-negative bacteria cell well.

Source: https://cdn1.byjus.com/wp-content/uploads/2018/11/biology/2018/05/19061322/Gram-Negative-Bacteria-cell-wall.png.

These LPS molecules serve as a defence mechanism against external threats, including antibiotics and detergents, thereby rendering Gram-negative bacteria notably resistant in clinical settings. The bilayer membrane structure not only enhances their rigidity but also impedes permeability to hydrophilic compounds, posing significant challenges in the effective treatment of infections caused by Gram-negative organisms. Consequently, a comprehensive understanding of the complex cell wall architecture of Gram-negative bacteria is essential for the development of novel therapeutic strategies capable of circumventing their inherent resistance mechanisms. The Gram-negative cell wall includes several components that can modulate host immune responses. Notably, lipopolysaccharides in the cell wall provoke a potent inflammatory response upon recognition by the immune system, potentially leading to septic shock during severe infections (Figure 7.3).

Furthermore, the outer membrane of these bacteria includes porins — porin proteins facilitating the passage of small molecules and nutrients — as well as exclusion barriers against bulk antibiotics. The regulation of selective permeability is governed by various bacterial mechanisms that can be manipulated to enhance survival in toxic environments. Advances in detection methods, such as terahertz time-domain spectroscopy, have enabled more accurate identification of these bacteria based on cell wall characteristics, thereby significantly improving diagnostic capabilities in clinical microbiology (Berrier et al., 2012). Research into novel antimicrobial agents, including magnesium oxide nanoparticles (nMgO), aims to specifically target the distinct cell wall structure of Gram-negative bacteria. nMgO demonstrates potent antimicrobial activity by disrupting bacterial cell membranes and inhibiting biofilm formation, especially in drug-resistant strains of *Escherichia coli* and other pathogens. The synergistic activity of nMgO suggests that these nanoparticles could serve as potential alternatives in the fight against Gram-negative infections, particularly when conventional antibiotics are ineffective. By elucidating the mechanisms of nMgO action, such as the production of reactive oxygen species (ROS) and regulation of bacterial ion concentrations, researchers are uncovering new avenues for infection control. This underscores the significance of emerging materials science applications in medicine and guides the development of effective treatment strategies against Gram-negative bacterial infections (Grelling et al., 2018).*Escherichia coli*

7.1.2. Mechanisms of Pathogenicity

The pathogenic mechanisms of Gram-negative bacterial infections are complex and often involve advanced strategies for immune evasion. Central to these mechanisms are the Type III secretion systems utilized by most Gram-negative pathogens, including *Escherichia coli* and *Salmonella*. This system functions as a needle-like apparatus that directly injects virulence factors into host cells, thereby commandeering intracellular processes to the benefit of the bacteria. For example, effectors such as Nleb from *Citrobacter rodentium* disrupt key signalling pathways by modifying host proteins through glycosylation. This modification inhibits the NF-κb pathway, consequently impairing the host's innate immune response and allowing bacterial survival and proliferation within host tissues. Therefore, understanding the complex mechanisms of Type III secretion systems and their effectors is of great importance in developing targeted therapeutic strategies against these infections (Garrido et al., 2020). Moreover, critical protein functions in Gram-negative bacteria extend beyond infection and survival within the host environment. In *Pseudomonas aeruginosa*, essential periplasmic proteins such as LptH and LolA are vital for maintaining cell envelope integrity and, by extension, virulence. The process of lipopolysaccharide and lipoprotein delivery to the outer membrane mediated by these proteins underscores the significance of bacterial pathogenicity. Research indicates that LptH plays a crucial role in the bacterium's ability to cause disease in various animal models, highlighting its potential as a target for novel therapeutic interventions. Conversely, although the downregulation of LolA has some impact on bacterial virulence, its significance appears to be less substantial than that of LptH. This variation in pathogenic effect emphasises the necessity for further research into essential genes to identify new targets for infection treatment (Bragonzi et al., 2015). The pathogenicity of Gram-negative bacteria also frequently depends on their capacity to adapt to dynamic host environments through the regulation of virulence factors. An additional aspect of this adaptability is the deployment of multiple secretion systems, including the Type IV secretion system, which facilitates the transfer of DNA and regulatory proteins involved in host interaction. These secretion systems enable pathogens to modify the host environment and evade immune detection, with the intricacy of host-pathogen interactions being a key component. By manipulating host signalling pathways and immune responses, Gram-negative bacteria can induce chronic infections. As scientific investigations continue to elucidate these mechanisms, future therapies are anticipated to emerge, potentially halting the cycle of infection and improving the efficacy of current treatment regimens for Gram-negative bacterial infections.*Escherichia coli*

7.1.3. Common Species of Gram-negative Bacteria

The ecology of Gram-negative bacteria is diverse and encompasses numerous species associated with various human infections. Among the most prevalent species are *Klebsiella pneumoniae* and *Escherichia coli*. *E. coli* is a commensal bacterium of the intestinal tract, with the potential to become pathogenic, causing urinary tract infections and gastroenteritis, particularly in vulnerable populations. *Klebsiella pneumoniae* is an opportunistic pathogen responsible for nosocomial infections such as pneumonia and sepsis.

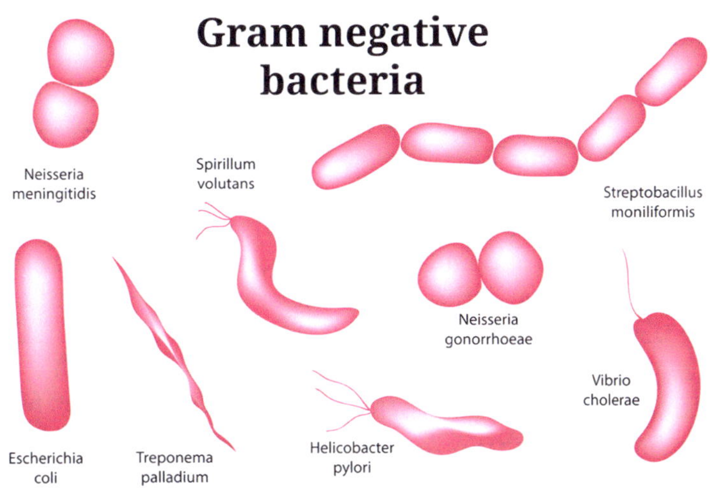

Figure 7.4. Examples of common Gram-negative bacteria.

Source: https://external-content.duckduckgo.com/iu/?u=https%3A%2F%2Fcdn4.vectorstock.com%2Fi%2F1000x1000%2F79%2F38%2Farrangements-of-gram-negative-bacteria-vector-23107938.jpg&f=1&nofb=1&ipt=06a41bbaf426a2e6b0c16d58d38f02478036a10bd4bad0459c95b2e27a6ce0b4.

The capacity of these organisms to develop resistance to multiple antibiotics enhances their clinical importance, complicating treatment regimens and leading to increased morbidity and mortality rates. Although *Pseudomonas aeruginosa* and *Acinetobacter baumannii* are also of significant clinical concern, other Gram-negative bacteria like *E. coli* and *Klebsiella pneumoniae* remain equally critical within the clinical setting. *Pseudomonas aeruginosa* exhibits resistance mechanisms and can survive in hospital environments as well as within immunocompromised hosts. It is a common etiologic agent of respiratory tract infections among patients with cystic fibrosis (see Figure 7.4).*Escherichia coliEscherichia coliEscherichia coli*

Similarly, *Acinetobacter baumannii* is increasingly recognised for its role in wound and ventilator-associated pneumonia infections and is frequently isolated in its drug-resistant form, particularly within intensive care units. The widespread distribution and adaptability of these bacteria necessitate prompt and effective infection control measures. Furthermore, the impact of Gram-negative bacterial infections extends beyond individual patients, presenting significant challenges to public health infrastructure and healthcare personnel. For instance, a case study conducted at Tygerberg Academic Hospital and Tygerberg Oral Health Centre revealed a notable discrepancy between Gram-negative staining and the actual culture results of Gram-negative organisms. Although the research identified that a high percentage of pus swabs stained positive for Gram-negative bacteria, only a subset yielded positive culture results, emphasising the importance of dependable diagnostic testing (Barnard, 2019). This paradox underscores the complexity of treating infections caused by Gram-negative organisms, which is attributable not only to their intrinsic resistance but also to diagnostic challenges. Consequently, this necessitates a reevaluation of current infection management strategies.Barnard, 2019

7.2. Transmission and Infection Pathways

The modes of infection and transmission of Gram-negative bacteria reflect their adaptive fitness under various environmental conditions. These bacteria frequently possess mechanisms to evade host defence systems, thereby facilitating infection. For example, *Salmonella enterica* serves as an exemplary model organism, demonstrating multiple strategies for immune evasion. As it traverses the digestive tract, it encounters adverse conditions such as low pH and antimicrobial peptides, to which it must adapt and proliferate despite these challenges. The bacterium's ability to modulate inflammatory pathways and interact with resident microbiota further elucidates its sophisticated infection dissemination strategies, thereby enabling persistent infection in the host despite initial immune responses (Bernal-Bayard & Ramos-Morales, 2017). Considerable research has also focused on the pathways through which Gram-negative pathogens establish infections, particularly via epithelial tissues. Nontypeable *Haemophilus influenzae* (NTHi) offers insight into another aspect of transmission, notably otitis media, which predominantly affects children. The pathogen efficiently invades human middle ear epithelial cells, where it may persist intracellularly, complicating host immune responses. Studies indicate that upon internalisation, NTHi can breach cellular membranes to survive freely within the cytoplasm. This intracellular survival mechanism hampers the epithelial cells' ability to produce β-defensin 2, a vital immune molecule involved in combating infections, thereby demonstrating the bacterium's ability to manipulate host defence mechanisms (Lee et al., 2014). Both NTHi and *Salmonella* exemplify the complex strategies employed by Gram-negative bacteria during infection and transmission. They have developed various adaptations to evade or even exploit host immune responses. For instance,

Salmonella's capacity to activate dendritic cells and manipulate T and B lymphocytes enhances its ability to evade adaptive immunity. Similarly, NTHi 's exploitation of cytoplasmic pathways illustrates how these bacteria invade and manipulate cellular processes to ensure their survival. An understanding of these intricate transmission and infection pathways is crucial in developing effective therapeutic strategies to eradicate Gram-negative bacterial infections, thereby reducing their impact on public health (Lee et al., 2014; Bernal-Bayard & Ramos-Morales, 2017).

7.2.1. Modes of Transmission

Modes of transmission for Gram-negative bacterial infections are fundamental to their dissemination and the identification of control measures. These modes are predominantly direct person-to-person contact and indirect transmission via contaminated objects and surfaces. For example, bacteria such as *Escherichia coli* are excreted in the feces of infected individuals, thereby contaminating food and water sources. Additionally, aerosols generated during medical procedures can facilitate the spread of such pathogens, underscoring the critical importance of proper hygiene practices in both clinical and public environments.

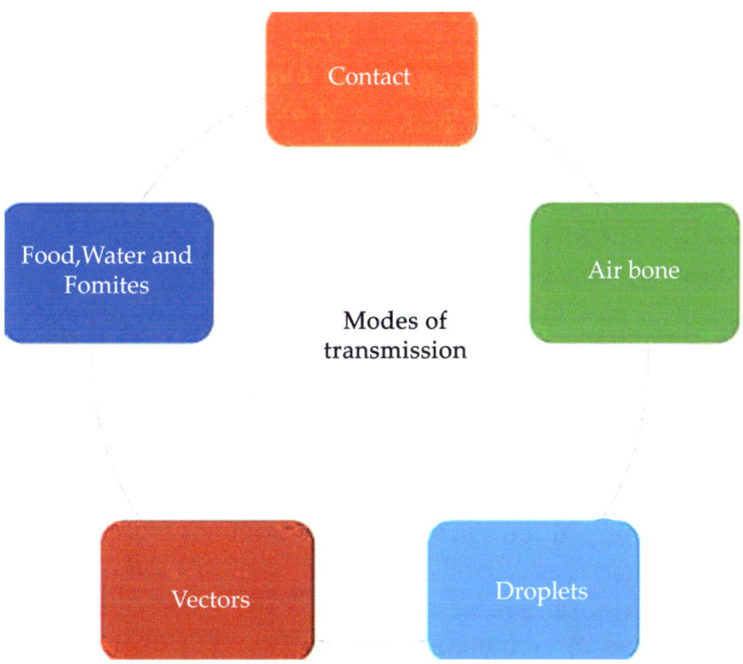

Figure 7.5. Modes of transmission.

Source: https://ars.els-cdn.com/content/image/3-s2.0-B9780323953887000048-f02-01-9780323953887.jpg.

The study of healthcare-associated infections highlights the vulnerability of susceptible populations, including those immunocompromised, thus necessitating ongoing research into transmission patterns and prevention strategies. Environmental factors also play a significant role in the spread of Gram-negative bacteria. Water pollution, especially in areas with inadequate sanitation facilities, creates a conducive environment for pathogen transmission. For instance, the presence of Gram-negative bacteria in water can lead to outbreaks when such untreated water is consumed or used for washing food. Monitoring environmental reservoirs, such as soil and aquatic systems, provides valuable insights into potential sites of infection dissemination. Furthermore, the emergence of resistant strains due to environmental exposure emphasises the urgent need for innovative antimicrobial solutions. Current research employing novel detection methods aims to enhance the rapid identification and control of Gram-negative bacterial pathogens (Berrier et al., 2012) (Figure 7.5).

In addition to direct contact and environmental pathways, vector transmission also plays a role in the dissemination of certain Gram-negative infections. Some bacteria are carried by specific insects, such as ticks and mosquitoes, and are transmitted to human hosts through bites. This mode of transmission exemplifies the complex dynamics of interactions within ecosystems, which may lead to outbreaks of infection, particularly in endemic regions. Nanobiotic interventions involving the deployment of antimicrobial nanoparticles have been proposed as a means to address such vector-borne transmissions (Burgu et al., 2017). Research into these innovative strategies holds promise for effective intervention against the persistent challenge of infections caused by Gram-negative bacteria, with an emphasis on exploring transmission routes in conjunction with technological advancements in intervention measures.

7.2.2. Entry Points into the Human Body

The pathways through which Gram-negative bacteria invade the human body serve as significant regulators of infection routes and subsequent disease manifestation. These bacteria employ several physical barriers, notably the mucous membranes and skin, which function as primary defences against pathogens. Incisions resulting from cuts, abrasions, or punctures compromise these surfaces, providing opportunities for opportunistic Gram-negative organisms such as *Escherichia coli* and *Pseudomonas aeruginosa* to invade the body. Additionally, the respiratory tract constitutes a major portal of entry, whereby the inhalation of contaminated particles can lead to severe infections, particularly in immunocompromised hosts. Recognising that these entry portals facilitate bacterial colonization and infection underscores the importance of maintaining skin integrity and respiratory hygiene to prevent Gram-negative bacterial infections. A secondary critical entry point is the gastrointestinal tract, often accessed by Gram-negative bacteria through ingestion of contaminated food and water. Once ingested, these pathogens can adhere to and invade the intestinal lining, causing gastroenteritis characterised by diarrhoea, vomiting, and systemic illness. The rise of antibiotic-resistant Gram-negative bacteria has heightened the necessity for effective infection control solutions, as therapeutic options become increasingly limited. This issue is exemplified by the high incidence of hospital-acquired infections caused by Gram-negative organisms utilising this route of entry, which underscores the importance of food safety and adequate sanitation measures to prevent such infections. The susceptibility of the gastrointestinal tract necessitates a comprehensive infection control approach that encompasses public health interventions and personal precautions. Furthermore, the urogenital tract is a significant route of entry for Gram-negative bacteria, especially in cases of urinary tract infections (UTIs). Studies have demonstrated that such infections typically originate from bacterial ascent through the urethra into the bladder, potentially progressing to complicated disease states if left untreated. Anatomical differences in females, notably the shorter urethra, predispose women to higher rates of UTIs, providing an easier route of bacterial entry. Clinically, managing these infections requires vigilant consideration of antimicrobial resistance. Recent research emphasises the importance of selecting appropriate antibiotics and adhering to correct treatment durations to prevent resistance development, as exemplified by comparisons between enrofloxacin and traditional therapies in uncomplicated UTIs in animals, with implications for antibiotic efficacy more broadly (Chew et al., 2012). Understanding these entry points and infection dynamics underscores the necessity of addressing Gram-negative bacterial threats through effective and multidimensional strategies.

7.2.3. Factors Influencing Infection Rates

When analysing the complex factors that influence infection rates attributable to Gram-negative bacteria, it is imperative to consider the interplay among host characteristics, environmental conditions, and pathogenic agents. Host factors such as age, comorbidities, and immune status significantly contribute to an individual's susceptibility to infection. For instance, elderly individuals with comorbidities are at heightened risk of developing infections due to compromised immunity. Likewise, surgical patients, particularly those with prosthetic devices, constitute high-risk groups. Such procedures expose individuals to bacterial colonization, as Gram-negative bacteria can readily proliferate in the presence of prosthetic devices. Consequently, understanding the vulnerabilities of hosts is crucial for the prevention and management of Gram-negative bacterial infections, as it allows for the targeted application of interventions that effectively mitigate such threats (Smith & Chetter, 2015). Environmental determinants also play a critical role in influencing infection rates related to Gram-negative bacteria. Sanitation practices, healthcare infrastructure, and antibiotic stewardship are vital factors that determine the prevalence of these infections. For example, hospital-acquired infections, including surgical site infections (SSIs), tend to be more common in facilities with inadequate hygiene and substandard infection control measures. The healthcare environment can either facilitate or hinder bacterial transmission. Moreover, the misuse and overuse of antibiotics can select for resistant Gram-negative strains, thereby exacerbating infection rates. Therefore, a comprehensive understanding of environmental influences enables the formulation and implementation of effective policies and practices to prevent infections within healthcare settings (Smith & Chetter, 2015). An additional vital aspect pertains to the specific virulence factors inherent to Gram-negative bacteria. These pathogens possess specialized mechanisms, such as biofilm formation and toxin secretion, to evade host defences. Biofilms, in particular, create protective niches that shield bacteria from host immune responses and antibiotic treatments. Elucidating these virulence factors is essential for developing targeted therapeutic and preventive strategies. Furthermore, the interactions between the human immune system and bacterial components, such as the role of lactoferrin-like compounds in modulating immune responses, are of considerable interest. Understanding such interactions underscores the complexity of infection dynamics and highlights the importance of personalised therapeutic approaches in combating Gram-negative bacterial infections.

7.3. Common Gram-negative Infections

The prevalence of Gram-negative infections presents a significant challenge to public health, with certain pathogens leading in clinical settings. Among these, *Acinetobacter* species are particularly noteworthy as critical contributors, especially in nosocomial infections. Characterised by their resilience under extreme conditions, *Acinetobacter* is frequently implicated in bloodstream infections and ventilator-associated pneumonia, predominantly affecting immunocompromised patients and individuals with prolonged hospital stays. Current research indicates that such infections may exhibit substantial antibiotic resistance, thereby complicating treatment and adversely affecting patient outcomes (Farooq et al., 2018). The organism's capacity to produce biofilms further complicates therapeutic strategies, as biofilms can shield bacteria from host immune responses and antimicrobial agents, underscoring the necessity for novel infection management approaches. Another prevalent Gram-negative bacterium is *Escherichia coli*, most commonly associated with urinary tract infections (UTIs). The emergence of Extended Spectrum β-Lactamase (ESBL)-producing strains has significantly impacted clinical management, as these enzymes confer resistance to many widely used antibiotics. ESBL-producing *Escherichia coli* strains have gained increased prominence due to their ability to persistently survive and form biofilms, which enhances their adhesion to uroepithelial cells and complicates eradication (Baho et al., 2019). Beyond UTIs, such isolates are implicated in more severe infections, including sepsis and intra-abdominal infections, underscoring the necessity for rigorous surveillance and the development of effective therapeutic strategies to combat resistant strains. *Klebsiella pneumoniae* is another formidable Gram-negative pathogen responsible for various infections, including pneumonia and septicemia. Its adaptability and resistance features make it one of the most challenging organisms encountered in healthcare environments. Recent studies reveal an alarming prevalence of multidrug-resistant *Klebsiella* strains, notably ESBL-producing and carbapenemase-producing variants, further constraining treatment options (Farooq et al., 2018). Additionally, its biofilm-forming ability increases the difficulty of achieving successful treatment outcomes, positioning *Klebsiella pneumoniae* as a potential target for innovative therapeutic interventions. Effective management of these infections necessitates a comprehensive understanding of their epidemiology, resistance mechanisms, and the development of synergistic treatment regimens to mitigate their impact on public health.

7.3.1. Urinary Tract Infections (UTIs)

Urinary tract infections (UTIs) represent some of the most prevalent infections encountered within clinical practice, significantly impacting patient quality of life and healthcare resources. Both Gram-positive and Gram-negative bacteria can be responsible for UTIs; however, the latter, particularly *Escherichia coli*, predominates within the pathogenic landscape. *E. coli* is implicated in approximately 80–90% of community-acquired UTIs, attributable to its capacity to adhere to urinary tract epithelial cells and its resistance to host immune responses. Such virulence factors are often preceded by the acquisition of antibiotic resistance among Gram-negative bacteria, rendering traditional treatment regimens less effective. The development of resistance is frequently associated with antibiotic misuse and biofilm formation, which can protect bacteria from antimicrobial agents and enhance their survival within the urinary tract, thereby presenting complex clinical management challenges. Characterisation of antimicrobial susceptibility patterns in Gram-negative bacteria responsible for UTIS has revealed concerning trends toward increasing resistance. A recent study investigating bacterial urinary tract infections in canines reported significant variability in bacterial antibiotic susceptibility, with *Escherichia coli* demonstrating differential resistance to widely used antimicrobials such as amoxicillin and trimethoprim-sulfamethoxazole, exemplifying the difficulties inherent in the successful treatment of these infections. Escherichia coli

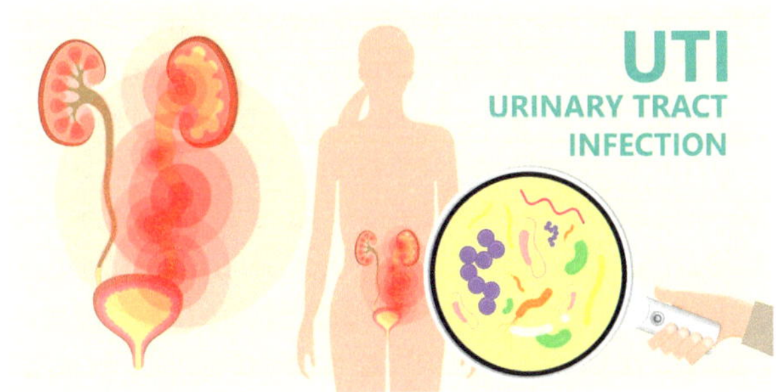

Figure 7.6. Urinary tract infections (UTIs).

Source: https://www.news-medical.net/images/Article_Images/ImageForArticle_553_16620069160399362.jpg.

Multi-drug-resistant *E. coli* and *Staphylococcus spp.* were mainly identified in complicated UTIs compared to uncomplicated ones, with a positive correlation between prior treatment and resistance development. Culture-based susceptibility testing is crucial because it enables clinicians to tailor antibiotic therapy, enhancing outcomes and preventing resistance. The increasing prevalence of extended-spectrum β-lactamase (ESBL)-producing bacteria complicates UTIs, especially for Gram-negative infections. ESBL enzymes, produced by bacteria like *Klebsiella pneumoniae*, break down common antibiotics such as penicillins and cephalosporins, limiting treatment options (Baho et al., 2019).

Innovative treatment approaches are vital; recent research explores alternatives like the anti-biofilm properties of compounds such as Manuka honey. Laboratory tests show that Manuka honey not only inhibits free-floating bacteria but also significantly reduces biofilm biomass of ESBL producers, making it a potential adjunct therapy for resistant UTIS. Continued research is essential for developing strategies to treat recurrent and complicated UTIs caused by resistant Gram-negative bacteria, ultimately improving patient care.

7.3.2. Respiratory Infections

Respiratory infections constitute a significant global health concern, frequently complicated by Gram-negative bacteria. These microorganisms are conventionally associated with both acute and chronic respiratory tract diseases, with their pathogenic potential evidenced by the increasing prevalence of antibiotic resistance. Regrettably, traditional therapeutic protocols for respiratory infections, especially within veterinary medicine, trail behind advancements achieved in human healthcare. The International Society for Companion Animal Infectious Diseases underscores the necessity for comprehensive guidelines to aid veterinarians in effectively managing bacterial respiratory infections, emphasising the importance of evidence-based antimicrobial selection. The complexity of the interaction between primary and secondary infections presents additional challenges in effective management, particularly in cases involving Gram-negative bacteria such as *Klebsiella pneumoniae* (Lappin et al., 2017) (Figure 7.7).

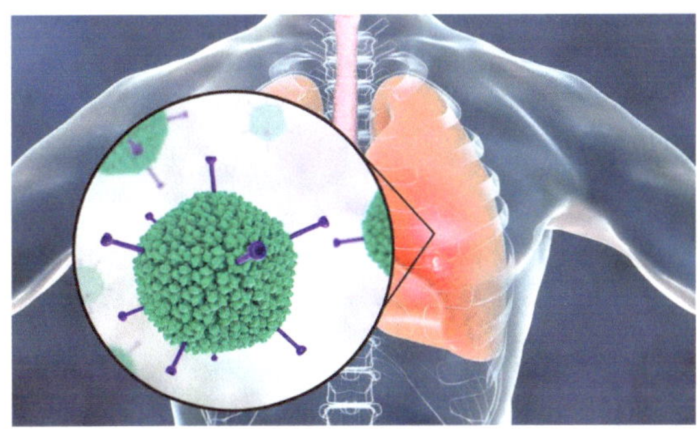

Figure 7.7. Respiratory infections.

Source: https://medicaldialogues.in/h-upload/2024/08/09/247073-respiratory-infection-50.webp.

Furthermore, chronic respiratory disease constitutes a significant public health concern, primarily attributable to pulmonary infections caused by Gram-negative bacteria. Evidence suggests that conditions such as COPD are adversely impacted by these pathogens, resulting in an increased frequency of exacerbations. Bronchoalveolar lavage has developed into an essential diagnostic technique utilized in detecting bacterial and fungal isolates in patients with chronic respiratory conditions. A pivotal study demonstrated that 35% of BAL samples yielded positive bacterial cultures, underscoring the predominance of Gram-negative bacteria, including *Acinetobacter baumannii*, in respiratory infections. This observation underscores the necessity for early and precise diagnostic procedures and susceptibility testing to guide clinical decision-making and enhance patient outcomes amidst the escalating challenge of antimicrobial resistance (Ahamed, 2017). The importance of Gram-negative bacterial infections extends beyond clinical manifestations; they compel healthcare systems to adapt and respond effectively.

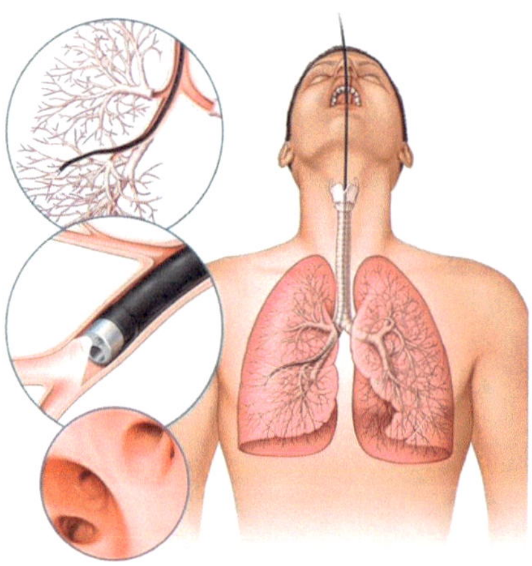

Figure 7.8. Bronchoalveolar lavage (BAL).

Source: https://drjeenamshah.com/assets/images/bal-service.jpg.

Given that many Gram-negative bacteria exhibit substantial resistance to conventional antimicrobial therapies, clinicians must rely on existing antibiograms reflecting local bacterial patterns to inform treatment strategies. The variability in antibiotic efficacy concerning regional resistance patterns necessitates vigilant monitoring to optimise treatment regimens. With Gram-negative pathogens frequently identified as principal causes of respiratory infections, the medical community faces the critical challenge of developing novel antimicrobial agents while simultaneously refining current treatment protocols. This balancing act is vital in combating the rising incidence of respiratory infections caused by these opportunistic bacteria, requiring concerted efforts across all healthcare sectors (Ahamed, 2017) (Figure 7.8).

7.3.3. Gastrointestinal Infections

Gastrointestinal infections caused by Gram-negative bacteria pose a significant public health concern worldwide. Among these pathogens, *Helicobacter pylori* is particularly notable due to its association with chronic gastritis, peptic ulcer disease, and gastric carcinoma. In addition to acute gastrointestinal symptoms, *H. pylori* infections have long-term health ramifications, thereby increasing morbidity among affected populations. The standard treatment typically involves a combination of antibiotics and proton pump inhibitors; however, escalating antibiotic resistance complicates therapeutic approaches. Evidence regarding the efficacy of colostral immune preparations against *H. pylori* suggests new avenues for alternative therapies. Notably, the synergistic effect of antibiotics and colostral antibodies has demonstrated substantial suppression of inflammation and bacterial colonization, underscoring the potential of adjunct therapies in combating these infections (Rokka, 2008). Another Gram-negative pathogen, *Campylobacter jejuni*, is responsible for one of the most prevalent gastrointestinal diseases, Campylobacteriosis, characterised by symptoms such as abdominal cramps, diarrhoea, and fever. This pathogen is primarily transmitted through ingestion of contaminated food or water, emphasising the importance of food safety and hygiene to prevent infection. Persistent infections with *C. jejuni* necessitate effective treatment strategies, especially considering the bacterium's resistance to certain commonly used antibiotics. Recent research has identified carvacrol, a natural compound extracted from oregano, as an effective agent against *C. jejuni*. In murine models, carvacrol has demonstrated remarkable capability in reducing pathogen loads and inhibiting the inflammatory response associated with infection. Such emerging evidence positions carvacrol as a prospective candidate for the treatment of campylobacteriosis and the prevention of related complications in both human and agricultural contexts (Bereswill et al., 2020) (Figure 7. 9).

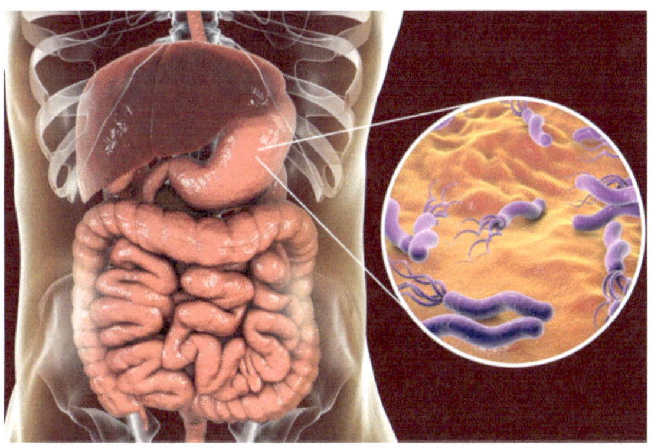

Figure 7.9. Gastrointestinal infections.

Source: https://www.infectiousdiseaseadvisor.com/wp-content/uploads/sites/16/2023/01/H-pylori-G-956351852-768x512.jpg.

The clinical significance of Gram-negative bacillary gastrointestinal infections extends into the broader public health framework, including zoonotic transmission and the risk of outbreaks. The convergence of animal and human health within the context of the One Health model underscores the importance of coordinated surveillance and innovative intervention strategies. For instance, with respect to *H. pylori* and *C. jejuni*, therapeutic approaches can be enhanced by incorporating dietary components and probiotics into treatment protocols, thereby presenting new opportunities to diminish infection severity and facilitate recovery. Furthermore, education regarding hygiene and food safety remains essential in reducing transmission rates within populations. Therefore, acquiring comprehensive knowledge of these infections and advancing research are imperative for designing effective control measures and ultimately improving health outcomes among populations at risk for Gram-negative bacterial infections.

7.4. Symptoms and Diagnosis

The clinical presentation of Gram-negative bacterial infections exhibits considerable variability depending on the specific pathogen and the site of infection. Common presenting symptoms include dyspnea, tachycardia, fever, chills, and localised pain, which may suggest more severe conditions such as sepsis. In cases of ascitic origin, patients may present with abdominal distension, marked tenderness, and features of hepatic encephalopathy if liver functionality is compromised. Given the nonspecific nature of these symptoms, an appropriate diagnostic approach is imperative. Typically, clinical assessment entails a comprehensive history-taking and physical examination, followed by targeted laboratory testing. It is important to recognise that some patients may yield negative results in standard culture tests; therefore, clinicians must remain vigilant for infection indicators even in the absence of traditional biomarkers, as corroborated by recent research emphasising the necessity for thorough diagnostic protocols in complex scenarios (Boaretti et al., 2016). Gram-negative bacterial infections are frequently elusive due to limitations inherent in routine microbiological procedures. Specifically, culture tests, despite their widespread use, tend to be negative in approximately 30–40% of ascitic fluid samples, which may lead to underdiagnosis in vulnerable populations such as individuals with cirrhosis. The application of culture-independent diagnostic methods is therefore essential to enhance detection sensitivity. Such methods include the identification of bacterial DNA, endotoxins, and other markers, which can furnish clinicians with valuable information regarding active infections. These molecular and biochemical techniques offer a more advanced understanding of infection severity, correlating the presence of bacterial markers with clinical outcomes. In modern healthcare practice, these sophisticated diagnostic tools are pivotal in advancing our comprehension of pathogen detection and its clinical significance (Boaretti et al., 2016). Ultimately, diagnosing Gram-negative bacterial infections remains challenging, especially considering the rising rates of antibiotic resistance; thus, the prompt and precise identification of causative pathogens is crucial. As demonstrated, the overuse of broad-spectrum antibiotics has unintentionally contributed to the emergence of resistant strains, complicating treatment regimens and impacting patient outcomes. The urgency of addressing this issue is particularly pronounced in developing and resource-limited nations, where the prevalence of resistant infections continues to escalate dramatically. This scenario underscores the importance of implementing vigilant surveillance methods capable of early infection detection and enabling the selection of appropriate therapeutic strategies, thereby improving patient prognosis. Adequate funding and research are vital to combat these infections and to strengthen global public health responses, representing a fundamental challenge within contemporary medicine.

7.4.1. General Symptoms of Gram-negative Infections

The nonspecific manifestations of Gram-negative bacterial infections can present in various ways, principally depending on the site of infection and the host's immune response. These include fever, chills, and malaise, as the host reacts to the invading organisms. In severe cases, patients may exhibit signs of systemic inflammatory response syndrome (SIRS), characterised by an increased heart rate, elevated respiratory rate, and abnormal temperature. The endotoxin release, typical of Gram-negative bacteria, exacerbates these symptoms, leading to increased clinical complications such as septic shock. It is crucial to understand the clinical presentation of these infections because early detection significantly influences treatment outcomes and informs measures to address the rising issue of antibiotic resistance, which is linked to the prevalence of multi-drug-resistant pathogens in most healthcare facilities, thereby necessitating specialized therapeutic interventions (Lillestolen, 2018).

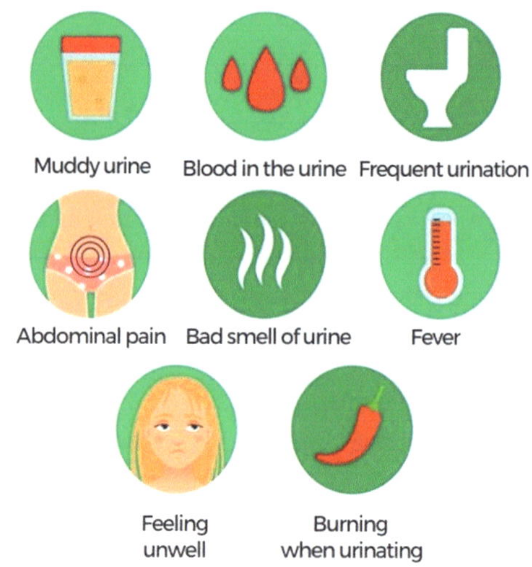

Figure 7.10. Urinary tract infections (UTIs) symptoms.

Source: https://external-content.duckduckgo.com/iu/?u=https%3A%2F%2Fecosh.com%2Fwp-content%2Fuploads%2Fsites%2F3%2F2021%2F08%2FUrinary_Tract_Infection_Symptoms_UTI_Symptoms.jpg&f=1&nofb=1&ipt=b3f4abd34acf228a2c5a7ac49e478b431aa64f03159df8a9a7f0e9cbf9801eee.

Infections caused by gram-negative bacteria tend to manifest symptoms varying according to the infection site within the body. For example, urinary tract infections (UTIS), commonly caused by *Escherichia coli*, are characterised by dysuria, polyuria, and lower abdominal pain. Conversely, respiratory infections, such as ventilator-associated pneumonia (VAP), typically present with cough, purulent sputum, and respiratory distress, especially in hospitalised patients. The high incidence of multidrug-resistant Gram-negative bacilli in these conditions contributes to the morbidity associated with respiratory infections, underscoring the importance of effective empirical treatment regimens. Recognizing these complex clinical presentations is vital for healthcare providers to develop appropriate management strategies and to anticipate the potential presence of resistant bacterial strains (Rosso-Fernández et al., 2015).

The implications of Gram-negative infections extend beyond immediate clinical manifestations. Patients frequently encounter complications that may impede recovery, such as secondary infections and chronic inflammation. The repercussions of such infections are significantly magnified in immunocompromised individuals, where systemic effects can increase vulnerability. Furthermore, the psychosocial consequences of chronic illness and repeated hospitalisations should not be overlooked, as patients may develop depression and anxiety related to their condition. Managing these complex effects necessitates an interdisciplinary healthcare approach that comprehensively addresses both physical recuperation and the psychosocial well-being of all parties involved. Public health initiatives and scientific research into the mechanisms of antibiotic resistance are essential to reduce the burden imposed by Gram-negative infections, underscoring the importance of thoroughly understanding their symptoms and broader impacts (Lillestolen, 2018).

7.4.2. Diagnostic Methods and Techniques

Infections caused by Gram-negative bacteria are primarily diagnosed through a comprehensive array of diagnostic methods and tests, aiming for precise identification and suitable treatment. Conventional culture techniques continue to form the fundamental basis of microbiologic diagnosis, whereby bacteria can be isolated and their susceptibility to various antimicrobials tested from specimens obtained at the infected site. Rapid identification techniques, such as mass spectrometry, are now in clinical use, substantially reducing the duration required to obtain results.

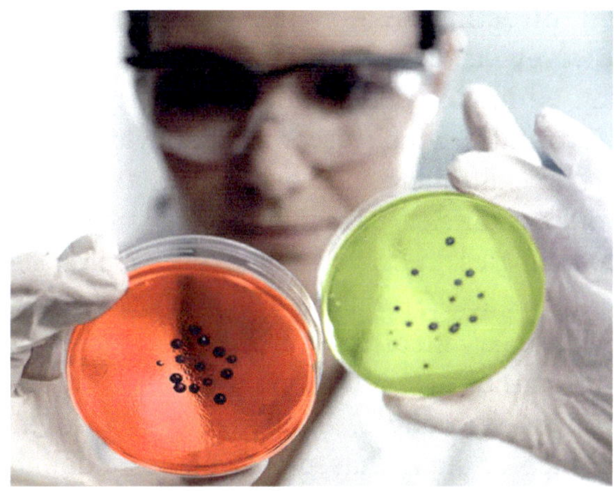

Figure 7.11. Diagnosis of Gram-negative bacterial infections.

Source: https://media.post.rvohealth.io/wp-content/uploads/sites/3/2022/09/gram-positive-negative-bacteria-thumb.jpg.

The prompt diagnosis afforded by these methods enables clinicians to commence appropriate antibiotic therapy at an earlier stage, which is vital in the context of the increasing prevalence of antibiotic-resistant Gram-negative bacteria. However, these traditional techniques are not without limitations, including the necessity for specific growth conditions and the lengthy duration of procedures, which can impede timely diagnosis and intervention. Molecular diagnostic tools, such as polymerase chain reaction (PCR) and next-generation sequencing (NGS), have demonstrated significant promise in the identification of Gram-negative bacteria. These advanced technologies facilitate direct detection of bacterial DNA from clinical specimens, offering faster turnaround times compared to conventional culture methods. PCR, in particular, can identify genes associated with antibiotic resistance and virulence, providing valuable information to inform targeted treatment strategies.

In particular, the rapid identification of resistant strains is vital for outbreak control and directing public health interventions. However, the utilisation of molecular techniques may be hindered by financial and equipment constraints, which are often unavailable to certain clinical facilities, especially in resource-limited countries. Consequently, although these technologies improve diagnostic capabilities, equitable access remains a significant concern. In veterinary medicine, the diagnostic approach to Gram-negative infections is also undergoing significant changes. Challenges such as the absence of standardised treatment guidelines mirror the difficulties faced in human health, where curing infections becomes increasingly complex. The International Society for Companion Animal Infectious Diseases has taken steps to address these issues by endorsing guidelines supported by rigorous data analysis and clinical methodologies (Lappin et al., 2017). These standards aim to assist veterinary practitioners in the appropriate use of antimicrobials, tailored to specific pathogens. Furthermore, the integration of mobile technology into clinical settings has implications for the containment of microbial contamination within healthcare environments. Studies have shown elevated microbial loads on equipment handled by medical personnel, underscoring the necessity for effective infection control practices within veterinary clinics as well (White et al., 2012). This emphasises the ongoing need for research and strict adherence to diagnostic and infection control protocols to effectively manage Gram-negative bacterial infections.

7.4.3. Challenges in Accurate Diagnosis

Proper recognition of Gram-negative bacterial infections is a critical challenge that can significantly influence patient outcomes. A major obstacle is the reliance on traditional laboratory testing, which often involves prolonged turnaround times that impede prompt treatment. Routine diagnostic procedures such as culture and sensitivity testing can take up to 28 hours to produce results, thereby delaying the administration of effective antibiotics. This issue is particularly urgent given the rapid evolution of resistance patterns among Gram-negative bacteria, driven by the indiscriminate use of broad-spectrum antibiotics. Innovative approaches, including advanced point-of-care diagnostic technologies, have the potential to substantially reduce these delays and optimise treatment efficacy. Nevertheless, recent studies indicate that the translational challenges associated with implementing such progress into clinical practice remain formidable, underscoring the necessity for rapid, sensitive, and cost-effective diagnostic tests (Barnes et al., 2018). Another significant barrier to accurate diagnosis is the misinterpretation of clinical signs. Notably, elderly patients often present with asymptomatic urinary tract infections (UTIs), leading to overdiagnosis and overtreatment (Beveridge et al., 2011). The lack of specific symptoms complicates the diagnostic process, as clinicians find it difficult to distinguish such infections from other underlying medical conditions. This challenge is compounded by routine urinalysis, which may produce unreliable results in this patient group. Additionally, asymptomatic bacteriuria presents a diagnostic dilemma; recent evidence unequivocally indicates that this condition does not necessarily require treatment. However, the risk of misdiagnosis remains high, often prompting clinicians to administer inappropriate antimicrobial therapy. This subtle interaction necessitates the development of novel guidelines aimed at enhancing diagnostic sensitivity and treatment protocols. Hospital-acquired infections, notably the rise in catheter-associated urinary tract infections (CAUTIs), introduce additional complexities in diagnosis. Given that Gram-negative bacteria readily colonise patients with urinary catheters, distinguishing between colonization and true infection becomes increasingly intricate. The challenge of accurate diagnosis is further amplified by the lack of a universally accepted set of criteria for CAUTIs, leading to variability in diagnostic approaches across different healthcare settings. Moreover, local antimicrobial resistance patterns necessitate frequent revisions of guidelines to reflect evolving clinical landscapes. The management of CAUTIs is best achieved through the application of narrow-spectrum antibiotics to prevent resistance development; however, accurate diagnosis remains critical to ensure optimal treatment outcomes. Overcoming these diagnostic challenges not only enhances patient care but also contributes to public health by mitigating the development of antibiotic resistance.

7.5. Treatment Options

Gram-negative bacterial infections, especially those caused by multidrug-resistant organisms, present significant challenges in the clinical setting. The emerging resistance patterns further complicate treatment modalities and underscore the necessity for innovative therapeutic strategies. Infections caused by carbapenemase-resistant *Klebsiella pneumoniae* (CR-Kp) have historically lacked effective treatments. However, extensive research has demonstrated that combination therapy is a promising approach, often yielding improved patient outcomes. Notably, combinations such as meropenem-colistin or tigecycline have become standard treatments. Their efficacy, however, is tempered by colistin's nephrotoxicity, prompting ongoing efforts to identify alternative pharmacotherapies. Given the threat posed by resistant strains, it is imperative to balance the use of effective medications against the risks of toxicity and the potential for further resistance development (Mascellino et al., 2017).

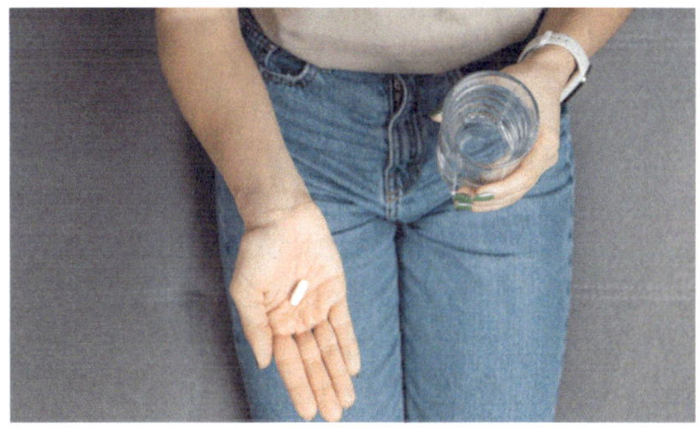

Figure 7.12. The oral administration of medication.

Source: https://www.clinicbarcelona.org/media/cache/960_jpeg/uploads/media/default/0012/70/059cf49267ec369e2eac9cd7f80c9cb38b976e11.png.

Concurrently, the advent of novel antibiotics in recent years has opened new avenues for treating Gram-negative infections. Agents such as ceftazidime-avibactam and ceftolozane-tazobactam specifically target resistant pathogens like CR-Kp and extensively drug-resistant *Pseudomonas aeruginosa*. These therapeutics mark a pivotal advancement in the antimicrobial arsenal, offering hope in cases where traditional antibiotics have failed. Moreover, evidence suggests that the concurrent use of these novel agents alongside conventional antibiotics can significantly reduce mortality rates among affected patients. Nonetheless, healthcare professionals need to recognize that resistance can develop more rapidly than new treatments are discovered. Therefore, prudent antibiotic use and responsible stewardship remain critical principles in combating Gram-negative bacterial infections and safeguarding the efficacy of future therapies (Jenner et al., 2017) (Figure 7.12).

To effectively address the challenge of treating Gram-negative bacterial infections, a comprehensive approach involving novel diagnostics, antimicrobial stewardship, and research innovation is imperative. In light of the global issue of antimicrobial resistance (AMR), collaboration between the public and private sectors is necessary to prioritise the development of new treatments and diagnostic tools. This encompasses not only the creation of new therapeutic options but also the facilitation of equitable access to these innovations across various healthcare settings. Interventions such as effective governance, public education campaigns, and incentives for research and development can mitigate the detrimental impact of AMR on global health. Furthermore, the implementation of intellectual property systems within incentive mechanisms can provide motivation for innovative responses while allowing for successful local deployment. By fostering a collaborative global effort, the medical community can unite to limit the spread of antibiotic-resistant infections and enhance patient outcomes (Jenner et al., 2017).

7.5.1. Antibiotic Therapies

Antibiotic resistance in Gram-negative bacteria constitutes a formidable challenge in current medicine, jeopardising treatment efficacy and patient outcomes. Gram-negative bacteria such as *Klebsiella pneumoniae* and *Acinetobacter baumannii* are increasingly associated with highly lethal infections and elevated mortality rates. Effective management of these infections necessitates the development of novel therapeutic strategies, particularly concerning carbapenem-resistant isolates. While traditional antibiotic therapies often fail against these resistant organisms, combination treatments have gained prominence. For instance, colistin-containing regimens — comprising agents like meropenem or tigecycline — have been identified as crucial in combating carbapenemase-resistant *Klebsiella*. However, nephrotoxicity associated with colistin presents a significant concern, requiring careful consideration by clinicians in selecting treatments that balance efficacy with safety, as evidenced by recent studies (Mascellino et al., 2017). In recent years, there has been a marked decline in the discovery of new antibiotics, further complicating therapeutic options against Gram-negative infections. Most new agents introduced since the 1980s are merely derivatives of existing classes, indicating an alarming stagnation in research progress. Scientific obstacles in drug development, coupled with regulatory challenges and limited pharmaceutical investment, have led to a substantial decline in the antibiotic development pipeline. Given the increasing sensitivity of resistance mechanisms to selective pressures from widespread antibiotic use, the urgent need for novel therapeutic agents remains critical. The significant deficiency in effective therapies underscores the importance of emphasising additional measures, including research into combination therapies and alternative modalities (PEW Charitable Trust Report, 2016). Combination antibiotic therapy is now widely accepted in treating resistant Gram-negative infections, offering the dual benefits of enhanced efficacy and reduced resistance development. Empirical evidence demonstrates that patients receiving combination regimens experience lower mortality rates relative to those receiving monotherapy. For example, the use of a double-carbapenem regimen in conjunction with colistin can be life-saving for patients infected with multidrug-resistant organisms. Furthermore, newer agents such as ceftazidime-avibactam and ceftolozane-tazobactam are being effectively employed against resistant pathogens, significantly enriching the clinician's therapeutic options. Ongoing collaboration between scientists and clinicians is crucial in addressing the challenges posed by resistant Gram-negative pathogens, necessitating timely and adaptable interventions to keep pace with evolving microbial resistance (Mascellino et al., 2017) (Figure 7. 13).

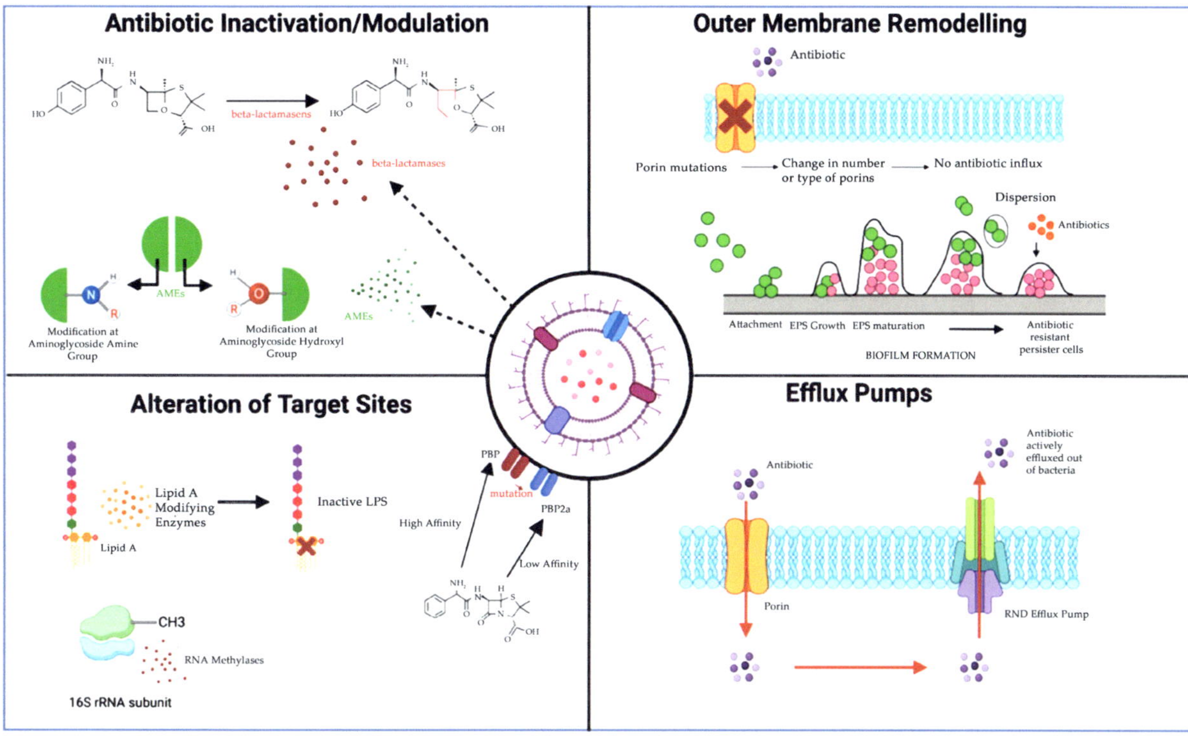

Figure 7.13. Overview of antibiotic resistance mechanisms in Gram-negative bacteria.

Source: https://www.mdpi.com/antibiotics/antibiotics-12-01590/article_deploy/html/images/antibiotics-12-01590-g003.png.

7.5.2. Resistance Mechanisms in Gram-negative Bacteria

The epidemic of antibiotic resistance in Gram-negative bacteria is driven by complex genetic interactions involving multiple drug resistance mechanisms that enable these pathogens to survive despite the presence of therapeutic agents. Among these mechanisms, the production of β-lactamases has become a primary factor contributing to resistance against β-lactam antibiotics such as penicillins and cephalosporins. Extended-spectrum beta-lactamases (ESβLs) are of particular concern due to their ability to hydrolyse a broad range of beta-lactam antibiotics, thereby conferring resistance to commonly used treatments. Furthermore, the emergence of carbapenemases, including KPC and NDM variants, indicates increasing difficulty in managing infections caused by Gram-negative bacteria, especially *Enterobacterales*. Beyond resistance transfer, these enzymes can disseminate between different bacterial species through horizontal gene transfer, significantly complicating infection control in clinical settings (Abu-Alsha'ar, 2022). Additionally, the capacity of Gram-negative bacteria to form biofilms compounds resistance further, complicating eradication efforts. Biofilms are structured populations of bacteria embedded within a protective extracellular matrix, shielding the organisms from both the host immune response and antibiotic activity. The formation of biofilms is associated with chronic infections, particularly on indwelling medical devices, where bacteria adhere and proliferate in highly resistant states, rendering treatment ineffective. This clinical challenge is exemplified by infections caused by Acinetobacter species, which possess diverse efflux pumps, carbapenemase enzymes, and biofilm-forming abilities. These features not only facilitate survival in hostile environments but also hinder the efficacy of conventional antibiotic therapies (Vo et al., 2023). To counteract these resistance mechanisms, novel strategies are being investigated to restore the effectiveness of existing antibiotics and to develop new therapeutic options. One promising approach involves adjunctive therapies, such as derivatives of phenothiazine, which are emerging as inhibitors of type IV pilus assembly — a critical factor in motility and biofilm development among Gram-negative pathogens. By disrupting biofilm formation processes, these compounds can enhance antibiotic efficacy against resistant bacteria. Additionally, advances in understanding the genomic and proteomic profiles of Gram-negative bacteria foster the development of targeted therapies designed to circumvent intrinsic resistance mechanisms. Continued research in this domain is essential to inform clinical practices and to improve treatment outcomes for infections caused by Gram-negative bacteria (Abu-Alsha'ar, 2022).

7.5.3. Alternative Treatment Strategies

Given that the emergence of antibiotic-resistant Gram-negative bacterial infections constitutes a significant global public health challenge, the development of novel therapeutic strategies has become increasingly essential to the field of medicine. These strategies are designed to address the limitations inherent in conventional antibiotic treatments, particularly in light of the epidemic spread of multidrug-resistant strains. Contemporary approaches aim not only to inhibit bacterial proliferation but also to interfere with the pathogen's capacity to establish infections. This paradigm shift underscores the importance of targeting bacterial virulence factors and biofilm formation, hallmark characteristics of Gram-negative bacterial pathogenicity. Utilising such mechanisms, researchers can develop viable treatment modalities that operate beyond the traditional antibiotic framework, thereby establishing an effective defence against these public health threats. The engineering of new materials, such as nanoparticles and hydrogels, has been highlighted as a promising avenue for alternative therapeutic interventions. These advanced materials possess novel antimicrobial properties capable of disrupting bacterial cellular processes or preventing biofilm development, ultimately enhancing treatment efficacy. For example, certain products exploit the capacity of nanoparticles to penetrate bacterial membranes or to interfere with critical signalling pathways associated with virulence, leading to a significant reduction in infection rates. Additionally, the application of surface coatings on medical devices is anticipated to significantly impact the prevention of catheter-related infections, which are frequent complications associated with Gram-negative microorganisms. By concentrating on such high-quality materials, researchers aim to effect a paradigm shift in the management and prevention of bacterial infections, thereby providing a vital countermeasure against the escalating threat of antibiotic resistance (Bassegoda et al., 2018) (Figure 7.14).

The imperative to implement second-line treatment protocols cannot be overstated, given the diminishing pipeline of antibiotics. As traditional antibiotics increasingly prove ineffective against resistant Gram-negative bacteria, the development of alternative medicinal solutions offers a viable response to this escalating health crisis. Most new antibiotics are merely derivatives of existing drugs, highlighting the urgent need for fundamentally novel, root-level innovations.

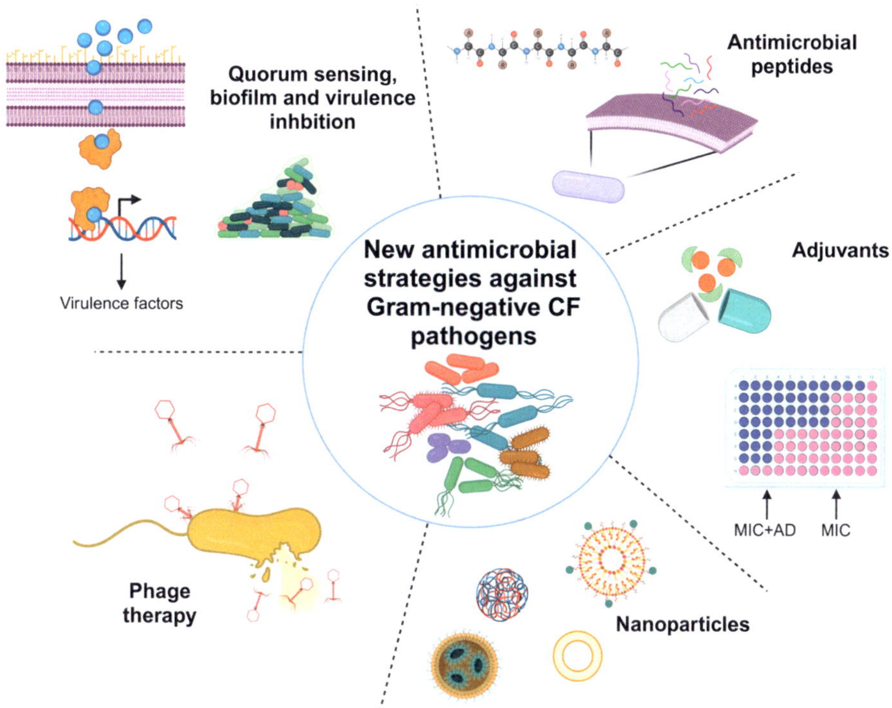

Figure 7.14. Alternative strategies to cope with multidrug-resistant CF pathogens.

Source: https://www.mdpi.com/antibiotics/antibiotics-13-00071/article_deploy/html/images/antibiotics-13-00071-g001.png.

By harnessing cutting-edge technologies and integrating them with current understanding of bacterial activity, researchers are establishing pathways toward more efficacious therapies. Besides protecting against the immediate threat posed by antibiotic resistance, this innovative strategy also holds promise for sustainable solutions in treating infections that have historically been challenging. While the scientific community broadens its focus within these promising fields, the primary goal remains the development of effective control measures for Gram-negative bacterial infections in an era of increasing resistance (PEW, 2016).

SUMMARY

The significance of Gram-negative bacterial infections extends beyond mere clinical symptoms to influence various aspects of patient health and treatment outcomes. These infections are notably resistant to antibiotics, owing to their advanced cellular structures and uptake mechanisms, making them challenging to treat. Current research indicates a notable link between lipid profiles and Gram-negative infections, revealing substantial alterations in the metabolic processes associated with sepsis, characterised by decreased levels of HDL and increased triglycerides — features typical of such infections. These findings support the necessity for a comprehensive treatment approach that addresses not only microbial eradication but also the metabolic disturbances induced by these pathogens (Wiguna et al., 2020). Consequently, understanding the interactions between Gram-negative bacteria and host physiology is essential in developing more effective therapeutic strategies. Furthermore, pathogen detection remains a clinical challenge, especially when relying solely on culture-based methods. Studies on cervico-facial sepsis demonstrate that, even when Gram-staining reports indicate the presence of Gram-negative bacteria, there exists a high likelihood of Undetected organisms. For instance, a subset of cases with Gram-negative staining results also yielded cultivable organisms (Barnard, 2019). Such diagnostic discrepancies can hinder optimal treatment, allowing infections to worsen and adversely affecting patient outcomes. Therefore, clinicians should adopt a proactive approach by employing advanced diagnostic techniques, such as molecular methods, to supplement traditional culturing procedures, thereby improving detection rates and enabling earlier, more effective intervention.

In conclusion, Gram-negative bacterial infections are complex entities characterised by distinct biological properties and significant health risks. Future research should focus on elucidating the intricate interactions between these bacteria and host immune responses, as well as refining diagnostic techniques to improve detection. These advancements would enhance understanding of the pathogenic mechanisms and inform the development of targeted therapies that consider microbiologic and metabolic factors. Given the rising prevalence of antibiotic resistance and associated complications, an interdisciplinary approach remains essential to effectively managing Gram-negative bacterial infections in clinical practice (Barnard, 2019; Wiguna et al., 2020).

The significance of investigating Gram-negative bacterial infections resides in their distinct structural features and the ensuing challenges they pose in treatment. Gram-negative bacteria are characterised by an outer membrane that confers a high degree of resistance to most antibiotics, rendering infections caused by these microorganisms particularly difficult to manage. This intrinsic resistance has been exacerbated by the overuse and misuse of antibiotics, leading to the emergence of antibiotic-resistant strains. Consequently, public health officials have emphasised the urgent need for effective strategies to combat such resistant microorganisms, especially in healthcare settings where these infections are prevalent. Despite scientific advancements through research, the development pipeline for new antibiotics has been markedly sluggish over recent decades. The slow discovery and development of novel antibiotics have raised concerns among health professionals, as most current agents are merely derivatives of earlier classes. These recurrent challenges in antibiotic discovery are further impeded by regulatory obstacles and a lack of sufficient financial incentives for pharmaceutical companies to invest in antibiotic research and development. Additionally, since nearly all antibiotics introduced in the 1980s belong to established classes, the landscape of drug resistance is evolving in a perilous manner, underscoring the necessity for new therapeutic options (PEW Charitable Trust Report, 2016). Resistance to antibiotics is an urgent issue not only in developed nations but also in low-income countries where healthcare facilities are often ill-equipped to address resistant infections. Gram-negative bacterial infections can result in severe complications and mortality, particularly among vulnerable populations. To deploy appropriate therapeutic interventions, a comprehensive understanding of the mechanisms underlying antibiotic resistance is essential. Adequate funding for research and a coordinated approach to antibiotic stewardship are vital in mitigating this multifaceted public health threat. As efforts to combat antimicrobial resistance are intensified, both developing and developed nations must prioritise collaborative initiatives, including enhanced surveillance, research funding, and public education programs, to curb the proliferation of resistant infections (Lillestolen, 2018).

CLOSER LOOK

ENTEROBACTERIACEAE

Enterobacteriaceae is a large and heterogenous family of facultatively anaerobic, Gram-negative rod-shaped bacteria that occur commonly throughout nature. They are widespread in various environments, including soil, water, and plants, but are most notably found in the normal flora of the intestines of animals and humans. The family members are oxidase-negative, glucose-fermenters, and nitrate reducers to nitrite and are, for the most part, motile via peritrichous flagella. The family consists of non-pathogenic commensals and significant pathogens and is therefore medically relevant in clinical microbiology (Figure 7.15).

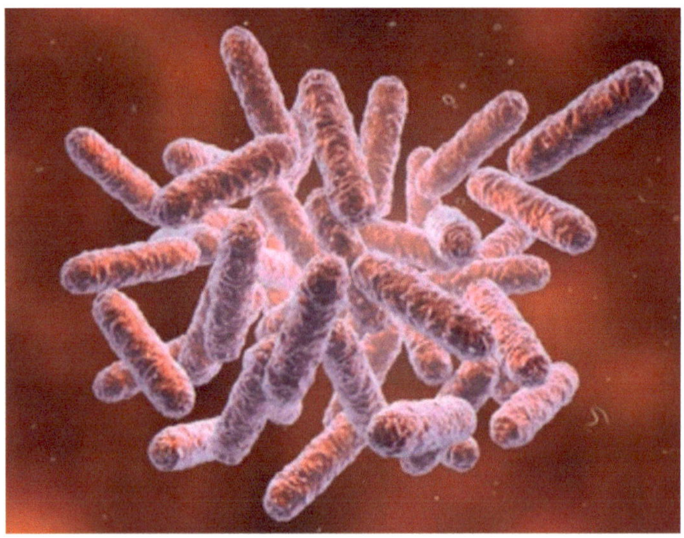

Figure 7.15. Illustration of rod-shaped, Gram-negative bacteria from the Enterobacteriaceae family, commonly associated with various infections in humans.

Source: https://www.shutterstock.com/image-illustration/enterobacteriaceae-gramnegative-rodshaped-bacteria-part-260nw-1041439810.jpg.

The family *Enterobacteriaceae* comprises over 30 genera and several hundred species, the most well-known being *Escherichia*, *Salmonella*, *Shigella*, *Klebsiella*, *Enterobacter*, *Citrobacter*, *Serratia*, *Proteus*, and *Yersinia*. *Escherichia coli* (*E. coli*) is the best-known member, varying from harmless gut strains to pathogenic forms that cause urinary tract infections, neonatal meningitis, and diarrheal diseases of all kinds. *Salmonella* and *Shigella* are renowned for causing food poisoning and dysentery, respectively. *Klebsiella pneumoniae* is among the most common causes of hospital-acquired infections, such as pneumonia, bacteremia, and liver abscess, with regular multidrug resistance.

Pathogenic *Enterobacteriaceae* employ numerous virulence determinants such as adhesins, invasins, toxins (e.g., Shiga toxin, heat-labile and heat-stable enterotoxins), capsules, and secretion systems that facilitate their ability to infect host tissues, evade immune defence mechanisms, and cause tissue damage. Others, like *Yersinia pestis*, the plague agent, possess sophisticated systems of intracellular survival and transmission by vectors.

Clinical significance is added by the fact that *Enterobacteriaceae* can pass genes horizontally, most importantly, antibiotic resistance genes. The spread of extended-spectrum beta-lactamases (ESBLs), carbapenemases (like KPC, NDM) and others among these microorganisms poses significant challenges within the healthcare setting. Surveillance, early diagnostics, and antimicrobial stewardship programs are critical to managing infections due to strains that are multidrug-resistant.

Laboratory isolation of *Enterobacteriaceae* typically involves culture on selective media such as MacConkey agar, biochemical reactions (e.g., lactose fermentation test, indole test), and increasingly, molecular methods such as PCR and MALDI-TOF mass spectrometry for rapid, precise identification.

REFERENCES

1. Berrier, A., Schaafsma, M. C., Nonglaton, G., Bergquist, J., & Rivas, J. G. (2012). Selective detection of bacterial layers with terahertz plasmonic antennas. *Biomedical optics express*, *3*(11), 2937–2949. https://doi.org/10.1364/BOE.3.002937(accessed on 16th July 2025).
2. Abu-Alsha'ar, A. F. T. (2022). *Antimicrobial drug resistance in Enterobacterales and the impact of biofilm on Staphylococcus aureus infections outcomes.* https://core.ac.uk/download/616597725.pdf (accessed on 16th July 2025).
3. Yopie Wiguna, Philia Setiawan, Prananda Surya Airlangga
4. (2020). *Hubungan profil lipid (kadar trigliserida, HDL, LDL, total kolesterol) dengan jenis infeksi bakteri pada pasien sepsis.* https://core.ac.uk/download/386326484.pdf (accessed on 16th July 2025).
5. Lappin, M. R., Blondeau, J., Boothe, D., Breitschwerdt, E. B., Guardabassi, L., Lloyd, D. H., Papich, M. G., Rankin, S. C., Sykes, J. E., Turnidge, J., & Weese, J. S. (2017). Antimicrobial use Guidelines for Treatment of Respiratory Tract Disease in Dogs and Cats: Antimicrobial Guidelines Working Group of the International Society for Companion Animal Infectious Diseases. *Journal of veterinary internal medicine*, *31*(2), 279–294. https://doi.org/10.1111/jvim.14627(accessed on 16th July 2025).
6. Araujo Garrido, J. L., Bernal Bayard, J., & Ramos Morales, F. (2020). *Type III secretion effectors with arginine N-glycosyltransferase activity.* https://core.ac.uk/download/299806865.pdf (accessed on 16th July 2025).
7. Baho, S., Czapnik, P., & Samarasinghe, S. (2019). Preliminary analysis of the anti-biofilm efficacy of manuka honey on extended spectrum β-lactamase producing *Escherichia coli* TEM-3 and *Klebsiella pneumoniae* SHV18, associated with urinary tract infections. https://core.ac.uk/download/228189014.pdf (accessed on 16th July 2025).
8. Barnard, N. (2019). *Prevalence of Gram-negative infections in cervico-facial sepsis.* https://core.ac.uk/download/289120735.pdf (accessed on 16th July 2025).
9. Barnes, L., Choe, J., Fitzgibbons, L. N., Fox, J., et al. (2018). *Smartphone-based pathogen diagnosis in urinary sepsis patients.* https://core.ac.uk/download/323062712.pdf (accessed on 16th July 2025).
10. Bartel, E. B., Bottero, D., Gaillard, M. E., Hozbor, D., et al. (2018). *Membrane vesicles derived from Bordetella bronchiseptica: Active constituent of a new vaccine against infections caused by this pathogen.* https://core.ac.uk/download/287882150.pdf (accessed on 16th July 2025).
11. Basheer Ahamed, M. (2017). Study of bacterial and fungal profile in bronchoalveolar lavage from chronic respiratory disease patients attending a tertiary care center in Thanjavur and molecular characterization for the commonest organism isolated. https://core.ac.uk/download/288215761.pdf (accessed on 16th July 2025).
12. Bassegoda, A., Ivanova, K., Ramon, E., & Tzanov, T. (2018). Strategies to prevent the occurrence of resistance against antibiotics by using advanced materials. *Applied microbiology and biotechnology*, *102*(5), 2075–2089. https://doi.org/10.1007/s00253-018-8776-0(accessed on 16th July 2025).

13. Bereswill, S., Escher, U., Heimesaat, M. M., Kehrenberg, C., et al. (2020). *Carvacrol ameliorates acute campylobacteriosis in a clinical murine infection model.* https://core.ac.uk/download/288114069.pdf (accessed on 16th July 2025).

14. Bernal-Bayard, J., & Ramos-Morales, F. (2018). Molecular Mechanisms Used by *Salmonella* to Evade the Immune System. *Current issues in molecular biology*, *25*, 133–168. https://doi.org/10.21775/cimb.025.133(accessed on 16th July 2025).

15. Beveridge, L. A., Davey, P. G., McMurdo, M. E. T., & Phillips, G., et al. (2011). *Optimal management of urinary tract infections in older people.* https://core.ac.uk/download/20450519.pdf (accessed on 16th July 2025).

16. Jenner, A., Bhagwandin, N., & Kowalski, S. P. (2017). *Antimicrobial resistance (AMR) and multidrug resistance (MDR): Overview of current approaches, consortia and intellectual property issues.* https://www.wipo.int/publications/en/details.jsp?id=4210 https://core.ac.uk/download/215505935.pdf (accessed on 16th July 2025).

17. Boaretti, M., Castellani, F., Lleo, M. M., Lucidi, S., et al. (2016). *Presence of multiple bacterial markers in clinical samples might be useful for presumptive diagnosis of infection in cirrhotic patients with culture-negative reports.* https://core.ac.uk/download/54526941.pdf (accessed on 16th July 2025).

18. Di Domenico, E. G., Farulla, I., Prignano, G., Gallo, M. T., Vespaziani, M., Cavallo, I., Sperduti, I., Pontone, M., Bordignon, V., Cilli, L., De Santis, A., Di Salvo, F., Pimpinelli, F., Lesnoni La Parola, I., Toma, L., & Ensoli, F. (2017). Biofilm is a Major Virulence Determinant in Bacterial Colonization of Chronic Skin Ulcers Independently from the Multidrug Resistant Phenotype. *International journal of molecular sciences*, *18*(5), 1077. https://doi.org/10.3390/ijms18051077(accessed on 16th July 2025).

19. Bragonzi, A., Fernandez Pinar, R., Imperi, F., Lo Sciuto, A., et al. (2015). *In vitro and in vivo screening for novel essential cell-envelope proteins in Pseudomonas aeruginosa.* https://core.ac.uk/download/54526511.pdf (accessed on 16th July 2025).

20. Chapin, A., Rule, A., Jensen, L. B., Schwab, K., Gibson, K., Mackiewicz, B., Buckley, T., et al. (2004). *Airborne multidrug-resistant bacteria isolated from a concentrated swine feeding operation.* https://core.ac.uk/download/pdf/3797183.pdf (accessed on 16th July 2025).

21. Smith, G. , & Chetter, I.(2015). *Infection in Prosthetic Material.* Surgery - Oxford International Edition, Volume 33, Issue 11, 559 – 564 (accessed on 16th July 2025).

22. Chew, D. J., Daniels, J. B., Irom, S., Keil, D., et al. (2012). *Evaluation of the efficacy and safety of high dose short duration enrofloxacin treatment regimen for uncomplicated urinary tract infections in dogs.* https://core.ac.uk/download/323068657.pdf (accessed on 16th July 2025).

23. PEW Charitable Trust Report (2016). *A scientific roadmap for antibiotic discovery: A sustained and robust pipeline of new antibacterial drugs and therapies is critical to preserve public health.* https://core.ac.uk/download/75785719.pdf (accessed on 16th July 2025).

24. Maria Teresa c, Massimiliano De Angelis and Alessandra Oliva (2017). *Multi-drug resistant Gram-negative bacteria: Antibiotic resistance and new treatment strategies.* Diagn Pathol Open 2017, 2:1 DOI: 10.4172/2476-2024.1000e106 (accessed on 16th July 2025).

25. Epstein, S. E., Westropp, J. L., & Wong, C. (2015). *Antimicrobial susceptibility patterns in urinary tract infections in dogs (2010–2013).* https://core.ac.uk/download/323068134.pdf (accessed on 16th July 2025).

26. Farooq, T., Nazir, A., Peerzada, B. Y., Sana, A., et al. (2018). *Study of prevalence and antimicrobial susceptibility pattern of blood culture isolates from a tertiary care hospital of North India.* https://core.ac.uk/download/543136128.pdf (accessed on 16th July 2025).
27. Grelling, N., Liu, H., Nguyen, N. Y. T., Rosario, K., et al. (2018). *Antimicrobial activities and mechanisms of magnesium oxide nanoparticles (nMgO) against pathogenic bacteria, yeasts, and biofilms.* https://core.ac.uk/download/323067341.pdf (accessed on 16th July 2025).
28. White S, Topping A, Humphreys P, Rout S, Williamson H. The cross-contamination potential of mobile telephones. *Journal of Research in Nursing*. 2012;17(6):582-595. doi:10.1177/1744987112458670
29. (accessed on 16th July 2025).
30. Zabielska, J., Tyfa, A., & Kunicka-Styczyńska, A. (2016). Methods for eradication of the biofilms formed by opportunistic pathogens using novel techniques – A review. *Acta Universitatis Lodziensis. Folia Biologica Et Oecologica*, *12*, 26–37. https://doi.org/10.1515/fobio-2016-0003(accessed on 16th July 2025).
31. Lee, Y. J., Lim, D. J., Moon, S. K., Oh, J. H., et al. (2014). *NOD2/RICK-dependent β-defensin 2 regulation is protective for nontypeable Haemophilus influenzae-induced middle ear infection.* https://core.ac.uk/download/323078660.pdf (accessed on 16th July 2025).
32. Lillestolen, D. (2018). *Infections Not Fought: Antibiotic Resistance in Underserved Communities.* https://core.ac.uk/download/158970352.pdf (accessed on 16th July 2025).
33. Vo, N., Sidner, B. S., Yu, Y., & Piepenbrink, K. H. (2023). Type IV Pilus-Mediated Inhibition of *Acinetobacter baumannii* Biofilm Formation by Phenothiazine Compounds. *Microbiology spectrum*, *11*(4), e0102323. https://doi.org/10.1128/spectrum.01023-23 (accessed on 16th July 2025).
34. Rokka, S. (2008). *Bovine Colostral Antibodies and Selected Lactobacilli as Means to Control Gastrointestinal Infections.* https://core.ac.uk/download/10928087.pdf (accessed on 16th July 2025).
35. Rosso-Fernández, C., Garnacho-Montero, J., Antonelli, M., Dimopoulos, G., Cisneros, J. M., & MagicBullet study group (2015). Safety and efficacy of colistin versus meropenem in the empirical treatment of ventilator-associated pneumonia as part of a macro-project funded by the Seventh Framework Program of the European Commission studying off-patent antibiotics: study protocol for a randomized controlled trial. *Trials*, *16*, 102. https://doi.org/10.1186/s13063-015-0614-4 (accessed on 16th July 2025).
36. Torrent Burgués, J. (2017). *Review on Bibliography Related to Antimicrobials.* https://core.ac.uk/download/81581543.pdf (accessed on 16th July 2025).

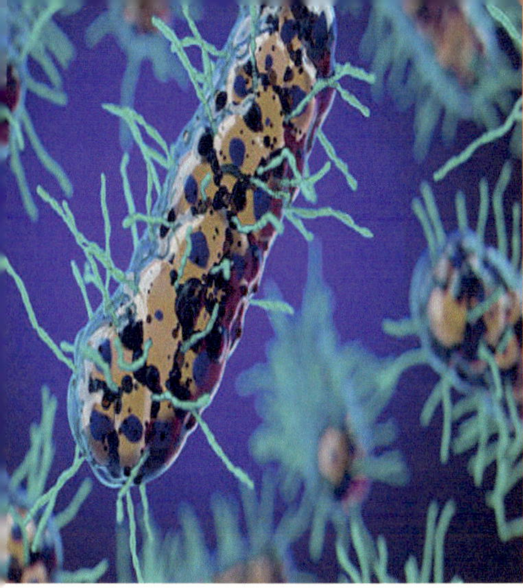

Chapter 8
GRAM-POSITIVE BACTERIAL INFECTIONS

Contents

Introduction

Barnard, 2019The infection caused by Gram-positive bacteria represents a critical area of investigation within microbiology and infectious disease research, due to the significant public health implications posed by these microorganisms. Gram-positive bacteria, characterised by a cell wall containing peptidoglycan that is substantially thicker than that of Gram-negative bacteria, include several pathogenic species capable of inducing severe infections, such as *Staphylococcus aureus*, *Streptococcus pneumoniae*, and *Enterococcus faecalis*. These bacteria typically reside benignly on human skin and mucosal surfaces but can become pathogenic under specific conditions, such as in immunocompromised hosts. To develop effective diagnostic tools and therapeutic regimens, it is essential to elucidate the mechanisms by which Gram-positive bacteria gain pathogenicity, namely, their ability to adhere to tissues, evade the host's immune response, and develop resistance to antibiotics. Recent studies have addressed the complexities associated with treating Gram-positive bacterial infections, particularly in light of the rising problem of antimicrobial resistance. The emergence of multidrug-resistant strains presents a formidable public health challenge, requiring a coordinated approach to infection management. Current therapeutic strategies are increasingly ineffective as these bacteria exhibit resistance to antibiotics, complicating treatment efforts. Evidence suggests that antibiotic misuse in various settings has contributed significantly to this resistance, underscoring an urgent need for novel medications and alternative treatment approaches. Furthermore, understanding the epidemiology and pathogenesis of Gram-positive infections is crucial for implementing effective public health measures. Research indicates that, even when Gram-negative pathogens are identified in cultures, the clinical impact of Gram-positive infections often surpasses that of their Gram-negative counterparts (Barnard, 2019). This underscores the importance of targeted intervention and surveillance to prevent outbreaks caused by Gram-positive bacteria. Public health campaigns combined with emerging diagnostic technologies can facilitate early detection and intervention. Ultimately, a comprehensive strategy integrating research, clinical practice, and public health initiatives is necessary to reduce the burden of Gram-positive bacterial infections and enhance health outcomes in affected populations.

Definition of Gram-positive Bacteria

These structural differences serve as the foundation for their classification, primarily elucidated by Hans Christian Gram through his Gram stain procedure. Gram-positive bacteria are characterised by their thick peptidoglycan cell wall, which retains the crystal violet dye during the Gram stain process. Their robust cell wall structure plays a significant role in the organism's pathogenicity and ability to withstand various environmental conditions.

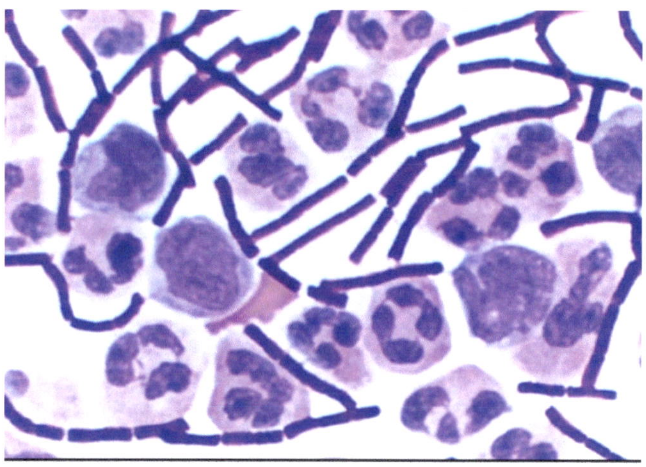

Figure 8.1. Rod-shaped, Gram-positive *Bacillus anthracis* bacteria in a cerebrospinal fluid sample stand out from round white blood cells, which also accept the crystal violet stain.

Source: https://en.wikipedia.org/wiki/Gram-positive_bacteria#/media/File:Gram_Stain_Anthrax.jpg.

The substantial peptidoglycan layer not only provides structural integrity but also acts as a barrier to certain antibiotics, thereby rendering infections caused by these bacteria particularly challenging to treat. Consequently, it is of paramount importance to understand the cellular characteristics of Gram-positive bacteria to develop effective therapeutic strategies against potential infections. Moreover, Gram-positive bacteria possess critical metabolic pathways that contribute to their virulence. These microorganisms tend to produce a variety of toxins and enzymes that enhance their pathogenic potential. For instance, some pathogens like *Staphylococcus aureus* produce enterotoxins leading to food poisoning or skin infections, while *Streptococcus pyogenes* can cause conditions ranging from mild sore throats to severe, life-threatening infections such as necrotising fasciitis. The capacity of these microorganisms to form biofilms further complicates treatment, as biofilms create protective niches, making it difficult for the immune system and antibiotics to eliminate established infections. This challenge is compounded by the ongoing development of antibiotic resistance, which continues to threaten the control of Gram-positive bacterial infections (Zabielska et al., 2016) (Figure 8.1).

The clinical significance of Gram-positive bacteria extends beyond their inherent biological properties. The rapid and precise identification of these organisms is of paramount importance in clinical microbiology, as prompt diagnosis directly influences therapeutic outcomes. Techniques such as terahertz time-domain spectroscopy have been investigated to augment the detection of Gram-positive bacteria, offering a more expedient alternative to conventional methods. This technological advancement underscores the importance of observable identification in microbial infections, where distinguishing between Gram types facilitates appropriate antibiotic selection and expedites patient recovery (Berrier et al., 2012). Consequently, acquiring comprehensive knowledge about Gram-positive bacteria is essential, not only for recognising their characteristics but also for addressing the heightened threat posed by infections they induce.

Importance of Studying Gram-positive Bacterial Infections

The importance of studying Gram-positive bacterial infections is highlighted by the fact that these organisms are widespread in clinical and community settings. Gram-positive bacteria, such as *Staphylococcus aureus* and *Streptococcus pneumoniae*, not only cause a range of infections but are also highly adaptable, making them difficult to treat. The emergence of antibiotic-resistant strains, especially methicillin-resistant *Staphylococcus aureus* (MRSA), emphasises the need for intensive research into resistance mechanisms. This can aid in developing new treatments that target these pathogens more effectively. Additionally, since Gram-positive bacteria tend to cause severe infections like pneumonia and skin infections, studying them is essential for guiding public health interventions and clinical practice, ultimately improving patient care and reducing infection rates in healthcare environments. Identifying Gram-positive bacterial infections also involves assessing their environmental and zoonotic significance. For instance, the use of non-therapeutic antibiotics in animal husbandry and agriculture can lead to the development of antibiotic-resistant Gram-positive bacteria, which may then enter the food chain. This presents a threat not only to livestock health but also to consumers who are exposed to resistant pathogens through contaminated meat products. Research has shown that air from animal feed operations contains multidrug-resistant bacteria and can serve as a route of exposure for humans, as demonstrated in studies of swine operation *Enterococcus* (Chapin et al., 2004). Therefore, environmental sources and transmission pathways of Gram-positive infections should be examined to mitigate public health risks. Furthermore, the broader impact of Gram-positive bacterial infections includes socioeconomic costs associated with healthcare provision. The financial burden of treating infections — especially those caused by resistant strains — can strain healthcare systems and influence health insurance costs. As Gram-positive bacteria are responsible for numerous costly hospitalisations and prolonged treatments, understanding these infections is vital for the efficient management of medical resources. Moreover, the development of new treatment approaches, such as human lactoferrin to manage infection and inflammation, exemplifies the potential of innovative techniques to enhance patient care (Rosa et al., 2017). By exploring the intersections of pathophysiology, resistance patterns, and clinical management, researchers are better equipped to develop strategies that not only cure infections but also reduce the economic costs associated with Gram-positive bacterial infections.*Staphylococcus aureusStaphylococcus aureus*

8.1. Characteristics of Gram-positive Bacteria

The characteristics of Gram-positive bacteria are primarily defined by their cell wall structure, which is quite different from that of Gram-negative bacteria. Gram-positive bacteria have a thick peptidoglycan layer that retains the crystal violet stain used in Gram staining, causing them to appear blue or purple under a microscope. This multilayered peptidoglycan not only provides structural integrity to the bacterial cell wall but also plays a crucial role in protecting against environmental stress. Moreover, the incorporation of teichoic acids into the peptidoglycan layer adds rigidity to the wall and may be involved in various cellular processes, such as surface adhesion and immune response modulation. Together, these structural features allow Gram-positive bacteria to thrive in diverse ecological niches and withstand different conditions. Structurally, Gram-positive bacteria possess a range of metabolic and pathogenic traits that significantly impact human health. Many Gram-positive genera, such as *Streptococcus* and *Staphylococcus*, serve as opportunistic pathogens, usually residing harmlessly within the human microbiota until environmental factors promote their pathogenic potential. For example, with compromised immunity or damaged skin, these bacteria can become invasive, causing infections that may lead to poor clinical outcomes. Some Gram-positive bacteria also produce exotoxins, which enhance virulence by damaging host tissues or disrupting normal physiological functions. Understanding these pathogenic mechanisms is essential for developing effective treatment protocols against Gram-positive bacterial infections, especially considering the rising issue of antibiotic resistance. The clinical importance of Gram-positive bacterial infections grows more alarming with the emergence of antibiotic-resistant strains. The slow progress in discovering new antibiotics, as recent literature indicates, underscores the difficulty of managing infections caused by resistant bacteria. Since almost all antibiotics approved over recent decades are derivatives of older drugs, options for treating Gram-positive infections are becoming increasingly limited. This challenge is compounded by the ability of Gram-positive bacteria to acquire resistance genes via horizontal gene transfer, rendering traditional treatments ineffective. As antibiotic resistance remains a critical public health concern, new strategies must be explored, including the development of novel antimicrobial agents and targeted therapies, to address the complex issues posed by Gram-positive bacterial infections effectively (Barnard, 2019; PEW Charitable Trust Report, 2016).

8.1.1. Cell Wall Structure and Composition

The cell wall of Gram-positive bacteria is essential for their structural integrity and virulence. It mainly consists of a thick peptidoglycan layer. This wall gives shape and rigidity, helping microorganisms withstand various environmental stresses. The peptidoglycan layer is made of glycan chains cross-linked by short peptides, forming a strong network that is notably thicker than that of Gram-negative bacteria. Moreover, teichoic acids — polymers of glycerol or ribitol phosphate — are crucial for cell wall function by affecting the surface charge and facilitating interactions with host cells. This complex structure not only provides protection but also makes treatment more difficult, as it can block the entry of some antibiotics that target cell wall synthesis. Additionally, the cell wall structure impacts the virulence and antibiotic resistance of Gram-positive bacteria. The dense peptidoglycan layer serves as a barrier to most antimicrobial agents; however, this also creates specific vulnerabilities, such as the targeting of enzymes involved in peptidoglycan cross-linking by penicillin, which is characteristic of Gram-positive bacteria. Recent advances include techniques like terahertz time-domain spectroscopy for differentiating bacterial species and classifying Gram status based on cell wall features, reflecting growing interest in non-invasive diagnostic methods in medicine (Berrier et al., 2012) (Figure 8.2).

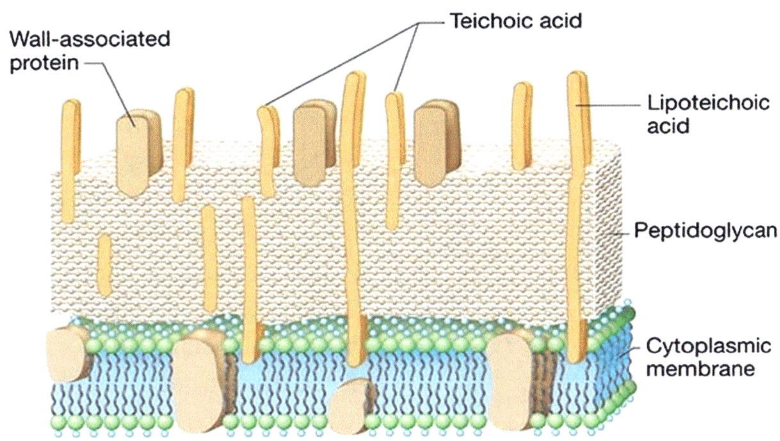

Figure 8.2. Cell wall of Gram-positive bacteria.

Source: https://microbenotes.com/gram-positive-cell-wall/.

These developments emphasise the significance of cell wall composition in developing effective treatment strategies against Gram-positive infections. The therapeutic landscape for Gram-positive bacterial infections is also shifting with the emergence of new antimicrobial agents such as magnesium oxide nanoparticles (nMgO). These antimicrobial nanoparticles have demonstrated activity against various Gram-positive pathogens by disrupting their cell wall organisation and biofilms. Research has shown that nMgO can kill the membranes of vulnerable bacteria, making them even more susceptible to other antimicrobial treatments (Grelling et al., 2018). Additionally, the different minimal inhibitory concentrations among strains highlight the need for tailored therapy approaches, as some strains may resist conventional antibiotics but still be sensitive to nanoparticle-based treatments. Ultimately, understanding the complexities of cell wall composition and structure is essential for developing more effective interventions against Gram-positive bacterial infections.

8.1.2. Staining Properties and Identification

The Gram-positive bacterial infections are primarily distinguished based on their unique staining properties, mainly demonstrated through the Gram stain technique. This differential staining method exploits structural features of bacterial cell walls to differentiate Gram-positive from Gram-negative bacteria. The thick peptidoglycan layer of Gram-positive bacteria retains the crystal violet stain, which appears purple under a microscope. This structural difference is significant for clinical diagnosis as it guides treatment options and the choice of effective antibiotics. Additionally, Gram-positive bacteria often display distinctive morphological features, such as cocci or bacilli shapes, which aid in their identification under a microscope. Besides the primary Gram stain, other staining techniques can facilitate easier identification of Gram-positive bacteria. Dyes such as methylene blue, eosin, and specific selective media enable the differentiation of various bacterial species by producing visible contrast and staining different cellular structures (Figure 8.3).

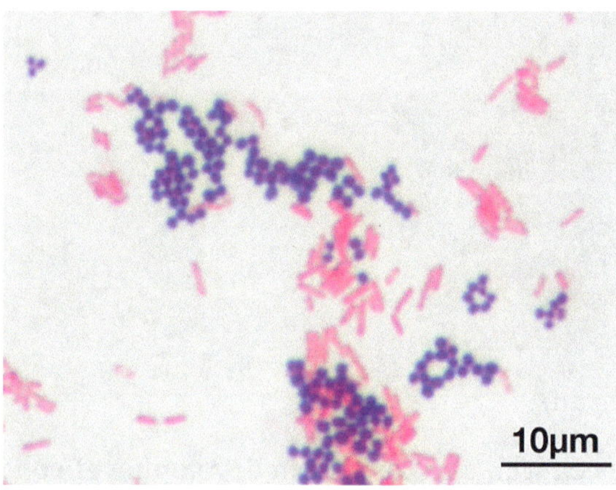

Figure 8.3. Violet-stained, Gram-positive cocci and pink-stained, Gram-negative bacilli.

Source: https://en.wikipedia.org/wiki/Gram-positive_bacteria#/media/File:Gram_stain_01.jpg.

For instance, the utilisation of specific chromogenic substrates can facilitate the differentiation of certain pathogens, such as *Staphylococcus aureus*, which exhibits distinctive colonial characteristics. The employment of this type of staining is particularly pertinent in the identification of opportunistic pathogens with Gram-positive infections. Such refinement processes enhance the precision of bacterial identification and are essential for guiding appropriate treatment strategies. In addition to staining properties, biochemical analyses are crucial for the identification of Gram-positive bacteria. Biochemical assays, including catalase, coagulase, and hemolysis patterns, offer supplementary levels of characterisation to complement staining data. For example, catalase testing differentiates staphylococci, which produce catalase, from streptococci, which do not. The combination of staining techniques and biochemical characteristics bolsters a definitive diagnosis of Gram-positive infections. Furthermore, recent advances in bacteriophage therapy targeting Gram-positive infections are emerging as innovative alternatives to conventional antibiotic treatments, as demonstrated in studies on the efficacy of bacteriophage techniques against biofilms in infections such as those caused by *Pseudomonas* (Arabski et al., 2016). Additionally, the development of novel antimicrobial compounds that specifically inhibit bacterial enzymes may further enhance therapeutic interventions in managing such infections (Phelan, 2016). *Staphylococcus aureus*

8.1.3. Common Genera of Gram-positive Bacteria

Gram-positive bacterial life encompasses a rich and diverse array of genera of crucial importance in human health and disease. The three most significant are *Staphylococcus*, *Streptococcus*, and *Enterococcus*. *Staphylococcus aureus*, recognised as one of the most virulent species, is well-known for causing skin infections, pneumonia, and sepsis, often demonstrating resistance to antibiotics, thus rendering treatment challenging. Conversely, species such as *Streptococcus pyogenes* and *Streptococcus pneumoniae* lead to conditions including pharyngitis and pneumonia, respectively, highlighting the clinical relevance of this genus in respiratory infections. *Enterococcus* species are commensals of the gastrointestinal tract that can opportunistically cause infections, particularly in immunocompromised individuals, with significant morbidity and mortality when other organ systems are affected. These genera emphasise the significance of Gram-positive bacteria in infectious processes, as an improved understanding of their mechanisms will augment clinical practice. The threat posed by Gram-positive bacteria extends beyond specific species; their capacity to form biofilms constitutes a critical virulence factor. Biofilm formation allows bacteria to adhere to surfaces, evade phagocytosis, and resist antimicrobial agents, thereby facilitating chronic infections. For example, *Staphylococcus epidermidis* biofilms are commonly implicated in medical device-related infections. Research indicates that biofilm development is frequently associated with the expression of particular virulence factors that enhance bacterial survival under stressful conditions (Figure 8.4).*Staphylococcus aureus*

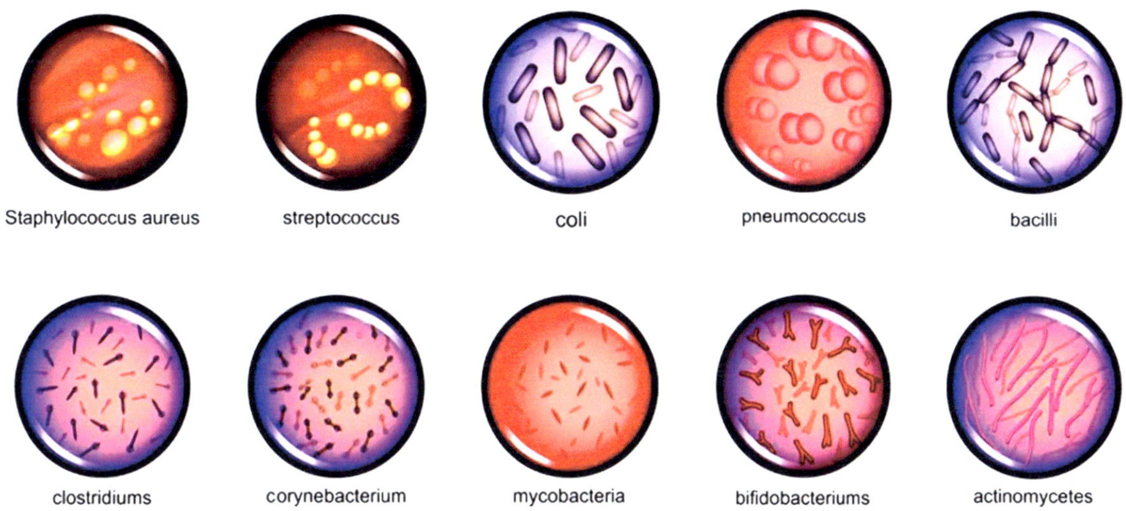

Figure 8.4. Common genera of Gram-positive bacteria.

Source: https://external-content.duckduckgo.com/iu/?u=https%3A%2F%2Fthumbs.dreamstime.com%2Fz%2Fgram-positive-bacteria-vector-illustration-microbiology-bacteriology-110426638.jpg&f=1&nofb=1&ipt=c6c229d8f52ed1bd2922074de140726bffb02b969602e3dc1ad988cd80df8221.

Furthermore, studies on the epidemiology of polymicrobial infections, which frequently include Gram-positive cocci, show a complex relationship between different bacterial populations in chronic infections. Such microbial interactions highlight the importance of understanding the ecology of Gram-positive bacteria for developing effective therapies and preventing repeated infections in patients. Recent work has highlighted the broader significance of Gram-positive bacteria in various clinical settings, particularly in managing biliary tract infections. A study examining bile cultures taken during endoscopic procedures found a predominance of Gram-positive bacteria within the biota. Specifically, *Enterococcus* and *Staphylococcus* genera were present alongside their Gram-negative counterparts, indicating their role in polymicrobial infections often complicated by biofilm formation. The presence of these genera together in biliary infections emphasises the need for new antimicrobial strategies to target resistant organisms. Additionally, understanding the susceptibility patterns of such microorganisms is vital because infections involve complex interactions between microbial communities that affect treatment outcomes. Therefore, gaining more knowledge about Gram-positive bacteria not only informs clinical practice but also forms the basis for developing therapeutic measures to effectively control bacterial infections.

8.2. Common Gram-positive Bacterial Infections

The impact of common Gram-positive bacterial infections is widespread and has significant consequences for human health, especially in healthcare facilities. Three of the most notorious culprits are *Staphylococcus aureus*, *Streptococcus pneumoniae*, and *Enterococcus*. *Staphylococcus aureus* is known for causing a range of infections from small skin abscesses to potentially fatal conditions such as sepsis and pneumonia. The emergence of methicillin-resistant *Staphylococcus aureus* (MRSA) has worsened the situation. This antibiotic-resistant bacterium makes treatment increasingly difficult, with early diagnosis and proper intervention being crucial. *Streptococcus pneumoniae* infections, which are most commonly responsible for pneumonia, meningitis, and otitis media, have also become a growing concern due to increasing antibiotic resistance rates. As these pathogens mutate, they present a major challenge to healthcare systems worldwide, requiring prompt responses and innovative strategies to minimise their impact on public health. Moreover, *Enterococcus* species, particularly *Enterococcus faecalis* and *Enterococcus faecium*, can cause life-threatening healthcare-associated infections such as urinary tract infections and endocarditis. Once thought to be harmless, these bacteria have shown increasing resistance to multiple antibiotic classes, heightening their threat in clinical settings. The rise of vancomycin-resistant *Enterococcus* (VRE) exemplifies the escalating danger of antibiotic resistance. Effective control of these Gram-positive infections is hampered not only by evolving resistance patterns but also by the dwindling pipeline of new antibiotics. The broad impact of these resistant Gram-positive pathogens is compounded by the slow pace of antibiotic development, which has visibly declined since the 1980s. This stagnation raises urgent concerns regarding future treatment options and underscores the pressing need for innovative solutions in antibiotic research and development (PEW Charitable Trust Report, 2016). The repercussions of common Gram-positive bacterial infections extend beyond individual health to broader public health issues. The rise of antibiotic-resistant strains has ignited fierce debate among healthcare professionals, policymakers, and researchers regarding resource allocation for public health initiatives and antibiotic stewardship programmes. The prevalence of infection caused by these Gram-positive bacteria in certain populations underscores the importance of research into resistance mechanisms. Studies conducted at Tygerberg Academic Hospital and elsewhere indicate that even in cases of cervico-facial sepsis involving Gram-negative organisms, the presence of Gram-positive pathogens often necessitates urgent action and expert treatment approaches (Barnard, 2019). Consequently, managing Gram-positive bacterial infections requires a comprehensive strategy that includes education, improved diagnostic protocols, and effective antibiotic stewardship to confront the mounting threat of antibiotic resistance in clinical practice.

8.2.1. Staphylococcus aureus Infections

Staphylococcus aureus infections are major causes of the syndrome of Gram-positive bacterial infection, characterised by a wide range of clinical presentations and increasing antibiotic resistance. *S. aureus* is a human skin and mucosal commensal that can coexist benignly on these sites in most individuals. However, when the integrity of the host's skin is compromised or their immunity is weakened, *S. aureus* can cause severe infections, including skin abscesses, pneumonia, and endocarditis. Since methicillin-resistant *Staphylococcus aureus* (MRSΛ) has emerged, treatment options for these infections are becoming more limited and challenging. Therefore, understanding the pathogenesis of *S. aureus*, such as its biofilm formation and environmental stress resistance, is essential for developing effective therapeutic strategies against associated infections. Biofilm formation plays a crucial role in *S. aureus* infections, especially as a significant barrier to treatment in cases involving implanted medical devices. Biofilms are clusters of bacteria embedded in an extracellular matrix that shields them, making them resistant to antibiotics and immune responses. Once biofilms form on a medical device, they are very difficult to remove, potentially leading to chronic infections and increased morbidity, particularly in immunocompromised patients. To effectively treat *S. aureus* infections, new mechanisms must be devised to disrupt biofilm formation and improve antibiotic efficacy. Recent research has explored methods to combat these biofilms, including using innovative antimicrobial materials and treatments that target biofilm matrices (Zabielska et al., 2016) (Figure 8.5).*Staphylococcus aureusStaphylococcus aureus*

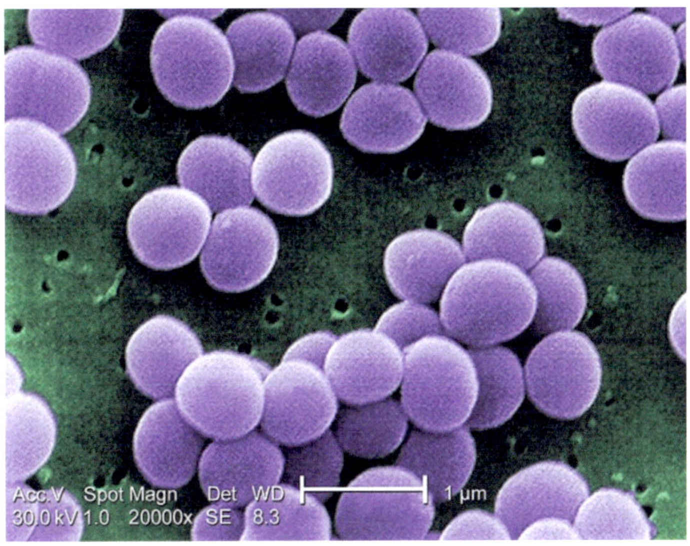

Figure 8.5. *Staphylococcus aureus.*

Source: https://en.wikipedia.org/wiki/Staphylococcus_aureus#/media/File:Staphylococcus_aureus_VISA_2.jpg.

These emerging strategies highlight the significance of continued research and development in the creation of interventions specifically aimed at *Staphylococcus aureus*. The challenge of antibiotic resistance poses a substantial obstacle to the effective treatment of *S. aureus*, thereby underscoring the critical need to discover innovative therapeutic solutions. The longstanding dependence on antibiotics has been critically scrutinised due to the emergence of multidrug-resistant strains, which have prompted researchers to investigate alternative methods for managing such infections. Progressive approaches include bactericidal agents with novel mechanisms of action, which may remain effective even against resistant organisms (Bassegoda et al., 2018). The advancement of engineered materials, such as nanomaterials and hydrogels, demonstrates the potential to introduce new antimicrobial activities, either by preventing infection onset or by reducing the impact of established biofilms. Ultimately, addressing the escalating challenge of antibiotic resistance in *S. aureus* infections will require a comprehensive effort involving ongoing research, the development of new therapeutic modalities, and the implementation of rigorous infection control measures within healthcare settings.

8.2.2. Streptococcus Pneumoniae Infections

Streptococcus pneumoniae is a Gram-positive coccus that is a significant pathogen causing a range of serious infections like pneumonia, meningitis, and bacteremia. The organism has a polysaccharide capsule that enhances its virulence by allowing it to evade the host's immune response. Clinically, *S. pneumoniae* is a major cause of community-acquired pneumonia and often results in significant morbidity among vulnerable populations such as young children, the elderly, and immunocompromised hosts. Evidence indicates that, among a sample of febrile adult patients, *S. pneumoniae* accounted for 15.2% of bloodstream infections and poses a high incidence and impact on public health, especially in areas with high HIV infection rates, as it increases the risk (Kabangila et al., 2012). The ability of *S. pneumoniae* to cause various diseases requires close monitoring and control strategies to manage its effects. Its pathogenicity is heavily influenced by various virulence factors, including its adhesion and invasion of host cells. Additionally, lipoproteins on the bacterium's surface play a critical role in its interactions and overall virulence. Research on a Δlgt mutant strain of *S. pneumoniae* shows that the loss of surface-localised lipoproteins causes severe deficiencies in cation acquisition, leading to impaired growth in nutrient-limited conditions and increased susceptibility to oxidative stress (Bidossi et al., 2012) (Figure 8.6).

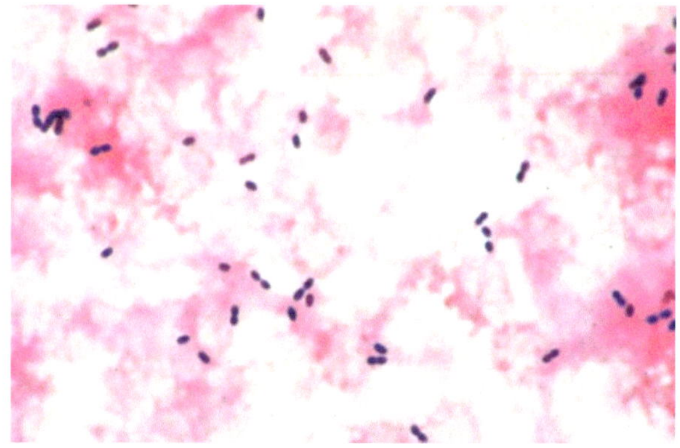

Figure 8.6. *Streptococcus pneumoniae* appear as Gram-positive diplococci.

Source: https://www.researchgate.net/figure/Streptococcus-pneumoniae-appear-as-gram-positive-diplococci-The-cells-are-somewhat_fig1_338792413.

These findings demonstrate not only bacterial mechanisms for deriving essential nutrients but also their effects within the broader context of infection. This advanced interaction between *Streptococcus pneumoniae*'s physiological requirements and its pathogenic potential underscores the importance of a comprehensive understanding of its biology in the development of effective therapeutic strategies. Due to the challenges posed by *Streptococcus pneumoniae*, particularly the emergence of antibiotic-resistant strains, effective prevention through vaccination remains a critical tool in combating infection. The pneumococcal vaccine has been demonstrated to reduce the incidence of invasive pneumococcal disease in most populations, thereby confirming its efficacy in preventing infections. Nevertheless, ongoing surveillance is essential, especially considering potential variations in vaccine coverage that may be incomplete. As Streptococcus pneumoniae continues to evolve, adapting to immune defences and therapeutic interventions, public health strategies must also adapt accordingly. Increased research into the pathogenic mechanisms and host interactions of *Streptococcus pneumoniae* will be pivotal in the development of novel vaccines and treatments, ultimately leading to improved control of Gram-positive bacterial infections and better health outcomes for affected populations.

8.2.3. Clostridium Difficile Infections

Among the wide range of Gram-positive bacterial infections, *Clostridium difficile* infections (CDIs) have gained significant attention due to their increasing incidence and clinical severity. *C. difficile*, an anaerobic spore-forming bacterium, is now recognised as the most common cause of nosocomial diarrhoea in Europe and North America. This has primarily been attributed to the indiscriminate use of antibiotics, which disturbs the gut microbiome's balance and creates an ideal environment for *C. difficile* colonization. The subsequent infections pose particular challenges in high-risk groups, such as individuals with underlying health conditions or immunocompromised states, further complicating clinical management. Hospitalised patients with extended stays, many receiving repeated courses of antibiotics for other infections, are at higher risk for CDI. Infection control and prevention practices in healthcare settings should be informed by knowledge of the epidemiology and risk factors associated with *C. difficile*. Furthermore, the virulence of *C. difficile* is primarily regulated by its toxins, which cause destruction of the intestinal epithelium and trigger an inflammatory response. Toxin A and Toxin B are the key virulence factors, leading to diarrhoea and colitis in affected patients. Not only do the toxins cause mucosal damage to the colonic lining, but they also provoke an overactive immune response, resulting in the clinical symptoms of CDI. Intriguingly, patients with cirrhosis of the liver are at increased risk of *C. difficile* infection because their compromised immune systems and extensive antibiotic use amplify this risk. Studies have demonstrated that immune dysfunction caused by cirrhosis (CAID) is the main factor behind the heightened susceptibility, and alterations in systemic and local liver immunity reduce the host's resistance to infection. Therefore, a nuanced understanding of toxin mechanisms and host-pathogen interactions is essential in addressing the CDI burden in high-risk populations (Dumitru et al., 2019) (Figure 8.7).

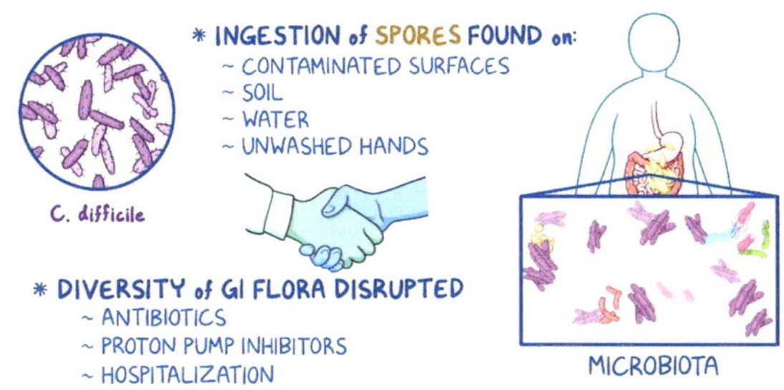

Figure 8.7. Clostridioides difficile infection.

Source: https://www.osmosis.org/_next/image?url=https%3A%2F%2Fd16qt3wv6xm098.cloudfront.net%2FJMGa1OZOS6ewuBHadpVf2_oYRBmQmKVN%2F_.jpg&w=3840&q=75.

Furthermore, the escalating trend of antibiotic resistance presents a significantly greater challenge in the management of *C. difficile* infections. The emergence of antibiotic-resistant strains, further facilitated by the inappropriate use of broad-spectrum antibiotics, complicates treatment procedures and contributes to heightened morbidity and mortality rates associated with CDIs. Antibiotic resistance remains a pervasive issue in most healthcare institutions, creating a cycle of ineffective treatments and recurrent infections in patients. This crisis is especially acute in developing regions, where limited access to antimicrobial stewardship programs and healthcare resources exacerbates the problem. Given these challenges, the pursuit of research and funding is integral to the development of innovative therapeutic approaches and the enhancement of patient outcomes. The threats posed by CDI and antibiotic resistance must be addressed through a multidisciplinary strategy that encompasses increased education on antibiotic usage, robust infection surveillance, and investment in novel therapeutic modalities (Lillestolen, 2018).

8.3. Pathogenesis of Gram-positive Bacterial Infections

The pathogenesis of Gram-positive bacterial infections is a complex process inherently connected to the unique structural features of these microorganisms. Gram-positive bacteria, such as *Staphylococcus aureus* and *Streptococcus pneumoniae*, contain a thick peptidoglycan layer that provides rigidity and structural stability. This characteristic enables them to survive in harsh environments while also aiding in immune evasion. Using a variety of virulence factors, including surface antigens and polysaccharides, these pathogens can adhere to host tissues, cause infections, and trigger inflammatory responses. When bacterial components interact with host immune cells, they initiate inflammatory processes, which can, paradoxically, lead to tissue damage and worsen disease symptoms, thus promoting disease progression and persistence. Additionally, the secretion of specific proteins is vital to Gram-positive pathogenicity.

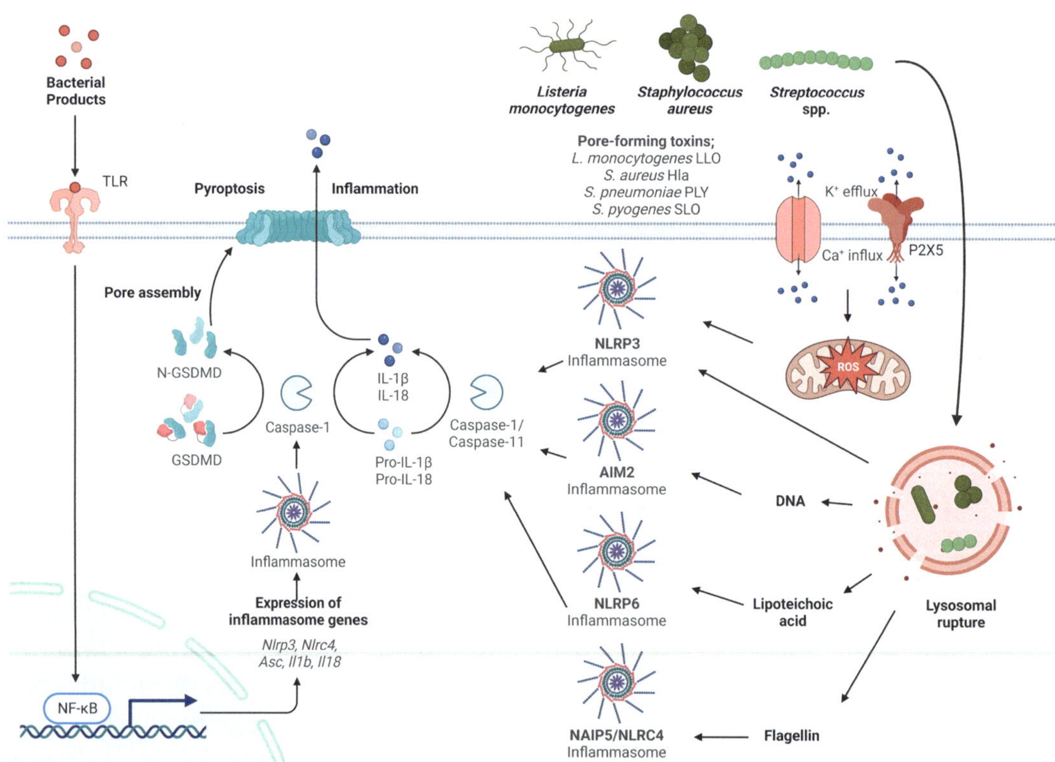

Figure 8.8. Inflammasome activation by Gram-positive bacteria.

Source: https://www.frontiersin.org/files/Articles/1075834/fimmu-14-1075834-HTML/image_m/fimmu-14-1075834-g001.jpg.

These secreted proteins modulate host immune responses and improve bacterial survival. For instance, research on *Mycobacterium tuberculosis* has shown that secreted proteins, such as Ag85B, follow complex secretion patterns that differ among bacterial strains, indicating a dynamic regulatory mechanism during infection (Bolz et al., 2019). Unlike Gram-negative bacteria, which use type III secretion systems to directly transfer virulence factors into host cells, Gram-positive bacteria usually use secreted proteins to indirectly modify host cell functions, aiding colonization and infection. This variability in protein secretion and expression highlights the adaptability of Gram-positive pathogens and presents challenges for diagnosis and effective treatment, given the variability in pathology associated with different bacterial strains. Understanding how Gram-positive bacteria cause disease is essential for developing targeted therapies and vaccines. The complex interaction between bacterial virulence factors and host immune responses calls for a coordinated research effort. Although advances in vaccine development against certain pathogens are promising, challenges remain in managing the diversity of immune responses triggered by different bacterial strains. The regulation of secreted proteins and their interactions with host cells is an important area for further investigation, especially regarding how these interactions influence infection outcomes (Garrido et al., 2020). Such insights could improve clinical interventions by identifying novel treatments that inhibit pathogenic processes and strengthen host immune defences, ultimately leading to better management of Gram-positive bacterial infections (Figure 8.8). *Staphylococcus aureus*

8.3.1. Mechanisms of Virulence

Understanding the mechanisms of virulence in Gram-positive bacterial infections is crucial for designing effective therapeutic interventions. The ability of the bacterium to adhere to host tissues is a key feature of virulence and a prerequisite for successful colonization. Gram-positive bacteria, such as Streptococcus pyogenes, possess numerous adhesion factors that enable attachment to epithelial cells and tissues. These adhesins not only help bacteria maintain their position within the host but also trigger inflammatory responses that can be exploited by the bacteria. Therefore, the fine line between adhesion and immune evasion highlights both the extent of bacterial pathogenesis and the importance of targeting these processes in therapy. Besides adhesion, Gram-positive bacteria also use a variety of virulence factors to evade the host immune response. For example, *S. pyogenes* employs proteinaceous virulence factors like M protein and streptolysins to escape phagocytosis and enhance survival within immune cells. These virulence factors disrupt normal immune functions and facilitate the growth and dissemination of severe infections such as necrotising fasciitis and toxic shock syndrome. Understanding these mechanisms not only sheds light on the pathogenicity of such bacteria but also emphasises the need for innovative approaches to boost immune responses or inhibit these virulence factors. The recent rise in antibiotic resistance necessitates a new approach to combat these stubborn pathogens. Additionally, the ability of Gram-positive bacteria to form biofilms significantly enhances their pathogenicity. Biofilms are complex communities of bacteria embedded within a protective matrix, enabling chronic infections — particularly on implanted medical devices and chronic wounds. Not only does the biofilm lifestyle shield bacteria from host immunity and antibiotics, but it also promotes inter-bacterial communication through quorum sensing, which increases their virulence as a collective. Interventions that disrupt the formation and stability of biofilms are vital for controlling Gram-positive bacterial infections. Trends in materials science, supported by recent literature, point towards promising new antimicrobial strategies that render bacteria producing biofilms vulnerable to attack, potentially reducing the infection load of these stubborn bacteria (Cevallos, 2008; Bassegoda et al., 2018).

8.3.2. Host Immune Response

The host immune response plays a crucial role in combating infections caused by various bacteria, such as Gram-positive bacteria. When confronted with these pathogens, the immune system deploys multiple layers of defense, beginning with physical barriers such as the skin and mucosal membranes, which prevent bacterial entry. The innate immune system responds promptly through well-coordinated mechanisms, including the activation of phagocytic cells like macrophages and neutrophils, which engulf and eliminate invading bacteria. Furthermore, the secretion of antimicrobial peptides and proteins, such as lactoferrin, is vital in initiating inflammation and recruiting immune cells to the infected site. Given that Gram-positive bacteria often possess distinctive cell wall structures, such as peptidoglycan, these components are recognized by the immune system, facilitating an effective response that limits bacterial proliferation and prevents systemic infection. Following the initial innate response, an adaptive immune response is activated, providing a more targeted response to Gram-positive bacterial infections. This system is characterised by specificity and immunological memory, involving the activation of T and B lymphocytes. T cells can orchestrate immune responses and assist in B cell activation, which leads to the secretion of antibodies against bacterial antigens. Interestingly, Gram-positive bacteria may exploit specific virulence factors that manipulate the immune response to persist within the host for extended periods. Of particular significance is their interaction with dendritic cells, as these antigen-presenting cells serve as a bridge between innate and adaptive immunity through the processing and presentation of antigens to naïve T cells.

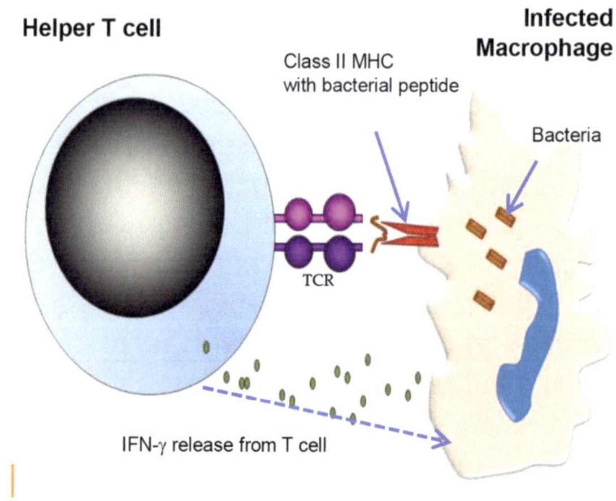

Figure 8.9. Immune responses to bacteria.

Source: https://www.immunology.org/public-information/bitesized-immunology/pathogens-disease/immune-responses-bacteria-0.

It is crucial to comprehend the complexity of these interactions for the advancement of therapeutic interventions aimed at augmenting the host's defense against pathogenic Gram-positive microorganisms. Moreover, interactions between the host immune system and Gram-positive bacteria offer valuable insights into potential treatment mechanisms. Given that lactoferrin has demonstrated antimicrobial and immunomodulatory properties, understanding its role as a component of host defense may lead to novel therapeutic approaches for combating infection. For example, the expression of lactoferrin receptors by human cholangiocytes has shown to promote cell proliferation, and supplementation has exhibited potential in restoring mucosal immunity during infection. As it is well established that pathogens utilize diverse mechanisms to evade immune defences, additional research is required to fully understand these interactions. A detailed examination of how Gram-positive bacteria evade or subvert specific immune mechanisms is essential for the development of targeted treatments that enhance immune responses, thereby potentially reducing the prevalence of related diseases and improving infection outcomes caused by these resilient microorganisms (Bernal-Bayard & Ramos-Morales; Valenti et al., 2018, 2017).

8.3.3. Factors Contributing to Infection Severity

In the examination of contributing factors to the virulence of Gram-positive infections, it is paramount to recognise the host' s immune response. The adaptive and innate immune responses determine clinical outcomes following pathogen exposure. When immune responses are compromised, as observed in patients with acute-on-chronic liver failure (ACLF), the risk of severe infection is significantly increased. Studies have demonstrated that immune paresis in these patients results in the accumulation of myeloid- derived suppressor cells (M-MDSCS), which inhibit T cell activation and diminish innate immune activity. This immunosuppression facilitates bacterial proliferation and correlates with increased mortality from secondary infections and heightened disease severity. Therefore, a comprehensive understanding of immune mechanisms is essential for assessing infection risk within vulnerable populations. An additional pivotal factor influencing infection severity is the presence of comorbidities that may impair immunity. Conditions such as diabetes mellitus, chronic liver disease, and obesity can compromise immune function, thereby elevating susceptibility to Gram-positive bacterial infections. For example, diabetic individuals often display dysfunctional neutrophils and impaired cytokine responses vital for effective bacterial clearance. The coexistence of inflammatory states with inadequate immune responses can exacerbate the severity of infections. Additionally, acute liver failure is associated with the release of inflammatory mediators such as interleukin-6 (IL-6), which can prolong patient vulnerability and adverse outcomes. Consequently, the management of coexisting conditions is crucial in reducing infection severity among affected patients. Iron metabolism is also a key factor in the severity of infections. Bacteria require iron for proliferation, and disruptions in iron homeostasis can significantly impair host defences against infection. Human lactoferrin (hLf) and bovine lactoferrin (bLf) exert inhibitory effects on bacterial growth due to their capacity to bind iron, thereby restricting pathogen nutrient availability. Moreover, in inflammatory states, bLf possesses anti-inflammatory properties capable of modulating immune responses, which is beneficial in cases of anemia of inflammation (AI). Excess iron renders the host increasingly susceptible to infections, a phenomenon observed in various clinical conditions. Mechanisms that regulate iron availability and bolster immune functions, such as bLf supplementation, present promising therapeutic potential in mitigating the severity of infections caused by Gram- positive bacteria, and may be advantageous in the treatment of acute and chronic inflammatory diseases.

8.4. Diagnosis of Gram-positive Bacterial Infections

The diagnosis of Gram-positive bacterial infections necessitates an interdisciplinary approach that incorporates both clinical evaluation and laboratory results. Clinically, the presentation of symptoms such as fever, localised pain, and swelling often initiates suspicion. Nonetheless, laboratory analysis — particularly Gram staining — serves as a crucial confirmatory method. This traditional yet straightforward technique classifies bacteria as either Gram- positive or Gram-negative based on cell wall properties. The detection of Gram-positive cocci, such as *Staphylococcus aureus* or streptococci, in purulent material can be strongly indicative of infection. However, clinicians must exercise caution, as Gram stains may sometimes yield false results. For example, in cervico-facial sepsis, a study revealed that although most specimens stained Gram-negative, few cultured Gram-negative bacteria, underscoring the necessity of employing advanced microbiological culture methods alongside staining (Barnard, 2019). Laboratory culture remains the definitive standard for accurate diagnosis of Gram- positive bacterial infections. Following Gram staining, specific cultures are conducted to isolate the pathogen, thereby enabling precise identification. Cultures also facilitate the determination of antibiotic susceptibility profiles, which are essential for guiding effective treatment. The emergence of antibiotic- resistant strains, notably methicillin-resistant *Staphylococcus aureus* (MRSA), complicates this process. Without susceptibility testing, healthcare providers may resort to empirical treatments that may prove ineffective. Furthermore, healthcare-associated infections frequently involve Gram- positive organisms; thus, clinicians must remain vigilant when obtaining patient histories, paying particular attention to prior antibiotic exposure and hospitalization, as these factors significantly influence infection dynamics (Merli et al., 2015). Consequently, ongoing research into infection and resistance patterns is vital for enhancing diagnostic techniques. Ultimately, accurate diagnosis of Gram-positive bacterial infections is critical to ensuring optimal treatment outcomes and reducing complications. Advances in laboratory technologies, such as molecular diagnostics including polymerase chain reaction (PCR), supplement traditional methods, enabling rapid pathogen detection from clinical samples. These improvements are especially valuable for early intervention in severe infections, where delays may result in additional morbidity. Nonetheless, practitioners must carefully interpret laboratory results to prevent misdiagnosis, particularly in cases involving polymicrobial infections or discordant Gram-negative findings. The integration of clinical evaluation, Gram staining, and culture techniques provides a comprehensive framework for the effective diagnosis of Gram- positive infections, underscoring the importance of continuous education and adaptation to current microbiological trends in clinical practice.

8.4.1. Clinical Symptoms and Signs

*Staphylococcus aureus*The clinical signs and manifestations of Gram-positive bacterial infections can vary significantly depending on the specific bacteria involved and the site of infection. The most common symptoms include fever, local infection, pain, and possibly systemic effects such as septicemia. For example, *Staphylococcus aureus* infections frequently present as skin abscesses or severe forms like pneumonia, and can quickly progress to sepsis if untreated. Conversely, infections caused by *Streptococcus* species may lead to pharyngitis or rheumatic fever. The main challenge lies in the non-specificity of these symptoms, which often results in misdiagnosis. Consequently, clinical assessment is essential to identify the primary infection, potential complications, and suitable treatment options. While Gram-positive infections are usually indicated by clinical signs, laboratory confirmation is often necessary. For instance, the presence of purulent drainage or local swelling combined with systemic signs such as fever can trigger further testing. In some cases, urine culture can detect pathogens like *Enterococcus*, particularly in urinary tract infections. However, a concern in elderly patients is the prevalence of asymptomatic bacteriuria, where patients exhibit vague symptoms and may unnecessarily receive antibiotics (Beveridge et al., 2011) (Figure 8.10).

This raises the issue of the validity of symptomatic presentation in elderly adults, highlighting the significance of sensitive diagnostic criteria that consider age-specific variables. The integration of clinical signs and laboratory data is crucial in differentiating true infections from contaminated samples and, consequently, in ensuring appropriate therapeutic interventions.

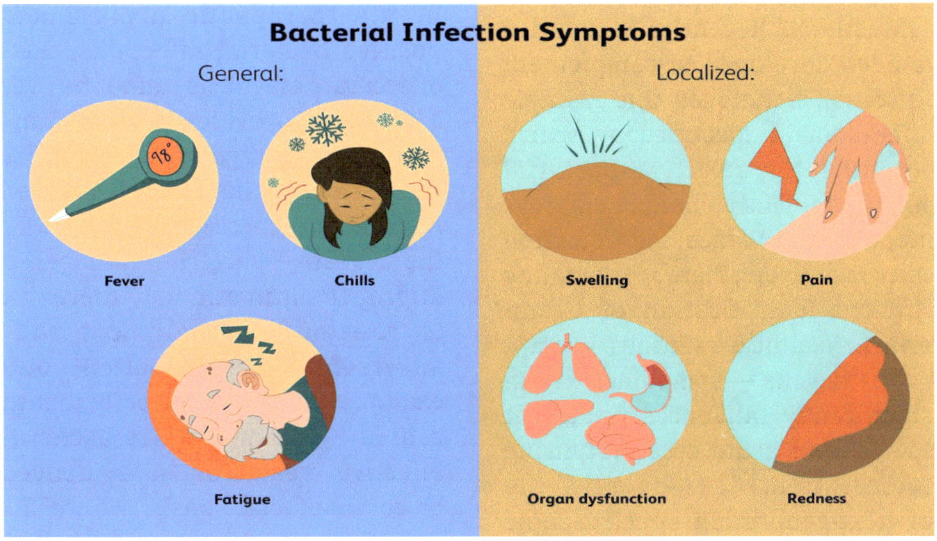

Figure 8.10. Symptoms associated with Gram-positive bacterial infections.

Source: https://external-content.duckduckgo.com/iu/?u=https%3A%2F%2Fwww.verywellhealth.com%2Fthmb%2FKwnReRJMLfmH9BZ15_i2YniYjME%3D%2F1500x0%2Ffilters%3Ano_upscale()%3Amax_bytes(150000)%3Astrip_icc()%2Fwhat-is-a-bacterial-infection-7705652_final-2f1b8b2429b2495c8333b584512d3afa.jpg&f=1&nofb=1&ipt=4c58893afed2e6b37cd6cf4c25b3156ae26f489e6b3080a7106bbd126c79be0d.

Moreover, individualised clinical signs may serve as indicators of specific infectious pathogens, thus providing valuable guidance for clinicians. Regarding urinary tract infections (UTIS), symptoms such as fever and dysuria may predispose individuals to underlying conditions, including potential Gram-positive bacterial infections like those caused by *Enterococcus* (Msaki et al., 2012). The identification of such signs can inform targeted treatment protocols, particularly in children, where febrile illnesses may result from multiple bacterial infections. Given the increasing emergence of multidrug resistance among Gram-positive bacteria, it is imperative to understand their clinical implications for effective management. Healthcare professionals must remain vigilant and stay informed about evolving resistance patterns and symptomatology to deliver appropriate and prompt treatment, thereby effectively combating these infections.

8.4.2. Laboratory Techniques for Identification

Identification of Gram-positive bacterial infections relies on a range of advanced laboratory techniques. Among these, Gram staining remains indispensable for the rapid differentiation of bacteria based on cell wall composition. Following this preliminary identification, further analysis can be conducted through biochemical tests, which assess specific enzymatic activities or metabolic processes characteristic of individual Gram-positive genera. Molecular methodologies, particularly polymerase chain reaction (PCR), have gained prominence due to their capacity to amplify specific DNA sequences, enabling precise identification even in samples with low bacterial density. Such approaches exemplify the multidisciplinary nature of clinical microbiology, which is essential for accurate diagnosis and effective treatment of bacterial infections. Recently, innovative methods have been developed to complement classical identification techniques. One example is terahertz time-domain spectroscopy, which offers the potential for selective bacterial species discrimination. This technique employs plasmonic antennas to enhance the detection sensitivity of microbial layers, thereby facilitating rapid and efficient identification of Gram-positive bacteria. In healthcare settings, prompt identification of pathogens — sometimes within minutes — significantly influences treatment outcomes, especially in acute cases requiring immediate intervention. Consequently, the integration of next-generation spectroscopic methods represents a paradigm shift, promising improved and expedited diagnostic capabilities in microbiological infections (Berrier et al., 2012).

The evolving landscape of diagnostic methodologies underscores the necessity of keeping pace with advancements in microbiology technology. As techniques such as terahertz spectroscopy increasingly replace traditional microbiological procedures, laboratories are better equipped to perform rapid and accurate pathogen identification. As these methods continue to develop, their incorporation into routine clinical practice will enhance diagnostic accuracy and patient care. Furthermore, these advancements highlight the importance of ongoing research and development in clinical microbiology to ensure that healthcare professionals have access to the most effective tools for combating Gram-positive bacterial infections. The availability of sophisticated identification techniques not only improves epidemiological data collection but also supports more personalised treatment strategies and infection management (Mkrtchyan et al., 2013).

8.4.3. Importance of Accurate Diagnosis

In the therapeutic management of Gram-positive bacterial infections, the significance of accurate diagnosis cannot be overstated. Such a diagnosis provides a foundation for effective treatment strategies, which is especially vital in the context of the escalating issue of antibiotic resistance. Incorrect or delayed identification of the causative bacterial pathogen can result in improper antibiotic use, thereby contributing to resistance development and potentially adversely affecting patient outcomes. For example, failure to correctly identify infections caused by Gram-negative bacteria may hinder effective treatment, as evidenced in studies of cervico-facial sepsis, where Gram-negative organisms were rarely isolated despite their presence in Gram stains (Barnard, 2019). Clinicians must prioritise the detection of clinical signs and the correct interpretation of laboratory results to confirm the presence of resistant strains. Furthermore, precise diagnosis is essential in improving prognoses, particularly among high-risk groups such as patients with cirrhosis or immunosuppression. Studies have indicated that bacterial infections often produce negative microbiological results despite clinical indications (Boaretti et al., 2016). This underscores the necessity of diagnostic approaches that integrate culture techniques with other methods, including molecular diagnostics, to detect bacterial DNA or other markers at an early stage. Such advancements would facilitate the identification of subclinical infections, enabling timely intervention that enhances clinical outcomes and reduces mortality. Employing comprehensive diagnostic strategies allows for a more sophisticated understanding and management of infections, tailored to the individual patient's clinical presentation. Ultimately, accurate diagnosis is not only critical for immediate clinical decision-making but also has significant and lasting public health and antibiotic stewardship implications. Inaccurate or delayed diagnosis can lead to ineffective treatment regimens, prolonging illness duration and increasing the risk of transmission within communities. Given that Gram-positive bacterial infections continue to burden healthcare systems, it is essential to upgrade diagnostic procedures to empower healthcare providers to make informed decisions swiftly. This system can minimise the risks associated with undiagnosed infections, optimise resource utilisation, and ultimately reduce healthcare costs. Emphasising precise diagnosis in the treatment of Gram-positive bacterial infections is a vital step towards enhancing patient safety, improving treatment quality, and mitigating the public health threat of antibiotic resistance.Barnard, 2019

8.5. Treatment Options for Gram-positive Bacterial Infections

Gram-positive bacterial infections are addressed through a comprehensive approach, primarily involving antimicrobial therapy. Antibiotics such as penicillins, cephalosporins, and vancomycin have constituted the foundation of treatment regimens for many years. These agents target the peptidoglycan cell wall characteristic of Gram-positive bacteria, resulting in the disruption of bacterial integrity and subsequent cell lysis. Nonetheless, the emergence of antibiotic resistance, notably among pathogens such as Methicillin-resistant *Staphylococcus aureus* (MRSA), highlights the necessity for continual vigilance and adaptation in therapeutic strategies. In veterinary medicine, similar principles apply, as evidenced by recent guidelines developed by expert working groups aimed at assisting veterinarians in the selection of suitable antimicrobials for respiratory diseases in companion animals, thereby reflecting an increased regard for treatment specifics across human and veterinary medicine (Lappin et al., 2017). Beyond traditional antibiotics, researchers are exploring alternative therapeutic agents, especially in response to rising resistance. Antimicrobial peptides such as Pep19–2.5 demonstrate promising potential through their ability to neutralise pathogenic organisms by exhibiting activity against both Gram-positive and Gram-negative bacteria. These peptides have shown significant activity by inhibiting vital cellular processes, such as phosphorylation involved in inflammatory responses. Importantly, preliminary data suggest that these peptides exhibit low cytotoxicity across various cell types and foster cellular migration, an activity that may enhance wound healing in skin infections. This innovative approach indicates that peptide-based therapies may serve as adjuncts to conventional antibiotics, offering a dual mechanism of action that not only targets bacterial pathogens but also supports host recovery from infections (Pfalzgraff et al., 2016). Overall, the landscape of Gram-positive bacterial infection management is transforming, addressing both the urgent need for effective antibiotics and the looming challenge of antibiotic resistance. As advanced treatment modalities, such as antimicrobial peptides, are studied more extensively, their integration with traditional antibiotic therapies could potentially lead to more effective management strategies. Such a combination of conventional and novel therapies holds promise not only for human medicine but also in veterinary practice, where protocols are being developed to optimise treatment approaches for bacterial infections in animals and to emphasise the importance of targeted antimicrobial therapy in achieving optimal patient outcomes (Lappin et al., 2017). Consequently, the future of combating Gram-positive bacterial infections will hinge on a thorough understanding of microbial resistance patterns and the development of innovative therapeutic strategies.*Staphylococcus aureus*

.

8.5.1. Antibiotic Therapies

The development of antibiotic therapies targeting Gram-positive infections has dramatically evolved over the past decades. Previously, the discovery of antibiotics such as penicillin was crucial in transforming the treatment of bacterial infections, playing a significant role in reducing death rates and improving patient survival. However, the rise of antibiotic resistance has become a clear obstacle in infection management. As bacteria grow more resistant to commonly used antibiotics, clinicians are increasingly forced to reconsider their empirical regimens. The slow pace of new antibiotic development is concerning, since most newly introduced drugs are variations of existing classes, offering limited options against resistant organisms. Additionally, the emergence of multidrug-resistant pathogens threatens the effectiveness of standard treatments, heightening the need for new approaches and drug development (PEW Charitable Trust Report, 2016). Evidence now highlights the pivotal role of antibiotic therapy in the development of multi-resistant infections, especially among vulnerable patient groups. For example, cirrhotic patients show a significantly higher rate of infections with multi-resistant pathogens, complicating antibiotic management. In a recent prospective study, isolates from 51% of cirrhotic patients were multidrug-resistant, underscoring the importance of enhanced epidemiological data and tailored empirical antibiotic regimens. Risk factors such as recent healthcare exposure are major influences shaping resistance patterns, implicating healthcare-associated infections in treatment failures. Awareness of these complexities underpins the need to inform clinicians about the intricate dynamics of Gram-positive bacterial infections and resistance (Merli et al., 2015). To combat the rising incidence of resistance, healthcare systems must prioritise the development of comprehensive global strategies to optimise antibiotic use. Implementing rapid diagnostic techniques can facilitate the timely identification of pathogens and their susceptibility, leading to more effective treatment. Furthermore, enhancements in antibiotic stewardship programmes are essential to promote judicious use of existing therapies and prevent further resistance. Preventive measures, including vaccination and strict infection control protocols, are also vital in reducing resistant Gram-positive bacterial infections. Through fostering interdisciplinary collaboration among healthcare professionals, researchers, and policymakers, the medical community can strengthen its response to the dual challenge of Gram-positive bacterial infections and resistance, ultimately improving patient outcomes.

8.5.2. Challenges of Antibiotic Resistance

Antibiotic resistance represents a complex emerging issue that poses a substantial threat to global health, particularly concerning infections caused by Gram-positive bacteria. The once-reliable protective barrier offered by antibiotics is increasingly compromised due to the continual evolution of bacterial species. When Gram-positive pathogens develop resistance mechanisms, conventional treatment regimens, which were previously effective, become ineffective. This situation is exacerbated by the lack of development of new antibiotics, as their introduction has significantly declined since the 1980s, resulting in most available drugs being merely derivatives of older classes. This stagnation underscores the urgent need for renewed focus on antibiotic discovery to address the escalating threat of resistance and to sustain therapeutic efficacy against Gram-positive infections (PEW Charitable Trust Report, 2016). Furthermore, the overuse and misuse of antibiotics, in both human healthcare and veterinary contexts, contribute substantially to resistance development. Indiscriminate application of antibiotics in clinical settings and in agriculture — where they are used to promote growth — has led to the emergence of multidrug-resistant (MDR) organisms, complicating treatment efforts. Antimicrobial resistance (AMR) is most conspicuous in environments where antibiotics are overutilized, often unnecessarily, thereby undermining the effectiveness of existing antimicrobial agents and jeopardising healthcare systems. Recognising the interconnectedness of antibiotic stewardship, access, and resistance necessitates collaborative efforts across public and private sectors to ensure antibiotics remain potent weapons in combating Gram-positive bacterial infections (Jenner et al., 2017). Addressing the multifaceted challenges posed by antibiotic resistance requires comprehensive strategies encompassing research, policy formulation, and education. Innovation in diagnostics and the development of region-specific vaccines are vital to revitalising the antibiotic pipeline. Simultaneously, governance and international cooperation must be prioritised to address resistance holistically. These initiatives should include increasing awareness about the consequences of antibiotic misuse and establishing robust frameworks to promote responsible prescribing practices. By fostering a culture of stewardship and ensuring equitable access to essential treatments, the global community can mitigate the impact of antibiotic resistance on Gram-positive infections, thereby safeguarding public health for the long term (PEW Charitable Trust Report, 2016; Jenner et al., 2017) (Figure 8.11).

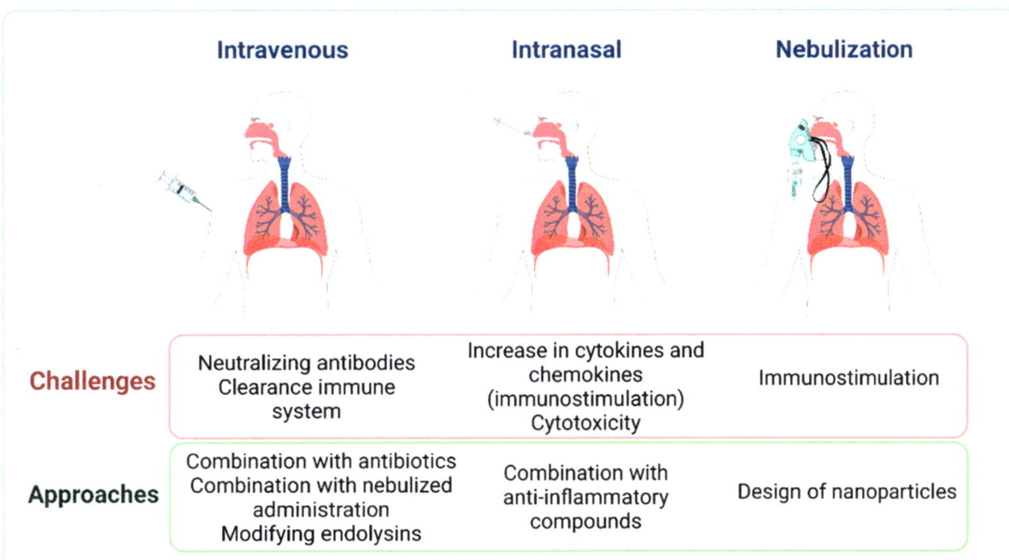

Figure 8.11. Different possibilities for delivery of phage therapy for the treatment of pneumonia caused by Gram-positive bacteria.

Source: https://www.mdpi.com/2079-6382/10/8/1000.

8.5.3. Alternative Treatment Strategies

The issue of antibiotic resistance, particularly concerning Gram-positive infections, has garnered significant interest in alternative therapeutic strategies. Traditional antibiotic treatments are increasingly ineffective due to the rapid emergence of resistant strains, commonly referred to as superbugs. In response to this urgent need, researchers are exploring innovative techniques aimed at countering bacterial virulence and biofilm formation, both of which are central to persistent infections. Promising laboratory-scale approaches include the use of bactericides that operate via mechanisms distinct from those of conventional antibiotics. The latest advancements feature engineered materials, such as nanoparticles and hydrogels, which exhibit novel antimicrobial properties capable of inhibiting resistant bacterial proliferation and preventing the dissemination of infections. These advancements not only address current infections but also serve a preventive role against potential future epidemics, thereby supporting public health initiatives. Another highly promising alternative treatment is phage therapy, which utilizes bacteriophages — viruses that specifically infect bacteria — to eliminate Gram-positive pathogens. The feasibility of phage therapy is increasing as awareness grows regarding the limitations of traditional antibiotics against resistant strains. Given their ability to target and destroy specific bacterial cells, bacteriophages offer a compelling approach to treating infections caused by highly resistant bacteria. Furthermore, research indicates that phages can enhance the efficacy of existing antibiotics, inhibit biofilm formation, and contribute to the development of new biological therapeutic modalities as adjuncts to conventional treatments. This multifaceted approach aims not only to eradicate bacteria but also to mitigate the development of antibiotic resistance. Consequently, phage therapy emerges as a promising strategy with the potential to become a vital tool in combating Gram-positive bacterial infections. Additionally, the development of immunotherapies presents a promising frontier in the fight against Gram-positive bacterial infections. By harnessing the body's immune system, these approaches seek to bolster natural defences rather than relying solely on antimicrobial agents. For instance, monoclonal antibodies can be engineered to specifically bind to bacterial cells, facilitating their destruction by immune cells. This method not only reduces the likelihood of resistance development but also provides a targeted means of pathogen elimination. Recent studies underscore that immunotherapeutic agents have demonstrated considerable effectiveness in reducing morbidity and mortality associated with severe bacterial infections. This paradigm shift aligns with the demand for sustainable treatments, especially as conventional antibiotics become less effective, thereby underscoring the importance of investigating alternative therapeutic strategies as integral components of modern medical practice (PEW Charitable Trust Report, 2016; Bassegoda et al., 2018).

8.6. Prevention and Control Measures

Effective prevention and control strategies are crucial in reducing the impact of Gram-positive bacterial diseases, which have become a significant public health concern in increasing numbers. The introduction of antibiotics revolutionised infection treatment; however, the rise in antibiotic-resistant microorganisms necessitates strategic intervention in prevention efforts. Proper education on antibiotic use is vital, as indiscriminate misuse has led to the emergence of resistant bacteria. As noted by Lillestolen (2018), despite increased understanding of resistance mechanisms, the fight is far from over. Promoting appropriate prescription practices among clinicians and raising public awareness about adhering to prescribed antibiotic dosages can effectively decrease unnecessary drug exposure, thereby helping to contain resistance. Besides careful antibiotic use, maintaining good hygiene practices is essential in managing Gram-positive bacterial infections. Strict sanitation in hospitals and community settings can lower transmission rates, including frequent handwashing, disinfection of medical equipment, and surface cleaning — especially in hospitals with higher infection rates. As explained by Klaas & Zadoks (2018), livestock industries must prioritise management and hygiene practices to control environmental pathogens. By fostering clean environments and providing infection control training, health systems can develop strategies that effectively reduce infection outbreaks, alleviating the burden of Gram-positive bacteria on public health. Vaccination is also a key element in preventing Gram-positive bacterial infections. While vaccine development targeting specific pathogens progresses unevenly, some vaccines protect against causative agents of environmental mastitis, such as *Escherichia coli*. However, vaccine development for Gram-positive bacteria remains at the experimental stage, as documented by Klaas & Zadoks (2018). Increased investment in vaccine research and development offers a proactive approach to disease management. These efforts should also aim to improve diagnostic technologies for accurate pathogen identification, enabling targeted interventions. Through focused vaccine research, coupled with enhanced diagnostics and patient education, health authorities can shape effective control strategies, ultimately reducing the prevalence and incidence of Gram-positive bacterial infections.

8.6.1. Vaccination Strategies

Vaccination strategies constitute a vital element in combating Gram-positive bacterial infections, especially in light of the escalating issue of antibiotic resistance. These approaches not only aim to prevent disease but also serve to reinforce the immune response against specific bacterial pathogens. The development of vaccines targeting mechanisms of bacterial adherence has gained considerable importance, given the significant role adherence plays in pathogenesis. By inhibiting the initial steps of binding necessary for infection and colonization, vaccine formulations can substantially reduce the risk of disease. Furthermore, advances in technology, including the application of novel antivirulence therapies, offer new prospects for vaccine development against Gram-positive bacteria, highlighting the urgent need for innovative approaches as resistance and treatment challenges intensify (Cusumano et al., 2016). In the context of environmental mastitis caused by Gram-positive bacteria, vaccination represents a practical strategy for management, considering the widespread issue within dairy herds. Amid increased regulatory scrutiny and challenges associated with traditional antimicrobial controls, particularly concerning antibiotic resistance, preventive measures such as vaccination have become increasingly critical. Vaccines currently available for coliform mastitis have demonstrated efficacy; however, for Gram-positive pathogens such as *Staphylococcus aureus*, only promising candidates exist, which still require further validation in clinical settings. It is essential to enhance education and communication between veterinarians and farmers to facilitate the adoption of vaccination strategies, potentially leading to a substantial decline in the prevalence of these diseases. Such proactive measures not only promote animal welfare but also align with societal pressures to minimise antimicrobial use in agriculture (Klaas & Zadoks, 2018) (Figure 8.12).

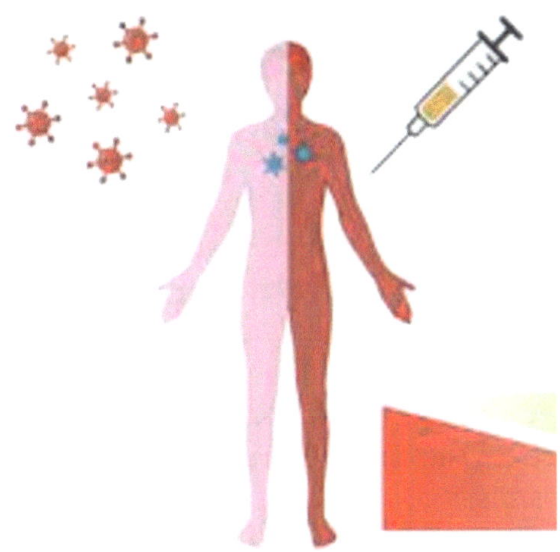

Figure 8.12. Vaccination strategies represent a pivotal component in the fight against Gram-positive bacterial infections.

Source: https://encrypted-tbn0.gstatic.com/images?q=tbn:ANd9GcQDEMDtHrzzYXix8hEP3kih06ox5xMhEEBWPjwtYt9_8njmFrSrj4O0agK40PE11chrj1Q&usqp=CAU.

Ongoing research in the fields of development and vaccine creation must be complemented by comprehensive strategies that address the multifaceted nature of Gram-positive bacterial diseases. These strategies should encompass improved diagnostic procedures for the precise isolation of pathogens, thereby facilitating the development of targeted vaccines capable of effectively attacking specific strains. Investigations into the mechanisms by which Gram-positive bacteria evade immune responses are also vital to inform future vaccine development. A deeper understanding of the complexities of host-pathogen interactions will significantly enhance the creation of vaccines that elicit stronger and more durable immunity. Furthermore, given the persistent threat posed by emerging antibiotic resistance, the integration of successful vaccination strategies into both veterinary and human public health initiatives will be crucial in combating Gram-positive bacterial infections and safeguarding animal and human populations (Cusumano et al., 2016).

8.6.2. Hygiene and Sanitation Practices

The relationship between sanitary habits, hygiene, and the prevention of Gram-positive bacterial infections is of paramount importance. Handwashing, waste disposal, and sterilisation of equipment constitute essential hygienic practices that serve as a barrier against bacterial transmission. Gram-positive bacteria, such as *Staphylococcus aureus*, tend to proliferate in environments characterised by poor hygiene, thereby facilitating infection dissemination. The implementation of rigorous hygiene protocols within healthcare facilities has contributed significantly to the reduction of infection rates. Inadequate sanitation not only increases the risk of disease spread within hospitals but also worsens pre-existing medical conditions among vulnerable populations. Educating the public on the importance of hygiene can substantially diminish infection risks by cultivating habits that interrupt transmission cycles. Community participation in hygienic practices is also crucial for effective public health management. Educational campaigns aimed at raising awareness about the significance of handwashing, proper food handling, and access to clean water are instrumental in decreasing the incidence of Gram-positive infections. Combining educational efforts with practical demonstrations enhances understanding and reinforces adherence to best practices. Public health policies should incorporate such educational initiatives and ensure consistent messaging to communities, including those in low-income areas, regarding the vital role of hygiene in disease prevention. Improved community perceptions of hygiene can lead to more vigorous infection control measures and ultimately reduce morbidity and mortality associated with Gram-positive bacterial infections.

Furthermore, the role of sanitation in managing antimicrobial resistance cannot be overstated. The misuse and overuse of antibiotics in human medicine and agriculture, coupled with inadequate sanitation, create environments conducive to the development of resistant bacterial strains. Evidence indicates that sanitation improvements can effectively mitigate the spread of resistant microorganisms (Lillestolen, 2018). Increasing awareness of the One Health approach, which recognises the interconnectedness of human, animal, and environmental health (Dar et al., 2015), underscores the importance of integrated strategies. By strengthening sanitation and hygiene practices, societies can not only prevent the transmission of Gram-positive infections but also contribute to more effective management of antimicrobial resistance, thereby preserving the efficacy of existing antibiotics for a longer period.*Staphylococcus aureus*

8.6.3. Public Health Initiatives

Public health interventions play an essential role in managing the escalating threat of Gram-positive infections, especially amid rising antibiotic resistance. The increase of Gram-positive pathogens such as *Staphylococcus aureus* and *Streptococcus pneumoniae* underscores the necessity of effective public health measures rooted in prevention, surveillance, and education. Robust public health programs can mitigate the dissemination of these infections by advocating for the prudent use of antibiotics, thereby curbing the development of resistance. Raising awareness among healthcare professionals and the public about the importance of judicious antibiotic use is crucial to address the growing challenge posed by Gram-positive bacterial infections, which constitute a substantial obstacle to global health systems. Besides educational efforts, research dedicated to the development of novel therapeutics and diagnostic tools is vital for the efficacy of public health interventions against Gram-positive infections. The stagnation in antibiotic research and the emergence of resistant pathogens highlight the urgent need for innovative paradigms in research and development. Public health authorities must collaborate with private sector entities to facilitate the development of new antibiotics and alternative interventions, as current strategies often prove insufficient. Significant investment is required to initiate research efforts aimed not only at creating new treatments but also at enhancing the efficacy of existing medications. Both public initiatives and private innovation are pivotal in addressing the current deficiencies in combating Gram-positive infections and the rising tide of resistance. Furthermore, comprehensive governance and stewardship are integral components of public health strategies designed to prevent Gram-positive bacterial infections. Antimicrobial resistance constitutes a global challenge that transcends national borders and necessitates international cooperation. Countries must collaboratively formulate policies focused on antibiotic stewardship while ensuring equitable access to lifesaving medicines. This includes fostering environments conducive to research and development and promoting sustainable prescribing practices within healthcare systems. An effective public health strategy must support a globally coordinated framework that respects local needs while aligning with international efforts to prevent resistance development. Failure to harmonise such initiatives may result in widespread adverse health outcomes, emphasising the importance of sustained public health efforts in combating Gram-positive bacterial infections and antimicrobial resistance (PEW Charitable Trust Report, 2016; Jenner et al., 2017).

SUMMARY

In summarising the realm of Gram-positive bacterial infections, it is evident that comprehending their clinical significance is essential for developing effective management and therapeutic strategies. Gram-positive bacteria such as *Staphylococcus* and *Streptococcus* species are commonly implicated in various infections that may pose serious clinical challenges, especially in immunocompromised individuals. The distinction between Gram-positive and Gram-negative bacteria also forms the basis for defining treatment protocols, as existing research has identified differences in patient outcomes and microbial responses. Notably, Gram-positive infections present unique challenges, including patterns of antibiotic resistance, which complicate both diagnosis and therapy. Moreover, the relationship between Gram-positive infections and systemic conditions such as sepsis underscores the importance of comprehensive knowledge regarding lipid profiles in infected patients. Evidence from research indicates that alterations in lipid metabolism, particularly concerning high-density lipoprotein (HDL) and triglyceride levels, correlate with the severity and progression of these infections. For example, studies have demonstrated that patients with Gram-negative infections are more prone to significant lipid profile disturbances compared to those with Gram-positive infections, potentially impacting clinical outcomes such as organ failure and mortality (Wiguna et al., 2020). These findings highlight the significance of lipid assessments in the management of sepsis and bacterial infections. Ultimately, the complex nature of Gram-positive infections necessitates a multifaceted approach that integrates microbiological insights with comprehensive health evaluations. As ongoing research continues to explore the complications associated with such pathogens, clinicians must remain vigilant in updating their strategies to mitigate these issues. This encompasses not only the administration of effective antimicrobial therapies but also the formulation of thorough treatment protocols that consider underlying metabolic conditions and patient-specific risk factors. Further investigation into the role of lipid profiles during infections may yield vital knowledge to improve patient management and optimise treatment methodologies across diverse clinical scenarios (Barnard, 2019).Barnard, 2019

The field of Gram-positive bacterial infections offers a promising avenue for future research, particularly concerning the differential outcomes based on the timing of infection. Existing studies indicate inherent variations between first-hit and second-hit infections, specifically in bacterial organisms. For instance, data demonstrate that Gram-negative bacteria are associated with higher mortality rates in initial infections compared to Gram-positive bacteria, raising questions about the determinants contributing to these outcomes (Morgan et al., 2016). Investigating the genetic, microbiological, immunological, and environmental mechanisms that differentiate such infections could be instrumental in enhancing risk stratification protocols in clinical practice. This, in turn, has the potential to improve intensive care unit patient management and outcomes, emphasising the importance of understanding the complexity of bacterial behaviour in both acute and chronic infections. An additional vital area for future research involves adopting a comprehensive global perspective on Gram-positive bacterial infections, especially in developing regions. The approximately one million neonatal deaths annually attributable to invasive bacterial infections highlight an urgent need for epidemiological data specific to community-acquired infections in these regions (Ahmad et al., 2011). Understanding the prevalence and patterns of Gram-positive infections among neonates born in home or community settings can inform therapeutic strategies and guide the development of management protocols. Research in this domain not only contributes to reducing neonatal morbidity and mortality but also supports the formulation of targeted vaccination programs and treatment algorithms tailored to the challenges of low-resource settings. Consequently, examining the epidemiological characteristics of Gram-positive infections is crucial for effective public health initiatives. Finally, characterising the mechanisms underlying antibiotic resistance among Gram-positive bacteria should be a primary focus of future investigation. Despite the ongoing threat posed by resistant strains to existing treatment regimens, elucidating the genetic mutations and environmental pressures responsible for resistance provides a foundation for novel therapeutic approaches. The implications of such resistance are extensive, as they complicate the treatment of both initial and subsequent infections, as evidenced by variations in mortality rates across different bacterial species (Morgan et al., 2016). Collaborative efforts among researchers, clinicians, and public health professionals are essential to establish comprehensive surveillance systems and to employ advanced genomic tools for tracking resistant strains. Addressing these issues through future research efforts has the potential to significantly impact the global fight against Gram-positive infections, ultimately leading to improved patient outcomes and public health strategies.

CLOSER LOOK

LISTERIA MONOCYTOGENES

Listeria monocytogenes is a Gram-positive, facultatively anaerobic, rod-shaped bacterium and the causative agent of listeriosis, a life-threatening foodborne illness. It is non-sporing, catalase-positive, and has tumbling motility at room temperature due to having peritrichous flagella. Contrary to any of the foodborne pathogens, L. monocytogenes can grow at refrigerator temperatures (up to 0°C), and therefore it is a source of severe risk in chilled and ready-to-eat foods.

This microbe is widespread in the environment and is present in soil, water, plant material, and animal gut. It usually infects milk, soft cheese, cooked deli meats, raw vegetables, raw unpasteurized milk, and processed foods. Due to its resistance to cold, high salt, and low-acid conditions, L. monocytogenes poses a unique challenge to the food industry and requires extreme hygiene in food processing and storage.

Listeriosis is primarily seen in risk groups such as pregnant women, newborns, the elderly, and immunocompromised individuals. In healthy individuals, the infection may not be symptomatic or result in mild flu-like illness. However, some severe manifestations of the disease occur in risk groups such as septicemia, meningitis, encephalitis, and pregnancy loss. Newborns develop listeriosis by getting it transplacentally or at the time of birth and can develop preterm labor or stillbirth (Figure 8.13).

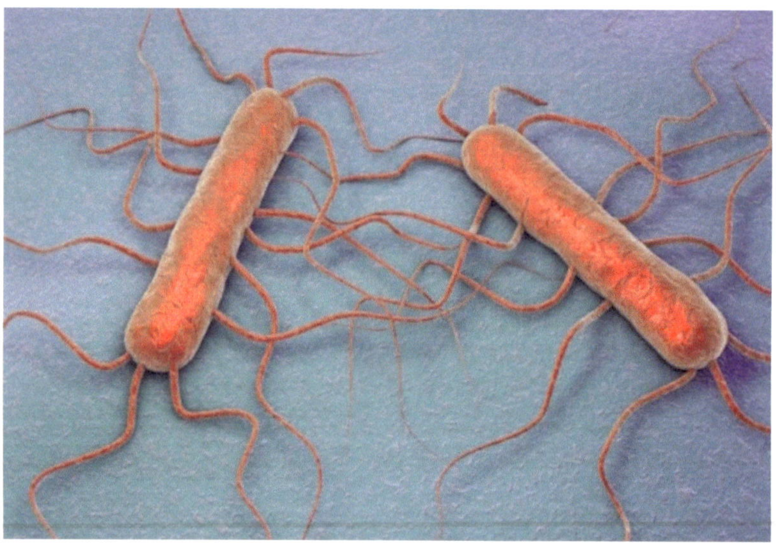

Figure 8.13. 3D illustration of motile, rod-shaped bacteria with flagella, enabling movement across surfaces. Such structures are characteristic of various pathogenic bacteria.

Source: https://www.news-medical.net/image-handler/picture/2021/9/shutterstock_400088737.jpg.

Pathogenicity of *L. monocytogenes* results from several virulence factors. These include internalins (InlA and InlB), responsible for the entry of bacteria into host cells, and listeriolysin O (LLO), a hemolysin that forms pores and enables the bacterium to escape into the cytoplasm from the phagosome. Upon entry into the cytoplasm, the bacterium exploits the host actin to travel and disperse from cell to cell, evading extracellular immune mechanisms. This intracellular existence makes L. monocytogenes very hard for the host to eradicate.

Diagnosis of listeriosis is usually achieved by the recovery of the organism from blood, cerebrospinal fluid, or amniotic fluid. Culture with subsequent biochemical examinations and molecular techniques like PCR confirms the identification. Early diagnosis is essential, particularly in invasive infections.

Treatment is by prompt antibiotics, using ampicillin (with gentamicin) as the first choice. Prevention involves good handling of food, avoiding high-risk foods during pregnancy, and strict control of the food industry.

References

1. Valenti, P., Rosa, L., Capobianco, D., Lepanto, M. S., Schiavi, E., Cutone, A., Paesano, R., & Mastromarino, P. (2018). Role of Lactobacilli and Lactoferrin in the Mucosal Cervicovaginal Defense. *Frontiers in immunology*, *9*, 376. https://doi.org/10.3389/fimmu.2018.00376(accessed on 16th July 2025).

2. Dar, O. A., Hasan, R., Schlundt, J., Harbarth, S., Caleo, G., Dar, F. K., Littmann, J., Rweyemamu, M., Buckley, E. J., Shahid, M., Kock, R., Li, H. L., Giha, H., Khan, M., So, A. D., Bindayna, K. M., Kessel, A., Pedersen, H. B., Permanand, G., Zumla, A., ... Heymann, D. L. (2016). Exploring the evidence base for national and regional policy interventions to combat resistance. *Lancet (London, England)*, *387*(10015), 285–295. https://doi.org/10.1016/S0140-6736(15)00520-6(accessed on 16th July 2025).

3. Berrier, A., Schaafsma, M. C., Nonglaton, G., Bergquist, J., & Rivas, J. G. (2012). Selective detection of bacterial layers with terahertz plasmonic antennas. *Biomedical optics express*, *3*(11), 2937–2949. https://doi.org/10.1364/BOE.3.002937(accessed on 16th July 2025).

4. Cusumano ZT.Klein RD.Hultgren SJ.2016.Innovative Solutions to Sticky Situations: Antiadhesive Strategies for Treating Bacterial Infections. Microbiol Spectr4:10.1128/microbiolspec.vmbf-0023-2015.https://doi.org/10.1128/microbiolspec.vmbf-0023-2015(accessed on 16th July 2025).

5. Adams, D. H., Antoniades, C. G., Bernsmeier, C., Brenig, C., et al. (2017). *CD14$^+$ CD15$^-$ HLA-DR$^-$ myeloid-derived suppressor cells impair antimicrobial responses in patients with acute-on-chronic liver failure.* https://core.ac.uk/download/287649765.pdf (accessed on 16th July 2025).

6. Ahmad, A., Campbell, H., Jawad, I., Lukšić, I., et al. (2011). *Aetiology of community-acquired neonatal sepsis in low and middle income countries.* https://core.ac.uk/download/28973480.pdf (accessed on 16th July 2025).

7. Yopie Wiguna, Philia Setiawan, Prananda Surya Airlangga(2020). *Hubungan profil lipid (kadar trigliserida, HDL, LDL, total kolesterol) dengan jenis infeksi bakteri pada pasien sepsis.* https://core.ac.uk/download/386326484.pdf (accessed on 16th July 2025).

8. Alebouyeh, M., Alizadeh, A. H. M., Majidi, M. R. S., Sherafat, S., et al. (2016). Association of diverse bacterial communities in human bile samples with biliary tract disorders: A survey using culture and polymerase chain reaction-denaturing gradient gel electrophoresis methods. https://core.ac.uk/download/52205553.pdf (accessed on 16th July 2025).

9. Lappin, M. R., Blondeau, J., Boothe, D., Breitschwerdt, E. B., Guardabassi, L., Lloyd, D. H., Papich, M. G., Rankin, S. C., Sykes, J. E., Turnidge, J., & Weese, J. S. (2017). Antimicrobial use Guidelines for Treatment of Respiratory Tract Disease in Dogs and Cats: Antimicrobial Guidelines Working Group of the International Society for Companion Animal Infectious Diseases. *Journal of veterinary internal medicine*, *31*(2), 279–294. https://doi.org/10.1111/jvim.14627s(accessed on 16th July 2025).

10. Arabski, M., Briers, Y., Danis-Wlodarczyk, K., Drabik, D., et al. (2016). *A proposed integrated approach for the preclinical evaluation of phage therapy in Pseudomonas infections.* https://core.ac.uk/download/55746521.pdf (accessed on 16th July 2025).

11. Araujo Garrido, J. L., Bernal Bayard, J., & Ramos Morales, F. (2020). *Type III secretion effectors with arginine N-glycosyltransferase activity.* https://core.ac.uk/download/299806865.pdf (accessed on 16th July 2025).

12. Barnard, N. (2019). *Prevalence of Gram-negative infections in cervico-facial sepsis.* https://core.ac.uk/download/289120735.pdf (accessed on 16th July 2025).

13. Bassegoda, A., Ivanova, K., Ramon, E., & Tzanov, T. (2018). Strategies to prevent the occurrence of resistance against antibiotics by using advanced materials. *Applied microbiology and biotechnology, 102*(5), 2075–2089. https://doi.org/10.1007/s00253-018-8776-0(accessed on 16th July 2025).

14. Bernal-Bayard, J., & Ramos-Morales (2017). *Molecular mechanisms used by Salmonella to evade the immune system.* https://core.ac.uk/download/222572248.pdf (accessed on 16th July 2025).

15. Beveridge, L. A., Davey, P. G., McMurdo, M. E. T., & Phillips, G., et al. (2011). *Optimal management of urinary tract infections in older people.* https://core.ac.uk/download/20450519.pdf (accessed on 16th July 2025).

16. Jenner, A., Bhagwandin, N., & Kowalski, S. P. (2017). *Antimicrobial resistance (AMR) and multidrug resistance (MDR): Overview of current approaches, consortia and intellectual property issues.* https://www.wipo.int/publications/en/details.jsp?id=4210 https://core.ac.uk/download/215505935.pdf (accessed on 16th July 2025).

17. Bidossi, A., Cockayne, A., Dintilhac, A., Hamilton, A., Hiron, A., Kadioglu, A., Marra, A., et al. (2012). Effects of deletion of the *Streptococcus pneumoniae* lipoprotein diacylglyceryl transferase gene *lgt* on ABC transporter function and on growth *in vivo.* https://core.ac.uk/download/9648767.pdf (accessed on 16th July 2025).

18. Mkrtchyan, H. V., Russell, C. A., Wang, N., & Cutler, R. R. (2013). Could public restrooms be an environment for bacterial resistomes?. *PloS one, 8*(1), e54223. https://doi.org/10.1371/journal.pone.0054223(accessed on 16th July 2025).

19. Boaretti, M., Castellani, F., Lleo, M. M., Lucidi, S., et al. (2016). *Presence of multiple bacterial markers in clinical samples might be useful for presumptive diagnosis of infection in cirrhotic patients with culture-negative reports.* https://core.ac.uk/download/54526941.pdf (accessed on 16th July 2025).

20. Bolz, M., Cornelius, A., & Ernst, J. D. (2019). *Dynamics of Mycobacterium tuberculosis Ag85B revealed by a sensitive enzyme-linked immunosorbent assay.* https://core.ac.uk/download/323068033.pdf (accessed on 16th July 2025).

21. Pfalzgraff, A., Bárcena-Varela, S., Heinbockel, L., Gutsmann, T., Brandenburg, K., Martinez-de-Tejada, G., & Weindl, G. (2018). Antimicrobial endotoxin-neutralizing peptides promote keratinocyte migration via P2X7 receptor activation and accelerate wound healing in vivo. *British journal of pharmacology, 175*(17), 3581–3593. https://doi.org/10.1111/bph.14425(accessed on 16th July 2025).

22. Merli, M., Lucidi, C., Di Gregorio, V., Falcone, M., Giannelli, V., Lattanzi, B., Giusto, M., Ceccarelli, G., Farcomeni, A., Riggio, O., & Venditti, M. (2015). The spread of multi drug resistant infections is leading to an increase in the empirical antibiotic treatment failure in cirrhosis: a prospective survey. *PloS one, 10*(5), e0127448. https://doi.org/10.1371/journal.pone.0127448 (accessed on 16th July 2025).

23. Cevallos, M. E. (2008). *Streptococcus Pyogenes: A Versatile Human Pathogen.* https://core.ac.uk/download/51097354.pdf (accessed on 16th July 2025).

24. Chapin, A., Rule, A., Jensen, L. B., Schwab, K., Gibson, K., Mackiewicz, B., Buckley, T., et al. (2004). *Airborne multidrug-resistant bacteria isolated from a concentrated swine feeding operation.* https://core.ac.uk/download/pdf/3797183.pdf (accessed on 16th July 2025).

25. PEW Charitable Trust Report (2016). *A scientific roadmap for antibiotic discovery: A sustained and robust pipeline of new antibacterial drugs and therapies is critical to preserve public health.* https://core.ac.uk/download/75785719.pdf (accessed on 16th July 2025).

26. Rosa, L., Cutone, A., Lepanto, M. S., Paesano, R., & Valenti, P. (2017). Lactoferrin: A Natural Glycoprotein Involved in Iron and Inflammatory Homeostasis. *International journal of molecular sciences, 18*(9), 1985. https://doi.org/10.3390/ijms18091985(accessed on 16th July 2025).

27. Dumitru, A. E., Popoiag, R., Micu, S. I., Moraru, L., et al. (2019). *The burden of Clostridium difficile infection in patients with liver cirrhosis.* https://core.ac.uk/download/232440323.pdf (accessed on 16th July 2025).

28. Msaki, B. P., Mshana, S. E., Hokororo, A., Mazigo, H. D., & Morona, D. (2012). Prevalence and predictors of urinary tract infection and severe malaria among febrile children attending Makongoro health centre in Mwanza city, North-Western Tanzania. *Archives of public health = Archives belges de sante publique, 70*(1), 4. https://doi.org/10.1186/0778-7367-70-4(accessed on 16th July 2025).

29. Morgan, M. P., Szakmany, T., Power, S. G., Olaniyi, P., Hall, J. E., Rowan, K., & Eberl, M. (2016). Sepsis Patients with First and Second-Hit Infections Show Different Outcomes Depending on the Causative Organism. *Frontiers in microbiology, 7*, 207. https://doi.org/10.3389/fmicb.2016.00207(accessed on 16th July 2025).

30. Grelling, N., Liu, H., Nguyen, N. Y. T., Rosario, K., et al. (2018). *Antimicrobial activities and mechanisms of magnesium oxide nanoparticles (nMgO) against pathogenic bacteria, yeasts, and biofilms.* https://core.ac.uk/download/323067341.pdf (accessed on 16th July 2025).

31. Kabangila, R., Kataraihya, J. B., Kidenya, B. R., Meremo, A. G., et al. (2012). *High prevalence of non-typhoid Salmonella bacteremia among febrile HIV adult patients admitted at a tertiary hospital, North-Western Tanzania.* https://core.ac.uk/download/pdf/16666649.pdf (accessed on 16th July 2025).

32. Klaas, I. C., & Zadoks, R. N. (2018). An update on environmental mastitis: Challenging perceptions. *Transboundary and emerging diseases, 65 Suppl 1*, 166–185. https://doi.org/10.1111/tbed.12704(accessed on 16th July 2025).

33. Zabielska, J., Tyfa, A., & Kunicka-Styczyńska, A. (2016). Methods for eradication of the biofilms formed by opportunistic pathogens using novel techniques – A review. *Acta Universitatis Lodziensis. Folia Biologica Et Oecologica, 12*, 26–37. https://doi.org/10.1515/fobio-2016-0003(accessed on 16th July 2025).

34. Lillestolen, D. (2018). *Infections Not Fought: Antibiotic Resistance in Underserved Communities.* https://core.ac.uk/download/158970352.pdf (accessed on 16th July 2025).

35. Phelan, D. (2016). *Biochemical characterization of diamide inhibitors with N-acetylglucosaminidases LytG from Bacillus subtilis.* https://core.ac.uk/download/56740592.pdf (accessed on 16th July 2025).

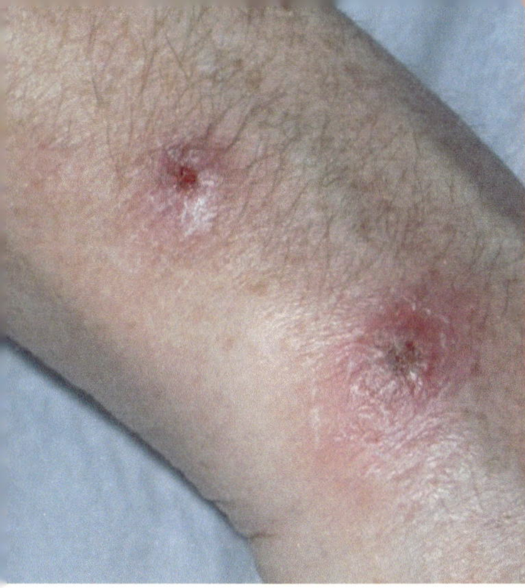

Chapter 9

MYCOBACTERIAL INFECTIONS

Contents

Introduction

Mycobacterial disease ranks among the foremost global health challenges owing to the extensive array of pathogens within the *Mycobacterium* genus. The most renowned among these is *Mycobacterium tuberculosis*, which is responsible for tuberculosis- an ailment that has afflicted humanity for centuries. Additionally, nontuberculous mycobacteria (NTM), including *Mycobacterium avium* and *Mycobacterium abscessus*, further complicate the landscape of mycobacterial diseases. These environmental bacteria are ubiquitous in water and soil and manifest a broad spectrum of clinical symptoms, particularly in patients with pre-existing pulmonary conditions, thus rendering diagnosis and treatment particularly challenging (Mortaz et al., 2017). Understanding the epidemiology and clinical implications of mycobacterial infections is essential for developing effective public health strategies. Notably, the clinical presentation of mycobacterial infections extends beyond pulmonary involvement. While pulmonary NTM infections pose significant concerns in patients with structural lung diseases such as cystic fibrosis or bronchiectasis, these organisms can also cause extrapulmonary infections involving lymph nodes, skin, soft tissues, and disseminated disease, particularly in immunocompromised individuals. For example, paediatric cases presenting with lymphadenitis due to NTM infections demonstrate that the pathogenic potential of these mycobacteria is not confined to adults with known risk factors (Mortaz et al., 2017).

The complexity inherent in mycobacterial diseases underscores the importance of a comprehensive understanding of host-pathogen interactions, especially since some patients may harbour NTM without any identifiable predisposing factors. This situation highlights the challenges faced by clinicians in diagnosing and treating such infections. Advances in molecular typing and microbiological techniques have markedly enhanced our understanding of mycobacterial pathogens; nevertheless, significant knowledge gaps persist. For instance, genetic analyses of *M. tuberculosis* strains have yielded valuable insights into transmission patterns and associations with specific disease manifestations, such as extrapulmonary tuberculosis (EPTB). The continual discovery of unclassified strains across various geographic regions emphasises the necessity for ongoing research to elucidate these pathogens and their clinical relevance. Moreover, limited understanding regarding the immunogenetic factors involved in NTM disease underscores the need for further investigation, as heterogeneity among strains may influence disease severity and treatment outcomes. Consequently, a multidisciplinary approach that integrates molecular advancements with clinical expertise is vital for the optimal management of mycobacterial infections.

Definition of Mycobacterial Infections

The term 'mycobacterial infections' pertains to infections caused by bacteria of the genus *Mycobacterium*, among which *Mycobacterium tuberculosis* is of paramount importance due to its role in the aetiology of tuberculosis (TB). Mycobacteria are distinguished by possessing a unique cell wall that is exceptionally rich in mycolic acids; these attributes confer resistance to conventional antibiotics. This inherent resistance, combined with their capacity to survive within host macrophages, poses significant challenges to their effective treatment and eradication. Within the genus *Mycobacterium*, aside from TB, there exist non-tuberculous mycobacteria (NTM), such as *Mycobacterium avium* complex and *Mycobacterium abscessus*, which are responsible for opportunistic infections, particularly in immunocompromised individuals. These infections present complexities in diagnosis and treatment, necessitating a deeper understanding of their biological nature and pathogenic mechanisms. This importance is underscored by global health initiatives aiming to diminish their impact (Legido-Quigley et al., 2012).

The epidemiology of mycobacterial infections intersects with social, environmental, and healthcare determinants. Tuberculosis remains a leading cause of morbidity and mortality worldwide, predominantly affecting resource-limited settings with restricted healthcare access. Factors such as HIV co-infection significantly elevate the risk of TB development, thereby complicating control efforts. Socioeconomic determinants, including poverty and malnutrition, also play a critical role in disease transmission by creating conducive environments for infection spread. The control of mycobacterial infections depends equally on medical interventions and strategies targeting social determinants that facilitate transmission. Innovative models, such as the integrated delivery of TB/HIV services, have been developed to enhance disease management through multidisciplinary approaches (Drummond & Brown, 2013) (Figure 9.1).

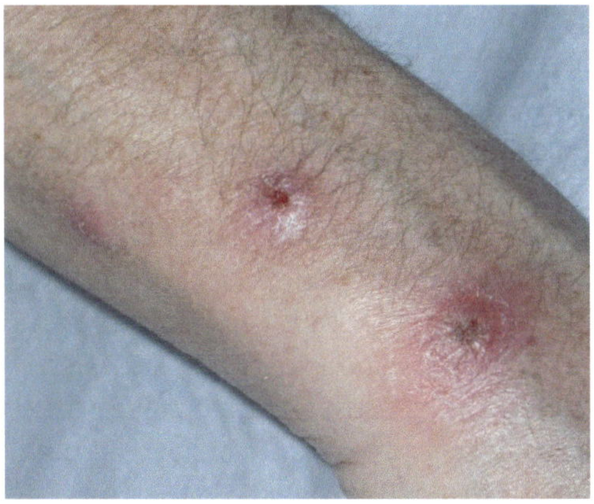

Figure 9.1. Mycobacterial infections.

Source: https://www.pcds.org.uk/imager/gallery/clinical/mycobacterial-infections/10817/Mycobacteria_marinumfish_tank1b_fee391183f15cb4d62773032fe0be92d.jpg.

Furthermore, the management of mycobacterial infections constitutes a complex challenge that necessitates meticulous procedures and prolonged antitubercular regimens. The treatment of tuberculosis (TB) with first-line agents involves a course of multiple antibiotics administered for no less than six months, which often encounters issues related to patient adherence and the development of drug resistance. This issue is especially pronounced in regions with a high prevalence of multidrug-resistant TB, where limited therapeutic options exacerbate morbidity and mortality rates. Although less common, infections caused by non-tuberculous mycobacteria also present significant therapeutic difficulties due to their unpredictable susceptibility to antibiotics and, in advanced cases, the potential requirement for surgical intervention. Consequently, ongoing research into novel therapeutic agents, enhanced understanding of bacterial resistance mechanisms, and the development of efficacious vaccines are essential components in the global effort to combat mycobacterial diseases (Legido-Quigley et al., 2012).

Importance of Studying Mycobacterial Infections

The significance of mycobacterial infection research spans from diagnostic and therapeutic applications to public health concerns and epidemiological insights. Mycobacteria, especially *Mycobacterium tuberculosis* and nontuberculous mycobacteria, have seen a sharp increase in incidence and drug resistance. The complexity of these infections, due to their multifaceted nature and diverse clinical presentations, necessitates extensive research. For example, the rising incidence of pulmonary infections caused by nontuberculous mycobacteria highlights the need for epidemiological studies to fully assess the impact of these pathogens on different populations (Yusti et al., 2018). Such knowledge is vital for public health initiatives aimed at preventing and controlling mycobacterial infections, particularly in resource-limited settings where confusion between tuberculosis and nontuberculous mycobacterial infections can lead to misdiagnosis. The emergence of drug-resistant mycobacteria also poses a significant threat to current treatment strategies, with implications for understanding the evolving landscape of therapy. Current research indicates that, even with molecular diagnostic tools, many healthcare systems still struggle to accurately differentiate between mycobacterial subspecies and species, especially in clinical laboratory settings (Zelazny & Olivier, 2015). This diagnostic gap affects not only individual patient management but also broader efforts to control mycobacterial infections. Better species and pathogen identification, alongside detailed knowledge of their unique virulence factors and resistance mechanisms, can inform treatment approaches and ultimately enhance patient care and public health responses. Beyond clinical practice, research into mycobacterial infections provides valuable insights into environmental and ecological factors influencing disease transmission. Various nontuberculous mycobacterial species may be acquired from environmental sources, complicating efforts to identify key triggers for disease onset (Yusti et al., 2018). Understanding the ecological niches of these pathogens is critical for pinpointing necessary preventive measures. Moreover, studying trends in mycobacterial infections, particularly among vulnerable groups such as those with chronic pulmonary disease or immunocompromised states, is important for predicting future health burdens (Zelazny & Olivier, 2015). Continued investigation into the multidisciplinary aspects of mycobacterial infections enables scientists to develop a more informed and adaptive approach to infectious disease management worldwide.

9.1. Types of Mycobacterial Infections

Mycobacterial infections are predominantly caused by organisms belonging to the genus *Mycobacterium*, characterized by their high virulence and slow growth mode. The most significant pathogen within this group is *Mycobacterium tuberculosis*, which is responsible for tuberculosis (TB), a disease that continues to pose a global health challenge. Although TB primarily affects the lungs, it can also disseminate to other sites, leading to widespread infections. In addition, *Mycobacterium leprae* is known to cause leprosy, a chronic infection affecting primarily the skin, peripheral nerves, and mucous membranes. While these two infections are the most recognised, they constitute only part of the broader spectrum of mycobacterial diseases, as non-tuberculous mycobacteria (NTM) can also induce illness, particularly in immunocompromised individuals. Diseases caused by NTM, such as *Mycobacterium avium* complex (MAC) and *Mycobacterium kansasii* infections, are increasingly identified, especially due to their association with pulmonary and extrapulmonary disease in patients with compromised immune systems. MAC, comprising *Mycobacterium avium* and *Mycobacterium intracellulare*, is commonly encountered in advanced HIV/AIDS cases and can lead to severe pulmonary complications similar to those observed in tuberculosis. Conversely, *Mycobacterium kansasii* can infect healthier individuals, presenting with respiratory symptoms and chronic cough. The rising incidence of these infections among immunocompromised groups underscores the importance of heightened awareness and tailored treatment approaches, given that their clinical presentations can mimic those of more common pathogens, thereby complicating diagnosis and management. Recent advancements in genomic analysis have elucidated the complexities of mycobacterial infections, particularly concerning within-host pathogen diversity. The development of tools such as ClassTR facilitates improved classification of *Mycobacterium tuberculosis* strains, enhancing our understanding of how genetic diversity influences clinical outcomes (Chindelevitch et al., 2015). Furthermore, research into other mycobacterial species, such as *Rhodococcus equi*, has uncovered significant adaptations that enable these organisms to thrive within host environments, often relying on horizontally acquired pathogenicity loci for virulence (Bentley et al., 2010). This broader perspective on mycobacterial infections extends beyond tuberculosis and leprosy, highlighting the critical importance of identifying diverse mycobacterial species and understanding their evolutionary mechanisms to inform public health strategies and therapeutic interventions.

9.1.1. Tuberculosis (TB)

Understanding the epidemiology of tuberculosis (TB) is crucial for addressing its role as a significant global health issue, particularly in the context of mycobacterial infections. TB is predominantly caused by *Mycobacterium tuberculosis*, a bacterium transmitted via airborne droplets when an infected individual coughs or sneezes.

The rising incidence of TB in various regions, notably the russian federation, is closely linked to comorbid conditions, including HIV infection. This co-occurrence exacerbates health impacts, necessitating specialized treatment and management of both conditions. Recent epidemiological research indicates that the concurrent occurrence of TB and HIV signifies a concerning trend; patients often present with complications that complicate treatment protocols, resulting in increased mortality rates among affected populations. Comprehending these dynamics is vital for developing effective public health strategies to combat TB, particularly in high-risk environments where the disease remains endemic (Zhdan et al., 2025).

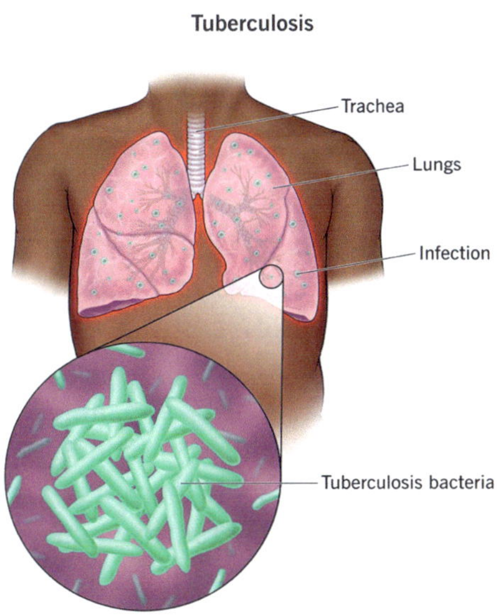

Figure 9.2. Your lungs are infected with tuberculosis bacteria when you have tuberculosis.

Source: https://my.clevelandclinic.org/-/scassets/images/org/health/articles/11301-tuberculosis.

Post-treatment trajectories of TB offer insights into mortality risks associated with this mycobacterial infection. Studies conducted within the United States reveal that individuals who have successfully completed TB therapy may still experience elevated mortality rates relative to the general population. A longitudinal study demonstrated that a small percentage of patients (7.3%) died due to various conditions, including cardiovascular diseases and cancers, especially within HIV co-infected subgroups. These findings emphasise the importance of ongoing monitoring and intervention following treatment, especially among populations with comorbidities. The observation that cured TB patients may endure long-term health consequences highlights the necessity for comprehensive care plans that address both the immediate effects of the disease and subsequent long-term sequelae (Gorvetzian et al., 2023) (Figure 9.2).

The intersection of tuberculosis (TB) with other diseases, such as HIV and chronic illnesses, complicates the landscape of mycobacterial infections. In the Voronezh region of Russia, studies indicate a significant correlation between TB and increasing trends of comorbid conditions, which necessitates a multifaceted public health response. Although reports suggest that the mortality rate attributable to TB declined during the study period, the overall increase in HIV infections has artificially inflated mortality statistics. While healthcare systems grapple with these challenges, understanding the social and demographic determinants that influence TB transmission and treatment adherence remains crucial. In the future, comprehending the interactions among TB, HIV, and other comorbidities will be vital for enhancing health outcomes and developing targeted programs that address the complexities of mycobacterial infections within diverse populations (Zhdan et al 2025).

9.1.2. Non-Tuberculous Mycobacterial Infections (NTM)

Non-tuberculous mycobacterial disease (NTM) is increasingly recognized within the field of infectious diseases, particularly owing to its association with diverse pulmonary and extrapulmonary conditions. NTM constitutes a group of environmental bacteria predominantly found in soil and water, accountable for a wide array of diseases in humans. Pulmonary NTM infections primarily affect individuals with underlying lung conditions such as bronchiectasis, chronic obstructive pulmonary disease (COPD), and cystic fibrosis. Furthermore, these pathogens can cause skin infections, lymphadenitis, and disseminated disease in immunocompromised hosts, including HIV-infected patients. The growing significance of NTM is evidenced by the increasing disease burden, now more frequently identified through advanced imaging and microbiological techniques, thereby necessitating enhanced provider education and awareness (Mortaz et al., 2017). Despite improved diagnostic capabilities, the treatment of NTM infections presents substantial challenges, chiefly due to the inherent antibiotic resistance exhibited by most of these organisms. Treatment regimens are complex, often requiring prolonged courses of multiple antibiotics; however, the tolerability and efficacy of such therapies can vary significantly among patients. Initiating treatment is often complicated by the potential for adverse side effects and the need to carefully balance clinical benefits against associated risks. Additionally, current guidelines issued by organizations such as the American Thoracic Society aim to facilitate the diagnosis and management of NTM-related diseases. Nevertheless, adherence to these guidelines remains suboptimal internationally, underscoring the importance of education and strict adherence to evidence-based practices to enhance patient outcomes (Chalmers et al., 2018) (Figure 9.3).

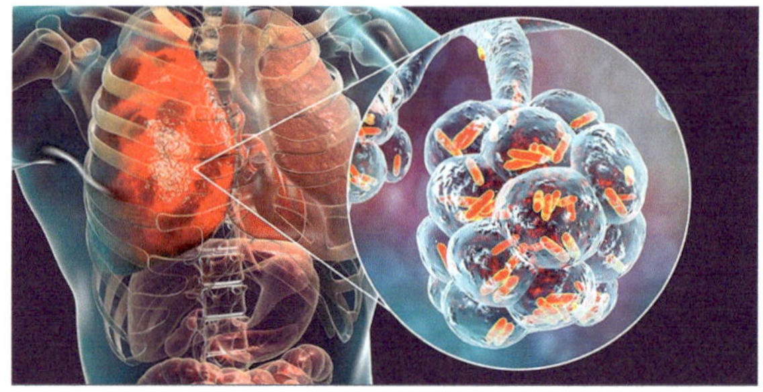

Figure 9.3. Non-tuberculous mycobacterial infections (NTM).

Source: https://uthealtheasttexas.com/sites/default/files/styles/services_node_image/public/sub-service-images/NTMLungDisease_subservice.jpg?itok=YbcCzZYm.

Furthermore, the epidemiology of non-tuberculous mycobacterial (NTM) diseases is undergoing evolution influenced by multiple factors, including demographic shifts such as population ageing, increased utilisation of immunosuppressive therapies, and advancements in the management of underlying health conditions, all contributing to a rise in case incidence. As awareness of NTM-related diseases expands, it is imperative to conduct comprehensive research into their epidemiology, clinical assessment, and treatment strategies. A multidisciplinary approach through interprofessional collaboration among physicians, microbiologists, and allied health professionals is crucial to ensure optimal management of NTM infections. Ongoing clinical trials are anticipated to yield valuable data concerning both emerging and existing therapeutic interventions, thereby enhancing understanding of these infections and supporting the development of appropriate care and management models (Chalmers et al., 2018).

9.1.3. Leprosy (Hansen's Disease)

Leprosy, or Hansen's disease, is most often caused by the bacillus *Mycobacterium leprae*, which has a particular affinity for the skin and peripheral nerves. This persistent granulomatous infection has historically been the target of stigma, often described as dying before dying due to the social exclusion that infected individuals face. The most significant public health challenge today is that leprosy remains endemic in many developing countries. Additionally, the presence of M. leprae and the limited control measures in place highlight the need for enhanced monitoring and preventive strategies, especially in areas inhabited by 9-banded armadillos, making disease control quite complex (Nicolle et al., 2024). Treatment for leprosy has evolved significantly over the years: since the early 1980s, multidrug therapy (MDT) has become the cornerstone of effective control. MDT employs antibiotics such as rifampin, dapsone, and clofazimine to efficiently eradicate the bacteria and prevent disability.

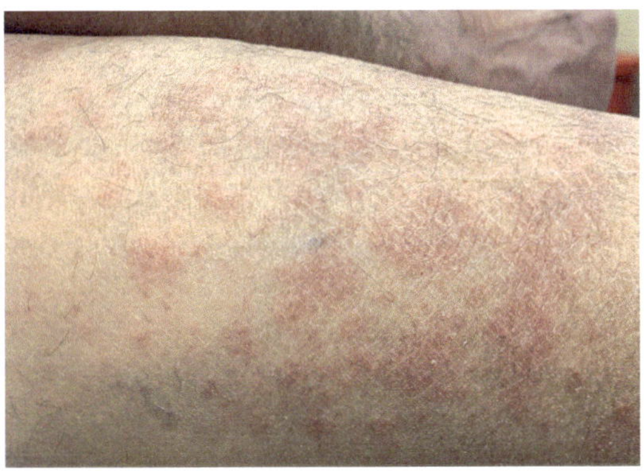

Figure 9.4. Hansen disease (leprosy).

Source: https://external-content.duckduckgo.com/iu/?u=https%3A%2F%2Fwww.mayoclinicproceedings.org%2Fcms%2Fattachment%2Fc5586bd8-76a2-4aee-b36d-9a4f329154de%2Fgr1_lrg.jpg&f=1&nofb=1&ipt=6cc138f83c1314d8e1aa776a941ac29cfa08144007cb4b1b0107280e4ef5fafb.

Case reports have demonstrated high recovery rates, underscoring the significance of early diagnosis and intervention. In specific regions, such as certain areas of Southern Georgia, locally acquired cases linked to contact with infected armadillos have prompted health authorities to reevaluate the associated risk factors of transmission. As the population of the nine-banded armadillo continues to grow, it is essential to ensure the availability of appropriate treatment facilities and awareness campaigns to prevent the re-emergence of this historically significant disease (Nicolle et al., 2024). Social stigma remains a substantial barrier to the eradication of leprosy. Patients diagnosed with this condition often face rejection from their families and communities, leading to social isolation. The psychological impact of leprosy can be as severe as its physical implications, resulting in mental health deterioration and diminished quality of life. Healthcare professionals must also prioritise community education efforts to dispel prevalent myths associated with the disease while concurrently addressing clinical challenges. Adopting a comprehensive approach to leprosy can enhance health outcomes and facilitate the reintegration of affected individuals into society by providing social support and emphasising the treatable nature of the disease (Srivastav et al., 2023).

9.2. Pathophysiology of Mycobacterial Infections

The pathophysiology of mycobacterial infections, particularly nontuberculous mycobacteria (NTM), exhibits intricate host- pathogen interactions that may significantly influence respiratory health. Mycobacterial species, such as *Mycobacterium abscessus*, are common opportunistic pathogens that predominantly flourish in immunocompromised individuals, including patients with cystic fibrosis (CF). The mutation of the CF transmembrane conductance regulator (CFTR) gene results in excessive mucus production and impaired mucociliary clearance, thereby creating an environment conducive to recurrent pulmonary infections. In these patients, the presence of NTM, especially in conjunction with other organisms like *Aspergillus fumigatus*, can further exacerbate lung inflammation and damage. Co- infection with *A. fumigatus* has been observed in affected individuals. Moreover, *A. fumigatus* can modulate immune responses, highlighting the complexity of pulmonary pathogen interactions and contributing to further declines in lung function and increased morbidity (Monin et al., 2018). Additionally, mycobacterial infections are challenging to diagnose and treat due to their resemblance to other respiratory comorbidities. Accurate diagnosis typically relies on the detection of mycobacterial species through culture and molecular techniques from clinical specimens. The case of *Mycobacterium gordonae* exemplifies the importance of comprehensive clinical and environmental investigations in suspected outbreaks. Although *M. gordonae* was identified in bronchoalveolar lavage samples, the patients did not meet the criteria for NTM lung disease, underscoring the necessity of distinguishing pathogenic from non-pathogenic mycobacterial species. This scenario highlights the complexity inherent in diagnosing mycobacterial infections and underscores significant considerations in clinical practice, particularly in hospital settings where environmental strains may mimic true infections (Scorzolini et al., 2016). Ongoing research into the pathophysiology of mycobacterial infections continues to elucidate their virulence factors and the dynamics of host immune responses. The immune system plays a vital role in controlling mycobacterial infections, with certain immune responses impacting clinical outcomes. For instance, type 1 and type 17 immune responses are pivotal in containing *M. abscessus* infection. These responses are regulated by transcription factors such as T-box 21 (Tbx 21) and retinoic acid receptor-related orphan receptor gamma t (Rorγt), which coordinate pulmonary immune responses. Such insights offer potential therapeutic targets and guide the development of improved treatment strategies, especially for infections resistant to conventional antibiotics. The interaction between pathogen virulence and host immunity remains an essential area of ongoing research, as efforts continue to identify effective interventions.

9.2.1. Mechanism of Infection

Understanding the pathogenesis of mycobacterial infections is crucial for developing effective therapeutic strategies and preventive measures. Most NTM infections are acquired through the respiratory system or skin breaks, and once inside the host, the bacteria evade the immune system by residing within macrophages that typically engulf and destroy pathogens. Mycobacteria disrupt host cell functions by employing mechanisms to avoid phagocytic killing, such as suppressing phagosome-lysosome fusion, which allows them to proliferate within immune cells.

This adaptation to the hostile environment of the host immune system makes controlling and treating mycobacterial diseases particularly challenging, as the bacteria survive despite the host's natural immunity. Consequently, understanding these mechanisms fully is essential for developing therapies and improving patient outcomes. The pathogenicity of mycobacteria is driven by specific genetic determinants and the host immune response. Some immunogenetic defects may predispose individuals to severe mycobacterial infections; for example, the identification of the first human mycobacterial susceptibility gene, associated with a mutation in the interferon gamma receptor 1 (IFNGR1) gene, highlights the role of genetic factors in infection susceptibility. Cases among young people on the small island nation of Malta demonstrate how virulent infections with this mutation can severely impair the immune response against intracellular pathogens (Figure 9.5).

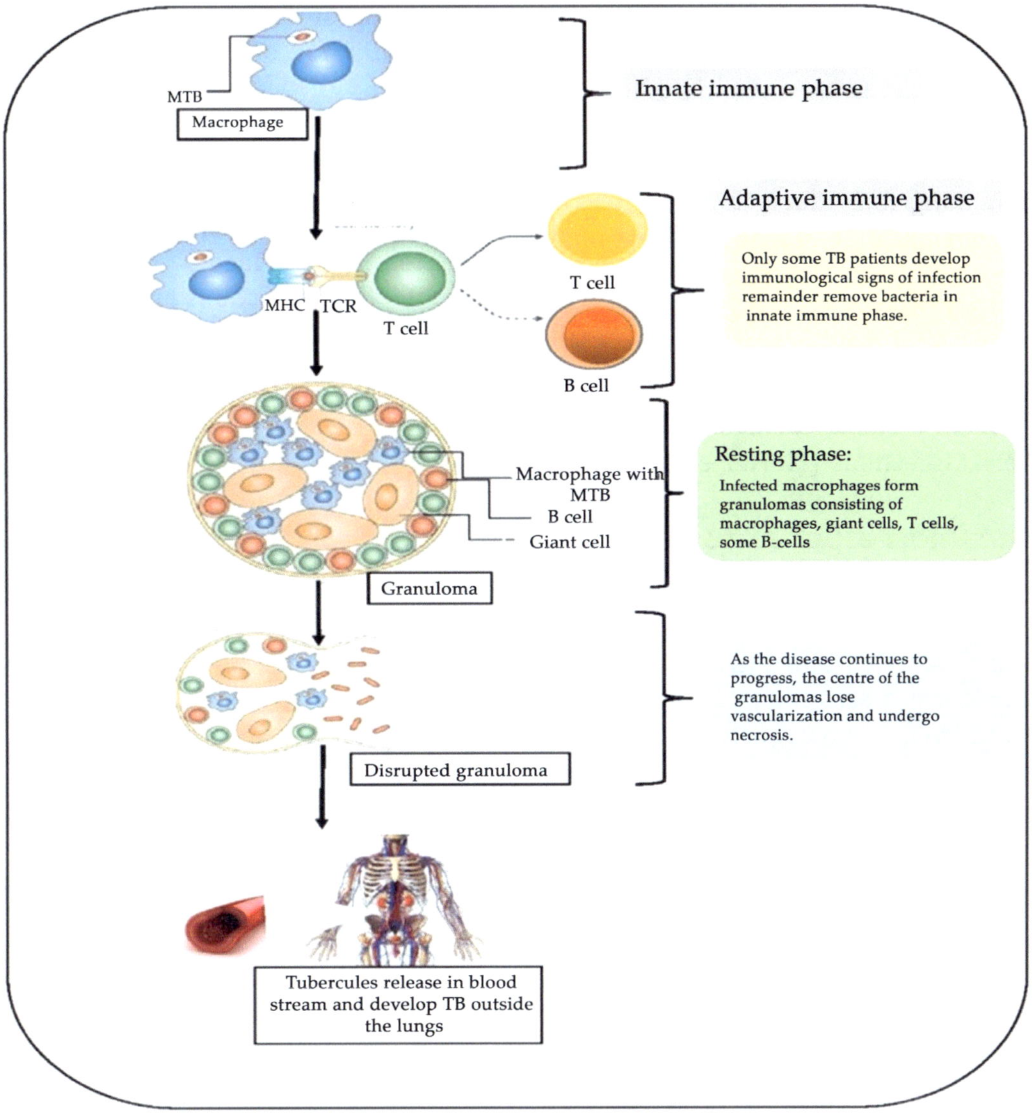

Figure 9.5. Basic mechanism of infection of *Mycobacterium tuberculosis*.

Source: https://www.researchgate.net/figure/Basic-mechanism-of-infection-of-Mycobacterium-tuberculosis_fig1_291952234.

The immunologic mechanism involving IFNGR1 is essential for activating macrophages to kill mycobacteria, demonstrating how genetic differences can influence an individual's susceptibility to mycobacterial diseases and highlighting the importance of further investigating host-pathogen interactions in mycobacterial infections (Anderson et al., 2012). Adding further complexity to the infection dynamics, environmental factors also play a crucial role in both the incidence and severity of mycobacterial infections. NTM, which is prevalent in water and soil, causes lung disease mainly in patients with pre-existing lung conditions such as cystic fibrosis and bronchiectasis that impair normal pulmonary function. The link between these chronic structural lung diseases and susceptibility to NTM underscores the importance of recognising environmental risk factors.

Individuals with increased susceptibility, such as those with chronic pulmonary disease or immunocompromised states, are more likely to develop severe clinical symptoms upon exposure to NTM. Moreover, the diversity of immune responses among individuals can result in a wide range of clinical presentations, from mild infection to extensive systemic involvement. Therefore, it is critically important to gain comprehensive knowledge of both environmental risk factors and genetic predispositions to develop effective management strategies for mycobacterial infections (Mortaz et al., 2017).

9.2.2. Immune Response to Mycobacterial Pathogens

The immune response against mycobacterial infection is a complex and intricate process, characterised by macrophage activation as its hallmark. When mycobacteria, such as *Mycobacterium tuberculosis* and nontuberculous mycobacteria (NTM), are exposed to the host body, the innate immune system is activated immediately. Macrophages play a crucial role by engulfing the bacteria through phagocytosis and attempting to destroy them. However, mycobacteria have developed sophisticated mechanisms to counter this attack. For example, they can inhibit the process of phagosome maturation, allowing them to survive and replicate within macrophages. This evasion not only leads to chronic infections but also presents challenges for the adaptive immune response, which subsequently recruits T cells and antibodies to eliminate the pathogens. The intracellular persistence of mycobacteria complicates treatment and underscores the importance of understanding the immunological processes involved (Mortaz et al., 2017). The unique features of mycobacterial infections further complicate the immune response. For instance, certain species, such as *Mycobacterium bovis* and *Mycobacterium avium,* employ different pathogenic strategies that influence the immune system's reaction. *M. bovis* is mainly responsible for bovine tuberculosis, whereas *M. avium* subspecies *paratuberculosis* (MAP) has been linked to Johne's disease in cattle. Since both pathogens survive and proliferate within macrophages, enabling them to evade the host's defence mechanisms, recent genomic research has provided significant insights into the complex interactions between mycobacteria and host macrophages (Figure 9.6).

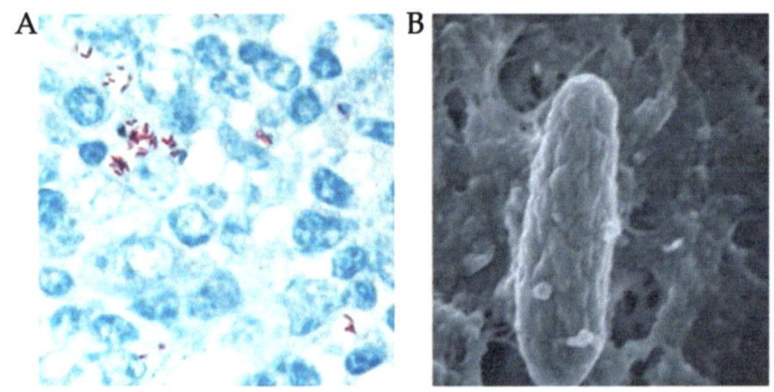

Figure 9.6. *Mycobacterium avium* subsp. *paratuberculosis* (MAP) properties.

Source: https://www.researchgate.net/figure/Mycobacterium-avium-subsp-paratuberculosis-MAP-properties-A-Acid-fast-stain-of_fig1_320875492.

An understanding of these interactions, namely cytokine responses and the generation of immunomodulatory signals, provides valuable insights into the various pathologies associated with such infections, thereby identifying potential therapeutic targets (Rue-Albrecht et al., 2014). The immune response against mycobacterium pathogens ultimately reflects the delicate equilibrium between host resistance and pathogen virulence. Although the initial immune response may effectively contain the infection, the survival mechanisms employed by mycobacteria can eventually lead to chronic disease and substantial morbidity. Factors such as host genetic predisposition, environmental influences, and co-morbid conditions may also modulate immune responses. For example, in patients with pre-existing structural lung disease or those who are immunocompromised, the likelihood of developing severe disease caused by non-tuberculous mycobacteria (NTMs) is markedly increased. Further research is necessary to deconstruct the complexity of mycobacterial infections, particularly through the investigation of genetic and immunological factors that predispose individuals to fatal outcomes. Developing a comprehensive understanding of these interactions will be instrumental in the development of effective vaccines and therapeutic strategies aimed at preventing mycobacterial infections and mitigating their impact on public health (Mortaz et al., 2017).

9.2.3. Factors Influencing Disease Progression

This discourse examines the progression of mycobacterial infections, including tuberculosis (TB), emphasising the complex interplay between environmental and individual factors. Central to this analysis are host immune responses, which are shaped by genetic determinants and psychosocial influences. Psychosocial stressors such as chronic stress and social isolation can significantly modulate immune function.

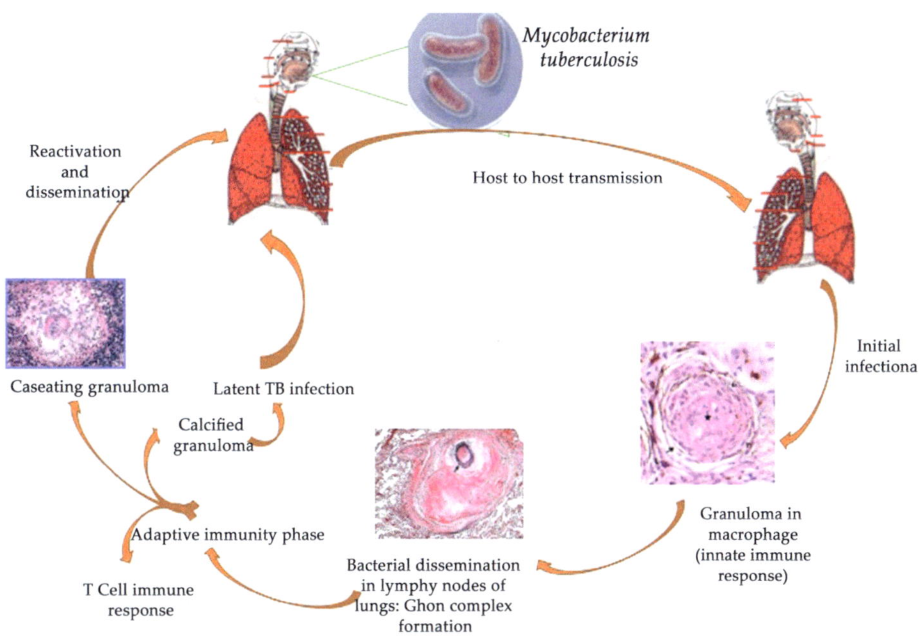

Figure 9.7. Disease progression of *Mycobacterium tuberculosis.*

Source: https://www.researchgate.net/figure/Disease-progression-of-Mycobacterium-tuberculosis_fig2_324524955.

For instance, individuals experiencing adverse psychosocial conditions often exhibit weakened immune responses, thereby reducing their resistance to infections, including TB. Moreover, existing literature indicates that social support mechanisms can mitigate negative health outcomes by enhancing immune function, potentially leading to improved prognoses for individuals at risk of disease progression (Jacobs & Ottinger, 2006). Consequently, understanding the intersection of psychosocial and biological factors is vital in the prevention and management of mycobacterial diseases. Environmental determinants, including exposure to pollutants and residential conditions, also markedly influence disease progression, particularly concerning mycobacterial infections. Factors such as overcrowding and air pollution may elevate infection risk and hasten the onset of overt disease. For example, residents of densely populated urban areas are more likely to encounter increased exposure to *Mycobacterium tuberculosis* due to heightened person-to-person transmission. Nutritional deficiencies, notably poor nutrition, can further augment susceptibility to mycobacterial infections by impairing immune functionality. Malnutrition has been associated with alterations in immune responses, rendering individuals more vulnerable to infections and affecting disease outcomes (Jacobs & Ottinger, 2006) (Figure 9.7).

Therefore, controlling environmental factors is essential to prevent the spread and impact of mycobacterial infections. The progression of these infections heavily depends on the type and availability of medical interventions. For example, vaccines like the BCG vaccine demonstrate how public health measures can influence disease pathways. However, responses to such vaccines can vary due to psychosocial factors and individual health conditions, necessitating adaptations in medical strategies. Effective public health approaches should account for these differences to optimise vaccine effectiveness and reduce the risk of worsening health after exposure. Additionally, treatment plans must consider host factors such as comorbidities and overall health, as these can influence treatment success and the likelihood of disease recurrence (Hayward et al., 2019). Overall, managing mycobacterial diseases requires integrating both medical and psychosocial considerations for effective prevention and treatment.

9.3. Epidemiology of Mycobacterial Infections

The epidemiology of mycobacterial diseases includes various species, most notably *Mycobacterium tuberculosis* and nontuberculous mycobacteria (NTM). *M. tuberculosis* remains a major global health issue, with millions of cases and deaths annually. It spreads through respiratory droplets from infected individuals, especially in crowded areas with limited healthcare resources. Despite advances in diagnostics and treatments, socioeconomic factors such as poverty, hunger, and high HIV prevalence continue to facilitate its spread. The interaction between social determinants and microbial pathogenesis underscores the importance of targeted public health measures for transmission prevention and improved patient outcomes. Recognising these trends is essential for developing effective vaccines and optimising healthcare resources. Besides *M. tuberculosis*, NTM are emerging as significant opportunistic pathogens, especially in people with pre-existing lung conditions. These bacteria, found in water and soil, cause pulmonary disease mainly in patients with structural lung issues like bronchiectasis and cystic fibrosis. NTM can also cause soft tissue infections and lymphadenitis in children, as well as disseminated infections in immunocompromised individuals, such as those with HIV. Their epidemiology is complex, as NTM often infects people without obvious risk factors, highlighting environmental exposure. Advances in imaging and microbiology have improved diagnosis and understanding of NTM diseases, but questions remain about immune responses and genetic factors influencing susceptibility (Mortaz et al., 2017). Mycobacterial infections in aquatic animals, particularly in striped bass off the Eastern Seaboard and Chesapeake Bay, have garnered interest. The species' susceptibility, along with infection rates in resident fish, suggests ecological impacts and highlights the role of environmental stress and host susceptibility. Monitoring these infections helps assess ecosystem health and biodiversity preservation. Since mycobacterial infections affect humans and wildlife, understanding their epidemiology is key to developing holistic strategies to control infections and protect biodiversity (Jacobs & Ottinger, 2006) (Figure 9.8).

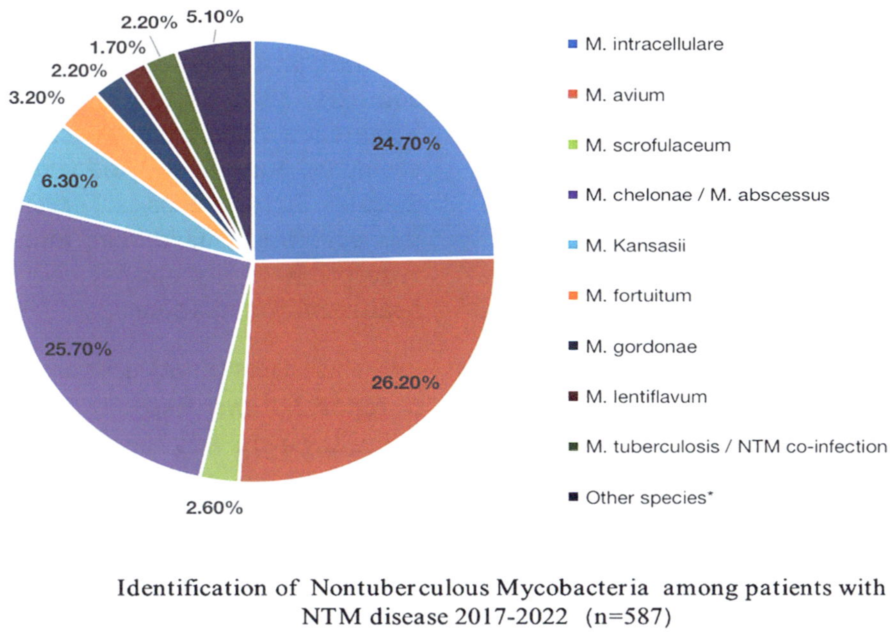

Figure 9.8. Identification of nontuberculous mycobacteria among patients with NTM disease.

Source: https://www.frontiersin.org/files/Articles/1282902/fcimb-13-1282902-HTML/image_m/fcimb-13-1282902-g003.jpg.

9.3.1. Global Prevalence and Incidence Rates

The global epidemiology of mycobacterial diseases, including tuberculosis (TB), is a complex scenario characterised by varying prevalence and incidence rates across different regions. TB remains a significant public health issue, with the World Health Organisation (WHO) estimating that there were approximately 10 million reported cases in 2019. The highest burdens are borne by low- and middle-income countries, a disparity attributable to a combination of socio-economic factors, healthcare accessibility issues, and the dual epidemic of HIV/AIDS. For example, integrated TB/HIV services are essential in mitigating the concurrent impacts of these conditions, as evidenced by numerous studies assessing various service integration models. Successful implementations depend on the synergistic collaboration of TB and HIV programs, which enhances early diagnosis and treatment opportunities, ultimately aiming to improve health outcomes within affected populations (Legido-Quigley et al., 2012). The prevalence of TB has exhibited diverse trends worldwide, influenced by factors such as public health interventions and socioeconomic conditions. In Malta and comparable regions, recent demographic studies of individuals born in Malta over the past 35 years show a decline in TB incidence. Such retrospective analysis reflects the effectiveness of public health initiatives aimed at TB control and prevention, indicating progressive strides toward the potential eradication of the disease within this demographic. Notably, age stratification during this period reveals that older populations exhibit higher prevalence rates, underscoring the necessity for targeted interventions that consider gender-specific vulnerability patterns (Ahmed et al., 2015). Furthermore, the global burden of mycobacterial infections is exacerbated by factors including migration, urbanization, and antimicrobial resistance. Recognising these dynamics underscores the importance of ongoing surveillance and research to identify emerging trends and challenges in disease management. Regions with unique epidemiological profiles require tailored strategies to effectively address the endemic nature of mycobacterial infections, integrating regional data into public health planning. Comprehensive responses should encompass multidisciplinary approaches, encompassing advanced diagnostics, vaccine research and development, and socio-economic interventions aimed at addressing the determinants of these diseases. Additionally, fostering international cooperation is pivotal in transforming the trajectory of mycobacterial infections worldwide, ultimately leading to improved health outcomes and a reduction in the global disease burden.

9.3.2. High-Risk Populations

Risk populations for mycobacterial infection reflect the nexus of social, economic, and health inequities that increase risk for these infections. Among the most significantly affected populations are HIV-positive patients. The compromised immune status of these patients tends to make them susceptible to opportunistic infections, including mycobacteriosis, which can lead to increased morbidity and mortality. A Malawian survey demonstrates the complexity of family planning among HIV-positive couples, with findings indicating that those HIV-positive individuals who reported knowing their status desired to end childbearing more than HIV-negative individuals. However, such knowledge was not then linked with increased use of contraception, suggesting barriers to knowledge that need to be overcome (Dube et al., 2012). Therefore, public health campaigns aiming to reduce the risk of infection among these groups must address broader issues of access to reproductive health services. Additionally, populations within specific geographical contexts, such as the Chesapeake Bay, face heightened risks owing to environmental and ecological burdens that influence mycobacterial disease. Striped bass, an essential species in this ecosystem, have been found to be highly susceptible to mycobacteriosis, affecting their health and populations.

This susceptibility has garnered interest due to reports of increased cases of lesions in fish, indicating a growing health concern that extends beyond individual species to impact entire aquatic ecosystems. The socioeconomic effects of declining fish resources resonate throughout commercial and recreational fisheries industries and highlight the complexity of managing health risks in interconnected ecosystems. Knowledge of these environmental determinants is key to developing effective interventions to safeguard such valuable resources from mycobacterial disease (Jacobs & Ottinger, 2006). Public health responses to mycobacterial disease must consider the multifaceted dynamics of high-risk groups. For example, interventions for HIV-positive individuals should not only focus on raising awareness of health status but also include robust support for access to reproductive health services and education about infection risks. Equally important is addressing environmental health issues for populations dependent on aquatic livelihoods, as their risks extend into their livelihoods. A multidisciplinary approach combining education, resource access, and environmental conservation can effectively reverse the impact of mycobacterial infection while promoting community well-being.

Stakeholder collaboration, involving medical professionals and environmental organisations, will be essential in shaping systemic reforms that address the integrated needs of high-risk populations.

9.3.3. Geographic Distribution of Infections

The global distribution of mycobacterial infections is markedly influenced by a variety of environmental and socioeconomic factors, exhibiting significant regional variability. Nontuberculous mycobacteria (NTM), a heterogeneous group of environmental organisms, are widespread across numerous ecosystems, particularly in water sources and soil.

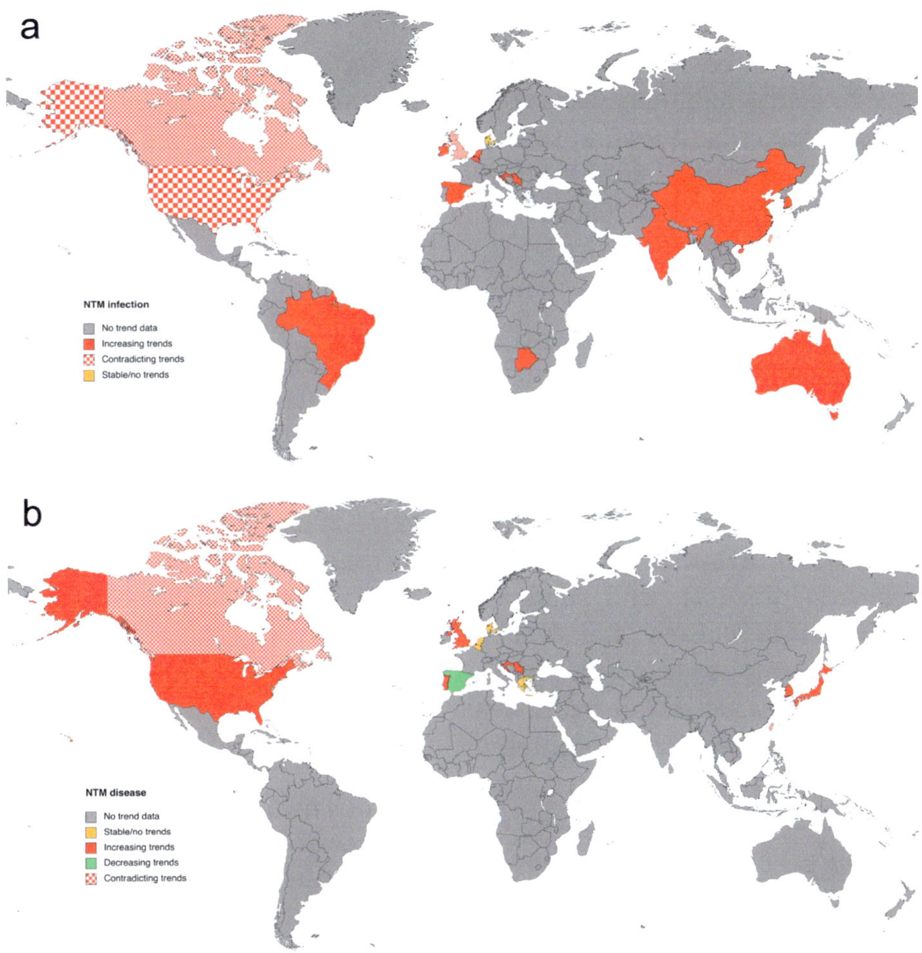

Figure 9.9. A world map of culture-based nontuberculous mycobacteria trend data. Trend data for NTM is presented in panels (a) and (b) for infection and disease (including microbiologically defined), respectively. Red colors represent increasing trends, yellow represents stable trends, green represents decreasing trends, and red-white checkered represents countries with contradicting trends (i.e., increasing, stable, and/or decreasing).

Source: https://www.ijidonline.com/cms/10.1016/j.ijid.2022.10.013/asset/398a2d83-8ab0-47e6-ac6f-27996c5fc631/main.assets/gr2.jpg.

Their prevalence is notable in environments with prolonged exposure, such as regions characterised by high humidity and warm climates, where these bacteria thrive. This ecological setting predisposes certain populations to NTM-related diseases, especially where pulmonary tissues are already compromised by pre-existing conditions. It is essential to comprehend how geographic factors impact the presence of such pathogens, as this understanding informs interventions targeting high-risk groups with structural lung diseases, including bronchiectasis and emphysema (Mortaz et al., 2017). Therefore, establishing correlations between geographical conditions and infection rates provides valuable insights for the prevention and control of these infections (Figure 9.9).

Furthermore, geographic patterns also reflect variations in healthcare access, which directly influence diagnosis and treatment rates for mycobacterial infections. For example, urban areas generally have better access to advanced medical facilities and diagnostic tools, enabling early diagnosis and control of conditions like tuberculosis and NTM infections. Conversely, rural or less developed regions often face shortages of information, diagnostic centres, and treatment facilities, which promote the spread of these infections. The epidemiological landscape is likely shaped by the intersection of geography, socioeconomic status, and healthcare infrastructure. Moreover, geographical differences may complicate national and international understanding of infection prevalence and risk factors, emphasising the need to develop locally tailored public health programmes that consider these spatial variations (Wilson et al., 2015). This analysis is vital for public health organisations striving to effectively counter the rising trend of mycobacterial infections. Additionally, climate change and urbanization have been shown to influence the distribution patterns of mycobacterial infections, mainly through effects on environmental reservoirs. Rising temperatures and increasingly unpredictable weather patterns may alter the supportive habitats of NTM and other mycobacteria, exposing new populations to these microorganisms. Urbanization tends to lead to changes in environmental landscapes, affecting water systems where NTM can thrive. The interface between human activity and the natural environment draws particular attention, with increased awareness of how human actions can modify disease processes. Another layer of complexity involves identifying immunogenetic factors that confer susceptibility to mycobacterial infections, which may be specific to certain locales. Consequently, geographic distribution is not only important for epidemiological surveillance but also for designing targeted interventions and ensuring healthcare systems are adequately prepared to manage these infections under evolving climatic conditions (Mortaz et al., 2017).

9.4. Diagnosis of Mycobacterial Infections

Diagnosing mycobacterial infections poses a substantial challenge within clinical practice, largely due to the diverse manifestations of such infections. Mycobacterial diseases, including tuberculosis (TB) and nontuberculous mycobacteria (NTM) infections, are frequently misdiagnosed, resulting in inappropriate treatment. In many low-resource settings, there exists a troubling tendency to over-diagnose malaria among febrile patients, thereby underestimating the prevalence of mycobacterial infections. A study conducted in northern Tanzania revealed that, although malaria was common and routinely monitored, it accounted for only a small proportion of fever cases; conversely, bacterial and mycobacterial diseases were grossly underestimated. This diagnostic discrepancy underscores the urgent need for improved diagnostic methods that adopt a systematic approach, considering a broad spectrum of potential febrile causes, particularly in resource-limited environments (Crump et al., 2013). Advances in diagnostic technology hold the promise of significantly improving mycobacterial infection detection. Conventional methods, such as culture and microscopy, often lack sensitivity and are time-consuming. Recently, mass spectrometry-based techniques have evolved as versatile tools for rapid identification of mycobacterial species. For instance, analysis of mycolic acids, a key component of mycobacterial cell walls, has proven particularly valuable. It has been demonstrated that electrospray ionisation tandem mass spectrometry can generate distinct profiles for different mycobacterial species, enabling reliable differentiation. A comparative study involving Polish patients found this method to possess higher sensitivity and specificity compared to existing diagnostic criteria, enabling the positive identification of TB within hours, thus facilitating timely clinical decision-making and effective management strategies (Szewczyk et al., 2013). Nonetheless, challenges remain regarding the widespread implementation of advanced diagnostic technologies for mycobacterial diseases. Access to sophisticated instruments, such as mass spectrometers, may be limited in low-resource healthcare facilities where traditional methods prevail. Consequently, a dual approach should be adopted, combining advanced techniques with simple diagnostic methods. Education and training of healthcare professionals are essential to enhance diagnostic accuracy and to ensure that differential diagnoses of febrile illnesses include mycobacterial diseases. A paradigm shift towards a diagnostic approach emphasising mycobacterial infections is necessary to improve patient outcomes and to reorganise public health strategies for more effective control of these widespread diseases. By bridging the gap between innovation and practical application, the diagnostic capacity for mycobacterial infections can be transformed, leading to improved disease management.

9.4.1. Clinical Symptoms and History

The clinical presentation of mycobacterial infection is notably diverse, reflecting the inherent challenges associated with both diagnosis and therapy. Such infections may manifest with a broad spectrum of respiratory and systemic symptoms, which can be indistinguishable from those caused by other infectious or non-infectious conditions. For example, pulmonary tuberculosis traditionally manifests with chronic cough, fever, night sweats, and weight loss, whereas extrapulmonary involvement varies depending on the affected organ system. Immunocompromised individuals, such as patients infected with HIV, may present with atypical symptoms, thereby complicating the diagnostic process. The level of adherence to antiretroviral therapy and the patient's CD4 immune status significantly influence both disease manifestation and symptomatology. Consequently, a comprehensive evaluation of clinical symptoms in conjunction with detailed history-taking is crucial for accurate diagnosis, particularly in patients with overlapping conditions such as sarcoidosis, where misdiagnosis is common (Mencarini et al., 2016). Moreover, the patient's medical history provides vital insights into the course and impact of mycobacterial infections. A thorough history can reveal potential exposures, previous infections, and overall health status that predispose an individual to mycobacterial disease. Historical information, including past tuberculosis infections and the efficacy of prior treatments, holds particular relevance. This assessment becomes more complex in patients with primary immunodeficiencies, such as X-linked hyper-IgM syndrome, wherein recurrent opportunistic infections, including mycobacterial infections, are frequently observed. Evaluation of familial predisposition and immune status further aids in clarifying the origins of symptoms and supports clinicians in devising appropriate therapeutic interventions. Therefore, assembling a comprehensive clinical history is essential for establishing a definitive diagnosis and guiding effective management of mycobacterial infections (Chen et al., 2014) (Figure 9. 10).

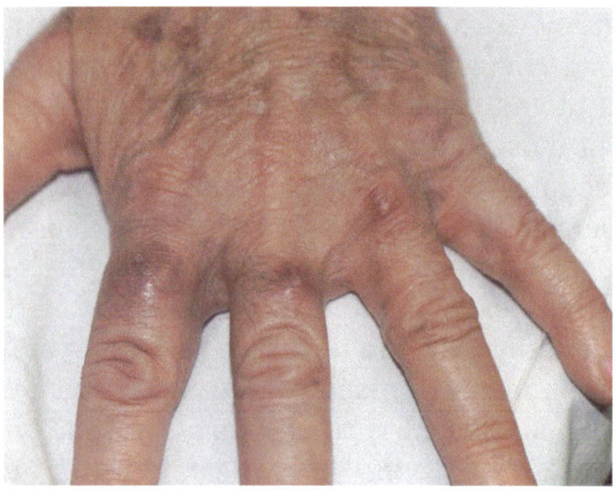

Figure 9.10. The clinical symptoms associated with mycobacterial infections.

Source: https://external-content.duckduckgo.com/iu/?u=https%3A%2F%2Fwww.dermatologyadvisor.com%2Fwp-content%2Fuploads%2Fsites%2F20%2F2019%2F03%2Fch757.fig1_.jpg&f=1&nofb=1&ipt=2905c867e89fe62cbb439ce19aa48577dc07398ab15fdd5fca99472b25a46b84.

Finally, information regarding the timing of symptoms and the history of the patient can give clues to the prognosis of mycobacterial infection. The pattern of recurrence of symptoms and chronicity will tend to reflect the immune response and the degree of disease development, particularly in the immunocompromised patient. For instance, in patients with a history of tuberculosis, a new presentation of the disease can not only be indicative of reactivation but also possibly co-infection with another causative agent of disease, complicating the treatment regimes. In addition, in broken treatment, even the risk of developing co-morbidities or developing strains may further complicate the patient's condition. Thus, longitudinal assessment of patient history and clinical signs is required to predict progression of the disease, guide the therapeutic interventions, and improve the outcome of the patient in mycobacterial infections. It is particularly crucial in a clinic where pathologies can overlap in possibility; hence, having the capability to grasp each patient's unique case becomes significant (Mencarini et al., 2016).

9.4.2. Laboratory Tests and Imaging Techniques

Diagnosis of mycobacterial infections primarily depends on laboratory methods and imaging techniques, which are essential for identifying and detecting causative organisms. Traditional laboratory techniques, such as acid-fast bacilli (AFB) smear microscopy and culture, remain the fundamental methods for diagnosing mycobacterial infections caused by *Mycobacterium tuberculosis* and non-tuberculous mycobacteria (NTM). These are complemented by newer molecular techniques, including polymerase chain reaction (PCR) assays, which offer rapid and specific detection of mycobacterial DNA. Although culture is considered the gold standard for definitive diagnosis, it is typically slow, making efficient imaging modalities crucial for early detection of infection and assessment of disease severity. Consequently, an integrated approach usually combines laboratory results with imaging findings to ensure accurate diagnosis and inform treatment planning in clinical practice. Imaging methods such as chest X-rays, computed tomography (CT), and magnetic resonance imaging (MRI) play significant roles in evaluating both pulmonary and extrapulmonary mycobacterial infections.

Chest X-rays are generally the initial imaging choice, revealing characteristic features like cavitating lesions or nodular opacities seen in pulmonary tuberculosis. Advanced imaging techniques, such as CT, provide detailed cross-sectional views that aid in assessing the scope of infection, guiding biopsies, and identifying complications like empyema or bronchiectasis. MRI can also be particularly useful in evaluating spinal infections, notably Pott's disease. Combining these imaging techniques with laboratory data enhances clinicians' ability to accurately stage infections and tailor therapeutic interventions according to the overall clinical picture, ultimately improving patient outcomes (Figure 9.11).

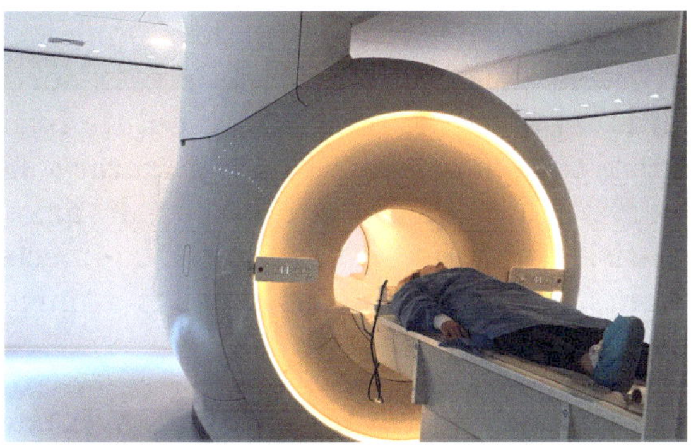

Figure 9.11. Magnetic resonance imaging (MRI) are instrumental in the evaluation of pulmonary and extrapulmonary mycobacterial infections.

Source: https://external-content.duckduckgo.com/iu/?u=https%3A%2F%2Fmrctcenter.org%2Fclinical-research-glossary%2Fwp-content%2Fuploads%2Fsites%2F8%2F2021%2F05%2Fmagnetic-resonance-imaging.png&f=1&nofb=1&ipt=e01b2fcd3df6119cab29bd7698b568e7c5e066e5f70ee7ec986687d25b1726af.

Emerging innovations in imaging devices and laboratory diagnostics are shaping the future of mycobacterial infection management. One notable advancement is positron emission tomography combined with computed tomography (PET/CT), which provides a significant advantage over traditional methods by visualising tissue metabolic activity to assess infection severity and treatment response. This technique can detect active disease before any structural damage occurs, enabling earlier intervention. Furthermore, improvements in radiopharmaceuticals are improving nuclear imaging, allowing non-invasive *in vivo* monitoring of mycobacterial infections. PET/CT has already proven effective in tracking drug delivery and pharmacokinetics, which is vital for developing successful treatments for mycobacterial diseases (Pawar et al., 2024). Collectively, these radiographic and laboratory innovations deepen our understanding of mycobacterial pathogenesis, leading to better management strategies and ultimately improving patient care and outcomes.

9.4.3. Challenges in Accurate Diagnosis

Mycobacterial diseases present significant diagnostic challenges, which considerably impact the promptness and appropriateness of treatment. The intricate group of mycobacteria, including *Mycobacterium tuberculosis* and numerous non-tuberculous species, compounds this complexity. Conventional diagnostic methods, such as smear microscopy and culture, rely on lengthy incubation periods, thereby delaying the detection of active infections. Such delays may lead to adverse clinical outcomes, particularly among immunocompromised individuals or patients with co-morbidities. Furthermore, these traditional techniques exhibit reduced sensitivity in patients with low bacterial loads, potentially resulting in false-negative results and misdiagnoses. Consequently, there is a pressing need for more effective diagnostic tools capable of rapid and accurate identification to improve management of mycobacterial diseases. Recent years have witnessed innovation in diagnostic approaches; however, several obstacles remain to be addressed. Emerging techniques, including mass spectrometry and molecular diagnostics, offer promising advancements in identifying *Mycobacterium tuberculosis* with enhanced sensitivity and specificity compared to conventional methods. For example, mycolic acid profiling has demonstrated an ability to classify mycobacterial species swiftly, generating distinctive profiles that could enhance clinical decision-making and patient care (Szewczyk et al., 2013).

Nevertheless, the deployment of such sophisticated technologies may be restricted in low-resource settings, where the necessary equipment and technical expertise may be unavailable or inadequately maintained. This disparity in diagnostic capacity contributes to unequal health outcomes across different regions, underscoring the imperative for interventions that facilitate equitable access to advanced diagnostic technologies. Additionally, the heterogeneous clinical presentation of mycobacterial infections further complicates accurate diagnosis. Symptoms are often non-specific and resemble those of recurrent respiratory infections, rendering misdiagnosis and inappropriate treatment more likely. Co-infections with other pathogens, such as human immunodeficiency virus (HIV), further obscure clinical assessments, making it difficult for healthcare professionals to attribute symptoms to a single etiological agent. Such overlapping clinical manifestations necessitate heightened clinical suspicion, a comprehensive understanding of mycobacterial pathology, and thorough diagnostic testing to ensure effective diagnosis and management. In the context of increasing antimicrobial resistance, the importance of accurate diagnosis is further amplified. This underscores the need to develop robust and diverse diagnostic techniques capable of capturing the nuanced presentations of mycobacterial infections (Tweyongyere et al., 2011).

9.5. Treatment Options for Mycobacterial Infections

The management of mycobacterial infections, such as tuberculosis (TB) and nontuberculous mycobacterial (NTM) disease, necessitates a multidisciplinary approach owing to the specificity of the pathogens involved. For TB, treatment predominantly involves a multi-drug regimen administered over an extended period, typically six months or longer, comprising isoniazid, rifampin, pyrazinamide, and ethambutol. This combination is designed to effectively eradicate the bacteria while concurrently minimising the development of drug resistance. Recent efforts are exploring additional strategies, including point-of-care testing, to enhance diagnostic accuracy and improve treatment outcomes, especially among high-risk populations such as HIV co-infected patients, where TB co-infection is common (Yoon et al., 2017).

Consequently, public health initiatives must focus on antibiotic stewardship and optimising diagnostic and therapeutic interventions to mitigate the challenge of drug-resistant strains. The treatment of nontuberculous mycobacterial infections, particularly those caused by species like *Mycobacterium avium* complex, may be more complex due to the heterogeneous susceptibility profiles of these organisms. Standard therapy generally involves a combination of macrolides, rifamycins, and ethambutol administered over a duration ranging from 12 to 24 months. Recent evidence suggests that integrating both pharmacologic and nonpharmacologic measures alongside conventional antibiotic therapy can significantly enhance patient outcomes. Given the prevalence of NTM in environmental reservoirs, notably water systems, surveillance programs and awareness campaigns are increasingly employed to underscore the influence of environmental factors on the aetiology and control of such infections (Nunes-Costa et al., 2016) (Figure 9.12).

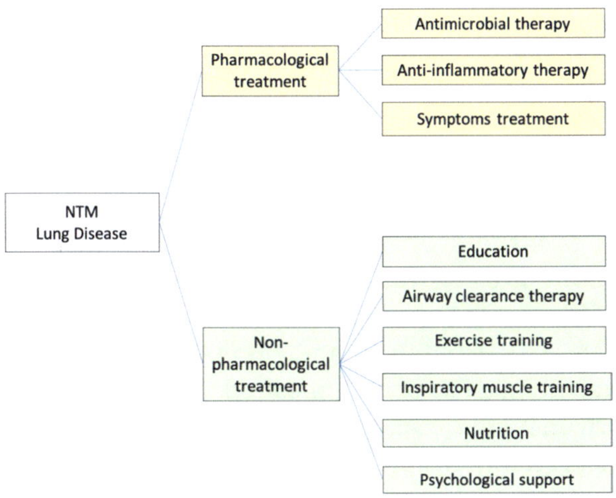

Figure 9.12. Comprehensive management of NTM pulmonary disease.

Source: https://media.springernature.com/lw685/springer-static/image/art%3A10.1007%2Fs15010-024-02183-3/MediaObjects/15010_2024_2183_Fig1_HTML.png.

This dual emphasis on environmental regulation and personalised treatment protocols is vital in addressing the rising prevalence of NTM disease worldwide. Furthermore, the field of mycobacterial infection therapy is undergoing significant evolution as researchers endeavour to discover novel therapeutic agents and methodologies. The advancement of adjunctive therapies, including immunomodulation and the application of newer drugs effective against resistant strains, is crucial in managing the resurgence of drug-resistant mycobacterial diseases. Recent clinical investigations are examining the efficacy of innovative compounds and combination therapies that could augment existing treatment protocols for tuberculosis (TB) and NTM infections. These developments have the potential to fundamentally transform the management of such infections, especially among immunocompromised populations. Ultimately, a coordinated strategy that integrates enhanced diagnostic techniques, individualised treatment plans, and judicious public health policies will be essential in combating the escalating threat of mycobacterial infections on a global scale.

9.5.1. Antibiotic Regimens for Tuberculosis

The treatment of tuberculosis (TB) mainly involves using specific antibiotic regimens aimed at targeting *Mycobacterium tuberculosis*, the bacterium that causes TB. The standard regimen usually includes a combination of at least four drugs: isoniazid, rifampin, ethambutol, and pyrazinamide, taken for six to nine months. This drug combination is important because it reduces the risk of developing new drug-resistant strains of the bacteria, which is a major concern in TB control. Strict adherence to the medication schedule is essential; failure to do so can lead to treatment failure and increase the risk of transmitting the infection to others. To support compliance, healthcare workers often use Directly Observed Therapy (DOT), where they supervise patients taking their medication, which helps improve treatment outcomes and lower the incidence of multidrug-resistant TB. Over recent decades, the rise of drug-resistant forms of *M. tuberculosis* has posed new challenges to TB management. Multidrug-resistant TB (MDR-TB) and extensively drug-resistant TB (XDR-TB) require alternative, more complex, and longer regimens. Treating these resistant strains involves second-line drugs, such as fluoroquinolones and injectable agents like amikacin. These treatments last between 18 and 24 months and require careful monitoring for side effects and response. Developing new drugs and formulations of existing medications remains a priority in addressing drug-resistant TB (Figure 9.13).

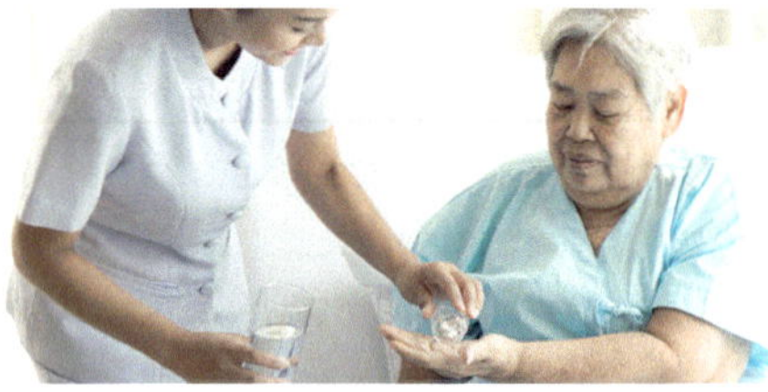

Figure 9.13. Directly observed therapy.

Source: https://external-content.duckduckgo.com/iu/?u=https%3A%2F%2Fwww.hamad.qa%2FEN%2FHospitals-and-services%2FCommunicable-Disease-Center%2FPublishingImages%2F020%2520Our%2520Services%2Fshutterstock_1053770519-856.jpg&f=1&nofb=1&ipt=fa1b9fa2e91471acdb802ad0466846165da51168957ff9a5d1b915d0228bbc98.

Notably, the incorporation of new diagnostic technology, namely molecular tests, facilitates more rapid detection of resistant strains, thereby enabling the timely adjustment of treatment regimens to optimise patient outcomes. The global health landscape also underscores significant disparities in access to effective tuberculosis (TB) treatment protocols. In low- and middle-income countries, where TB prevalence is generally highest, first-line and second-line antibiotics are frequently unavailable due to financial limitations and inadequate healthcare infrastructure. The presence of non-tuberculous mycobacteria (NTM), which complicates the clinical picture, further exacerbates these concerns. Given its increasing relevance, it is crucial to understand the relationship between NTM infections and *M. tuberculosis* infections. For instance, NTMS have been implicated in chronic pulmonary infections, particularly in patients with pre-existing lung conditions such as cystic fibrosis, necessitating systemic treatment regimens that consider both TB and NTMs. Adopting more aggressive antibiotic therapies that address co-infections will be essential in the global effort to combat mycobacterial diseases (Floto et al., 2015; Nunes-Costa et al., 2016.

9.5.2. Management of Non-Tuberculous Mycobacterial Infections

The management of non-tuberculous mycobacterial (NTM) infections presents considerable challenges, particularly in cases of pulmonary infections where predisposing factors complicate treatment. NTM are environmental organisms that predominantly infect patients with predispositions such as bronchiectasis and chronic obstructive pulmonary disease (COPD), often resulting in increased severity of illness. The rising incidence of NTM infections can be attributed to an ageing population and heightened use of immunosuppressive therapies, which increase susceptibility to these organisms. Regrettably, despite advancements in diagnostic imaging and microbiological techniques, there remains a lack of comprehensive understanding of the immunologic response to NTM. This uncertainty complicates clinical management, as healthcare professionals face difficulties in devising optimal treatment regimens within a fragmented system of knowledge and resources (Mortaz et al., 2017). Therefore, the most effective management strategies are those that involve a multidisciplinary approach through interprofessional collaboration among infectious disease specialists, pulmonologists, and microbiologists. Coordinated care is essential for addressing the complexities of NTM infections, which frequently necessitate long-term treatment involving complex drug regimens. Such therapies pose challenges, including inherent antibiotic resistance and potential severe side effects that may impair tolerability. Furthermore, initiating treatment requires a careful evaluation of risks and benefits, given that patient outcomes vary and some may experience suboptimal responses. Adherence to established guidelines, such as those endorsed by the American Thoracic Society and the Infectious Diseases Society of America, is crucial; however, global compliance remains notably low, thus hampering control efforts (Chalmers et al., 2018). Additional research into the epidemiology and therapeutic strategies for NTM disease is of paramount importance. Although acknowledgement of risk factors has increased, much remains to be understood regarding optimal treatment protocols. Ongoing randomised clinical trials are beginning to assess the efficacy of current and novel therapies and may provide vital guidance for clinical practice. As awareness of NTM-associated diseases advances, interdisciplinary collaboration and enhanced patient education will be imperative to improve outcomes. Ultimately, integrating research with clinical practice will empower healthcare providers to refine treatment paradigms, ensuring that patients receive comprehensive, individualised care tailored to their specific needs and circumstances to effectively manage non-tuberculous mycobacterial infections (Chalmers et al., 2018).

9.5.3. Emerging Therapies and Drug Resistance

The pattern of mycobacterial diseases, including infections caused by *Mycobacterium tuberculosis* and non- tuberculous mycobacteria, presents increasing challenges due to the emergence of drug resistance. Given that the incidence of non-tuberculous mycobacteria (NTM) infections is rising globally — propelled by aging populations and increased use of immunosuppressive therapies — the complexity of treatment has significantly escalated. Patients frequently encounter inherent antibiotic resistance, compelling clinicians to administer complex and often poorly tolerated drug regimens. The American Thoracic Society has recently promulgated guidelines intended to assist physicians in properly assessing NTM-related diseases; however, adherence remains suboptimal worldwide. This underscores the urgent need for heightened awareness and improved compliance with treatment protocols. The multifaceted nature of drug resistance necessitates a multidisciplinary approach, combining the expertise of various healthcare professionals to enhance patient outcomes and address the complex challenges posed by such infections (Chalmers et al., 2018). In response to the escalating threat of drug-resistant *Mycobacterium tuberculosis*, research efforts have increasingly focused on developing novel therapeutics aimed at enhancing treatment efficacy. Among these promising avenues are antimicrobial peptides (AMPs) — short, positively charged peptides that are integral to the innate immune response. AMPs offer several advantages over traditional antibiotics, including a reduced propensity for resistance development and broad-spectrum antimicrobial activity. Nonetheless, despite these potential benefits, advancing such therapeutic compounds from laboratory research to clinical application remains challenging due to technical hurdles related to optimising therapeutic properties and production processes. Addressing these issues could profoundly influence tuberculosis treatment protocols, particularly against multi-drug-resistant strains. Consequently, rigorous clinical trials and ongoing research are essential to evaluate the efficacy of AMPs and facilitate their integration into current treatment frameworks (Agerberth et al., 2016). The intricacy of treating mycobacterial infections underscores the importance of comprehensive awareness of emerging therapies and resistance mechanisms. As drug-resistant strains pose a severe public health threat, sustained research efforts are imperative. Innovative therapeutic strategies, such as combination therapy leveraging the synergistic effects of traditional antibiotics and novel agents, offer hope in combating resistant bacteria. Additionally, targeted therapies, improved vaccines, and advanced drug delivery systems are immediate priorities for research and development. Furthermore, fostering collaboration among clinicians, public health professionals, and researchers will significantly enhance the management of mycobacterial infections. Ultimately, future progress will depend on balancing novel drug development and alternative approaches with the evolving resistance landscape, thereby expanding the arsenal available to effectively counteract the impact of mycobacterial diseases (Chalmers et al., 2018).

9.6. Prevention and Control Measures

An interdisciplinary approach is essential for the control and prevention of mycobacterial infections, particularly regarding *Mycobacterium tuberculosis* and non-tuberculous mycobacteria (NTM). Vaccination remains a fundamental pillar in tuberculosis prevention, with the Bacillus Calmette-Guérin (BCG) vaccine serving as the primary intervention. Although BCG has limited efficacy in treating lethal forms of tuberculosis in infants, its effectiveness in adults remains inconsistent, indicating the necessity for the development of new vaccine candidates that can significantly enhance immunity beyond the neonatal period. As research progresses, solutions that build upon the success of BCG while integrating novel immunological insights are vital. Specifically, quantifying interferon-gamma (IFN-γ) responses to BCG and assessing differences across populations can facilitate the optimisation of vaccination strategies and improve overall immunogenicity, thereby contributing to better containment of tuberculosis in diverse settings (Finan et al., 2008). Beyond vaccination efforts, early detection and treatment programs are critical components of public health strategies against mycobacterial infections. Routine screening, particularly among high-risk groups such as individuals with underlying lung conditions or immunocompromised statuses, can enable timely intervention. For example, patients with bronchiectasis, pulmonary diseases, or a history of previous tuberculosis are at increased risk of NTM infections and should be subject to regular surveillance and prompt treatment upon diagnosis. Moreover, raising public awareness regarding the symptoms and transmission modes of tuberculosis and nontuberculous mycobacterial infections empowers communities to seek medical advice promptly. Proper application of diagnostic and treatment modalities can significantly diminish the incidence and prevalence of these infections, thereby enhancing overall health outcomes (Mortaz et al., 2017). Environmental factors also play a critical role in preventing mycobacterial infections. Understanding the environmental habitats of NTM, which include water and soil, can inform public health initiatives aimed at reducing exposure. Ensuring adequate water supply and sanitation facilities is a crucial strategy to mitigate NTM risks. Additionally, healthcare facilities must implement environmental controls as a priority, particularly in settings where patients are immunocompromised or at heightened risk of acquiring mycobacterial infections. Ongoing research endeavours to elucidate the complex interactions between host immunity and environmental exposure, and interdisciplinary collaboration remains paramount. Public health policy must integrate environmental sciences with clinical practice to develop a comprehensive strategy for the prevention and control of mycobacterial infections, thereby protecting vulnerable populations (Finan et al., 2008; Mortaz et al., 2017).

9.6.1. Vaccination Strategies

The significance of vaccination strategies in combating mycobacterial infections cannot be overstated, particularly for diseases such as tuberculosis and paratuberculosis. Current vaccines, including the Bacillus Calmette-Guérin (BCG) vaccine against tuberculosis, have demonstrated limited efficacy, underscoring the urgent necessity for the development of novel and improved vaccine formulations. The development of new vaccines capable of replacing or supplementing BCG is essential, as the existing vaccine does not offer comprehensive protection against the various strains of *Mycobacterium tuberculosis* responsible for the ongoing global epidemic. Innovative approaches, such as mucosal vaccine techniques, have emerged as promising alternatives, capable of eliciting more robust and localised immune responses, ultimately enhancing protection against mycobacterial infections, particularly among high-risk populations (Pinedo et al., 2018). The exploration of gene-manipulated and low-virulence derivatives of *Mycobacterium* to create effective vaccines presents an intriguing avenue of research. For example, studies on *Mycobacterium avium* subsp. *paratuberculosis* have identified certain strains, such as the low-virulence strain 1543/481, which lacks the capacity to elicit significant immune responses but shows promise as a live vaccine candidate. Conversely, the virulent strain 6611 exhibits high immunostimulatory properties, distinguishing it as a candidate for further evaluation in both live and inactivated vaccine formulations (Pinedo et al., 2018) (Figure 9.14).

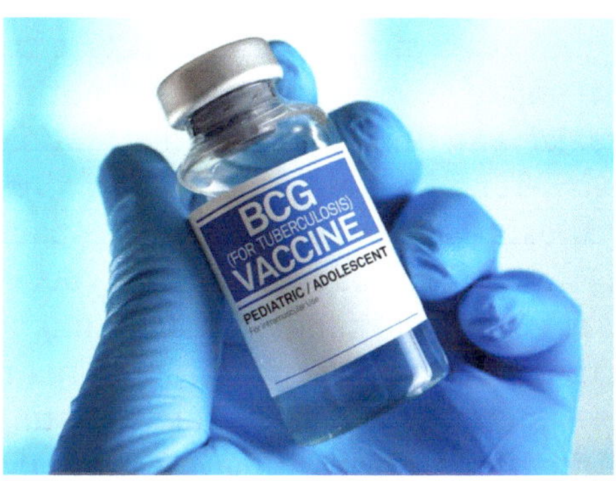

Figure 9.14. A gloved hand holds a vial of BCG vaccine, used for the prevention of tuberculosis in pediatric and adolescent populations.

Source: https://medicalupdateonline.com/wp-content/uploads/2024/04/AdobeStock_493765943-1000x667.jpg.

This immune response discrimination underscores the importance of selecting appropriate mycobacterial strains for use in vaccine development, given their direct impact on protective efficacy and the promotion of future research into personalized vaccination strategies. Additionally, the adoption of innovative delivery methods, such as mucosal routes of vaccination, may potentially augment vaccine effectiveness against mycobacterial infections. Since these are primarily respiratory infections, mycobacterial diseases offer the prospect that mucosal vaccines could immunize at the entry point of infection, potentially surpassing the efficacy of traditional systemic approaches. Current evidence indicates that mucosal vaccines could serve as a safe and effective means of combating tuberculosis; however, further refinement of delivery techniques and a clearer understanding of the underlying immunological mechanisms are required (Barclay et al., 2019). These ongoing advancements reflect a burgeoning appreciation for novel vaccination strategies that align with the complexities of mycobacterial diseases and ultimately contribute to improved global health outcomes.

9.6.2. Public Health Initiatives

Public health measures are of paramount importance in controlling mycobacterial infections, most notably tuberculosis (TB), which constitutes a significant global health challenge. These measures can be employed to decrease the prevalence and incidence of mycobacterial diseases and to elevate community awareness. Various initiatives — including vaccination campaigns, public education programs, and screening efforts — are conducted by government agencies and health organisations aimed at promoting early detection and prompt treatment. Through sustained efforts, public health authorities ensure that at-risk populations are informed about the signs and symptoms of mycobacterial infections, thereby facilitating early medical intervention. This preventive approach not only mitigates the burden of disease but also diminishes transmission rates within communities, contributing to the overall enhancement of public health outcomes in regions with high infection rates. Furthermore, reinforcing the efficacy of public health initiatives, policies addressing social determinants of health are equally crucial in combating mycobacterial infections. Factors such as poverty, healthcare accessibility, and education directly influence the likelihood of disease acquisition, including TB. Incorporating socio-economic interventions into public health models can improve access and continuity of care among vulnerable groups. For instance, public-private collaborations can promote resource sharing and improve healthcare delivery, particularly in rural areas with strained health systems. Implementing policies like the National Cancer Control Plan (NCCP), which focus on preventive measures such as lifestyle modifications and vaccination programs, not only enhances health outcomes but also reduces the long-term healthcare costs associated with advanced infection stages. Addressing these foundational issues enables public health programs to establish a resilient support network for individuals affected by mycobacterial infections. An additional critical component of public health strategies is the development and integration of research and surveillance systems. Evidence-based interventions informed by ongoing epidemiological research can lead to more effective prevention and control methods. For example, advancements in diagnostic technologies can significantly expedite and improve detection accuracy, facilitating easier treatment and reducing transmission risks. Moreover, investing in the education of healthcare professionals — equipping them with the necessary knowledge and skills — is essential for successful outbreak management. This not only enhances clinical practice but also ensures adherence to infection control guidelines. Ultimately, the success of public health interventions depends on a comprehensive approach that combines direct healthcare measures with attention to socio-economic determinants. Such an integrated strategy is vital for addressing the complexities of mycobacterial infections and for advancing the broader goal of public health improvement.

9.6.3. Importance of Early Detection and Treatment

Early detection and prompt treatment are crucial in managing mycobacterial infections, especially tuberculosis (TB), which remains one of the leading causes of death worldwide. *Mycobacterium tuberculosis* infection poses a significant challenge due to its virulence, which can cause irreversible damage unless identified quickly. Delayed diagnosis allows bacteria to replicate for longer, worsening clinical outcomes and increasing the risk of transmission. Additionally, understanding the immune response — particularly the role of type I interferons — emphasises how early intervention can prevent harmful effects of unchecked inflammation and bacterial growth. These risks can be mitigated through early treatment; therefore, effective screening and management form vital components of public health strategies aimed at preventing TB outbreaks and improving patient outcomes (Moreira-Teixeira et al., 2018). Besides tuberculosis, non-tuberculous mycobacterial (NTM) infections, such as those caused by *Mycobacterium gordonae*, also highlight the importance of early detection and treatment. Proper monitoring is essential to distinguish true infections from pseudo-outbreaks, as illustrated when clinical isolates were found without corresponding disease symptoms. An investigation into a pseudo-outbreak revealed that environmental factors contributed to diagnostic uncertainty, underscoring the necessity for rapid diagnostic capabilities in healthcare facilities. Routine environmental surveillance and strict adherence to protocols can greatly reduce misdiagnosis and ensure appropriate treatment. This preventive approach not only reduces unnecessary therapy but also emphasises understanding the clinical context of mycobacterial exposure (Scorzolini et al., 2016). Furthermore, initiating treatment early in mycobacterial infections is vital to improve patient outcomes and prevent disease progression. The disease course may be slow and asymptomatic initially, with delayed diagnosis often resulting in advanced stages of illness. Early antimicrobial intervention effectively reduces morbidity and mortality and helps prevent the development of drug resistance. As demonstrated, early treatment benefits individual patients and has a broader public health goal of limiting infection spread within communities. Consequently, a robust early detection system — supported by advances in molecular diagnostics and risk stratification — should form the backbone of healthcare policies for managing mycobacterial infections. With an active strategy, healthcare systems can enhance their capacity to control these diseases efficiently and effectively.

SUMMARY

Research on mycobacterial infections uncovers important insights into the complex interactions between host and pathogen, especially regarding genetic susceptibility. The discovery of a mutation in the interferon gamma receptor 1 (IFNGR 1) gene in Maltese children underscores the critical role of genetic factors in determining susceptibility to severe mycobacterial infections. This mutation exemplifies how specific genetic predispositions can influence the severity and progression of the disease, especially within populations exhibiting high endemicity. The findings indicate that while heterozygote carriers may exhibit relative resistance to less virulent strains, such genetic heterogeneity can increase vulnerability to more pathogenic mycobacterial strains, thereby complicating public health strategies and necessitating a multifaceted approach to management (Anderson et al., 2012). Additionally, ongoing research underscores the significance of genetic susceptibility in mycobacterial diseases, emphasising the importance of robust public health measures with tailored interventions that address the specific vulnerabilities of diverse populations within heterogeneous communities. These strategies include insights derived from genetic studies and epidemiological data to inform effective screening and treatment protocols. The importance of interdisciplinary collaborations, exemplified by studies supported by organisations such as the Wellcome Trust, demonstrates the vital role that collaborative efforts play in addressing complex health challenges. Furthermore, acknowledgement of authorship in such research enhances the value of collaborative strategies in combating mycobacterial infections and improving patient outcomes globally (Wilson et al., 2015). Ultimately, the persistent challenges posed by mycobacterial infections demand an integrated and coordinated response that equally advances medical innovation and public health initiatives. Identifying public health implications of genetic mutations such as IFNGR1 can facilitate the development of targeted interventions, vaccines, and preventive measures for high-risk groups. Data from recent studies not only deepen our understanding of these infections but also underscore the importance of integrating genetic information into clinical practice and public health policy. As the epidemiology of mycobacterial infections continues to evolve, establishing a comprehensive global awareness and response will be essential to effectively mitigate the impact of these formidable pathogens on human health (Anderson et al., 2012).

Knowledge regarding mycobacterial infections commences with a meticulous examination of their characteristics, modes of transmission, and associated diseases. Mycobacteria constitute a genus comprising several pathogenic species, notably *Mycobacterium tuberculosis*, which is the causative agent of tuberculosis (TB). The primary mode of transmission involves airborne particles expelled during coughing or sneezing by an infected individual. Social determinants such as poverty, densely populated environments, and limited access to healthcare significantly influence the incidence of mycobacterial infections. Current data reveal an alarming prevalence of TB in high-burden countries, necessitating appropriate intervention strategies. Furthermore, the global resurgence of TB and the emergence of drug-resistant strains underscore the urgent need for novel therapeutic agents and vaccines, as these factors complicate disease management and public health efforts. Research into mycobacterial infections also encompasses the identification of the pathogens' distinctive physiological traits. Mycobacteria are characterised by a cell wall rich in mycolic acids, which provides enhanced resistance to environmental stresses and antimicrobial agents. This structural feature enables their survival under adverse conditions such as hypoxia and nutrient deprivation within host tissues. Certain mycobacterial species have demonstrated a remarkable capacity to enter a nonreplicating state, rendering them more resistant to standard antibiotics. For example, the detection of nonreplicating tubercle bacilli prompts critical questions regarding treatment efficacy and mechanisms underlying chronic infection. Such persister-like populations, isolated from sputum samples, serve as valuable models for developing innovative approaches to optimise chemotherapy and elucidate transmission dynamics of TB, ultimately informing public health interventions (Garton et al., 2008). The implications of mycobacterial infections extend beyond individual health, impacting communities and healthcare systems worldwide. The economic burden associated with diseases like tuberculosis results in substantial losses due to decreased productivity and increased healthcare costs. Consequently, global health initiatives have been established to combat these infections through comprehensive strategies, including extensive screening, robust treatment protocols, and community-based public education campaigns. Collaboration among governments, non-governmental organisations, and healthcare professionals is essential to maximize the effectiveness of interventions and improve patient outcomes. Ongoing research remains crucial for understanding the biology, epidemiology, and socio-economic determinants of mycobacterial infections, thereby advancing control measures and addressing this pervasive global health challenge (Wilson et al., 2015).

CLOSER LOOK

EXTENSIVELY DRUG-RESISTANT TUBERCULOSIS (XDR-TB)

Extensively drug-resistant tuberculosis (XDR-TB) is a severe form of multidrug-resistant tuberculosis (MDR-TB) caused by Mycobacterium tuberculosis strains resistant to four key anti-TB drugs. To be exact, XDR-TB has been formally defined as resistance to isoniazid and rifampicin (the two most effective first-line drugs), any fluoroquinolone (such as levofloxacin or moxifloxacin), and one of the three second-line injectable drugs (amikacin, kanamycin, or capreomycin). The emergence of XDR-TB is a serious global public health hazard due to its cause by low treatment options, high treatment failure rates, and higher mortality (Figure 9.15).

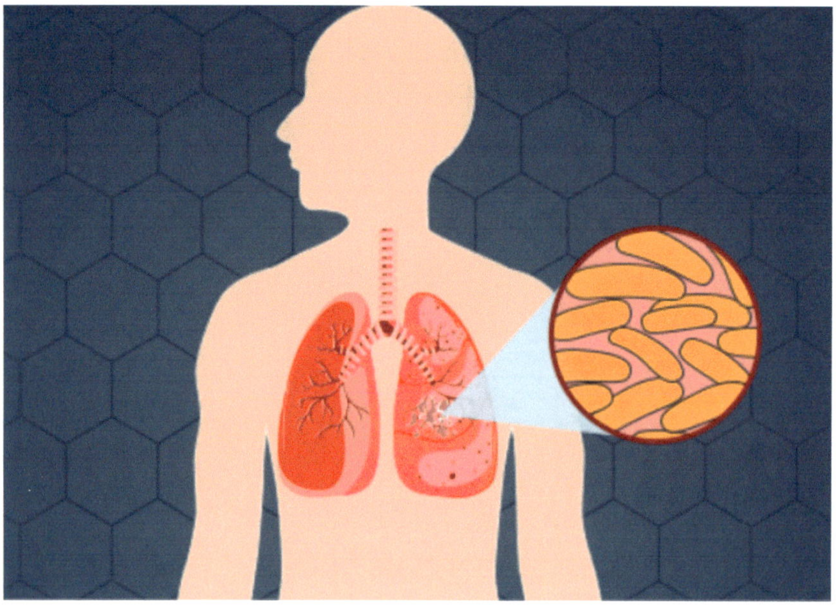

Figure 9.15. Illustration of a human respiratory system showing tuberculosis infection in the lungs, with a magnified view of *Mycobacterium tuberculosis*, the causative agent.

Source: https://cdn.sketchbubble.com/pub/media/catalog/product/optimized1/6/f/6f9a60742e10f346c9a2bcda206afa1f61c544c441d30c8b99b2123031e8c764/xdr-tuberculosis-slide1.png.

XDR-TB occurs primarily through inadequate treatment of TB, non-adherence to treatment, failure to conduct adequate diagnostic tests, or misuse of antibiotics. Person-to-person transmission of XDR-TB is also possible, especially in populous, poorly ventilated environments, e.g., prisons and hospitals. Anyone can contract XDR-TB, but individuals with compromised immune systems, such as individuals infected with HIV, are particularly vulnerable.

Clinically, XDR-TB is as symptomatic as drug-sensitive TB: chronic cough, fever, night sweats, weight loss, and weakness. But given its resistance to the best of drugs, it is harder, less effective, more toxic, and takes 18 to 24 months or more to cure. Treatment of XDR-TB includes second-line oral drugs combined with newer drugs like Bedaquiline and linezolid, and sometimes newer drugs like pretomanid. Treatment outcomes are far worse than for drug-sensitive TB, with cure rates for XDR-TB typically below 50%.

XDR-TB diagnosis requires advanced laboratory testing. Molecular techniques such as GeneXpert MTB/RIF can detect resistance to rifampicin quickly, while line probe assays and culture-based drug susceptibility testing (DST) can detect resistance to other drugs. Rapid and accurate detection is crucial to initiate appropriate treatment and prevent transmission.

XDR-TB preventive interventions are early detection and immediate treatment of drug-sensitive TB, good adherence to treatment, infection control in facilities, and contact tracing. BCG vaccine is some protection, with most of it being in children, and more research continues to come up with better vaccines against TB.

REFERENCES

1. Mortaz, E., Moloudizargari, M., Varahram, M., Movassaghi, M., Garssen, J., Kazempour Dizagie, M., Mirsaeidi, M., & Adcock, I. M. (2018). What Immunological Defects Predispose to Non-tuberculosis Mycobacterial Infections?. *Iranian journal of allergy, asthma, and immunology*, *17*(2), 100–109.(accessed on 16th July 2025).
2. Agerberth, B., Ahsan, F., Andersson, J., Andersson, M., Andries, K., Aoki, T., Asaduzzaman, S. M., et al. (2016). *Antimicrobial Peptides as Novel Anti-Tuberculosis Therapeutics.* https://core.ac.uk/download/55642138.pdf (accessed on 16th July 2025).
3. Chalmers, J. D., Aksamit, T., Carvalho, A. C. C., Rendon, A., & Franco, I. (2018). Non-tuberculous mycobacterial pulmonary infections. Pulmonology, 24(2), 120-131. https://doi.org/10.1016/j.pulmoe.2017.12.005(accessed on 16th July 2025).
4. Ahmed, W., Cacciottolo, J., Farrugia, B., Gauci, M., et al. (2015). *Tuberculosis in Malta: Thirty-Five Years of Epidemiological Trends in the Native Population.* https://core.ac.uk/download/46603551.pdf (accessed on 16th July 2025).
5. Nunes-Costa, D., Alarico, S., Dalcolmo, M. P., Correia-Neves, M., & Empadinhas, N. (2016). The looming tide of nontuberculous mycobacterial infections in Portugal and Brazil. *Tuberculosis (Edinburgh, Scotland)*, *96*, 107–119. https://doi.org/10.1016/j.tube.2015.09.006(accessed on 16th July 2025).
6. Wilson, G. J., Marakalala, M. J., Hoving, J. C., van Laarhoven, A., Drummond, R. A., Kerscher, B., Keeton, R., van de Vosse, E., Ottenhoff, T. H., Plantinga, T. S., Alisjahbana, B., Govender, D., Besra, G. S., Netea, M. G., Reid, D. M., Willment, J. A., Jacobs, M., Yamasaki, S., van Crevel, R., & Brown, G. D. (2015). The C-type lectin receptor CLECSF8/CLEC4D is a key component of anti-mycobacterial immunity. *Cell host & microbe*, *17*(2), 252–259. https://doi.org/10.1016/j.chom.2015.01.004(accessed on 16th July 2025).
7. Alvarado Pinedo, M. F., Colombatti Olivieri, M. A., Delgado, F. O., Gravisaco, G., et al. (2018). Protection efficacy of Argentinian isolates of *Mycobacterium avium* subsp. *paratuberculosis* with different genotypes and virulence in a murine model. https://core.ac.uk/download/287883333.pdf (accessed on 16th July 2025).
8. Garton, N. J., Waddell, S. J., Sherratt, A. L., Lee, S. M., Smith, R. J., Senner, C., Hinds, J., Rajakumar, K., Adegbola, R. A., Besra, G. S., Butcher, P. D., & Barer, M. R. (2008). Cytological and transcript analyses reveal fat and lazy persister-like bacilli in tuberculous sputum. *PLoS medicine*, *5*(4), e75. https://doi.org/10.1371/journal.pmed.0050075(accessed on 16th July 2025).
9. Yoon, C., Semitala, F. C., Atuhumuza, E., Katende, J., Mwebe, S., Asege, L., Armstrong, D. T., Andama, A. O., Dowdy, D. W., Davis, J. L., Huang, L., Kamya, M., & Cattamanchi, A. (2017). Point-of-care C-reactive protein-based tuberculosis screening for people living with HIV: a diagnostic accuracy study. *The Lancet. Infectious diseases*, *17*(12), 1285–1292. https://doi.org/10.1016/S1473-3099(17)30488-7(accessed on 16th July 2025).
10. Anderson, S. T., Attard Montalto, S., Felice, A., Hibberd, M., et al. (2012). *The role of the A C395 IFNGR1 mutation in determining susceptibility to intracellular infection in Malta.* https://core.ac.uk/download/46602324.pdf (accessed on 16th July 2025).
11. Mencarini, P., Bellagamba, R., Oliva, A., Ghirga, P., Giancola, M. L., Corpolongo, A., Ascoli Bartoli, T., De Nardo, P., Baiocchini, A., Del Nonno, F., Narciso, P., & Nicastri, E. (2016). Pulmonary

tuberculosis followed by sarcoidosis in an HIV-infected patient: A case report and a simplified diagnostic flowchart for diagnosis and treatment of sarcoidosis. *Respiratory medicine case reports*, *19*, 150–154. https://doi.org/10.1016/j.rmcr.2016.09.006(accessed on 16th July 2025).

12. Legido-Quigley, H., Montgomery, C. M., Khan, P., Atun, R., Fakoya, A., Getahun, H., & Grant, A. D. (2013). Integrating tuberculosis and HIV services in low- and middle-income countries: a systematic review. *Tropical medicine & international health : TM & IH*, *18*(2), 199–211. https://doi.org/10.1111/tmi.12029Ayub, N. I. F. (2015). *Molecular genotyping of Mycobacterium tuberculosis associated with extrapulmonary tuberculosis.* https://core.ac.uk/download/159615815.pdf (accessed on 16th July 2025).

13. Barclay, W. R., Stylianou, E., McShane, H., Paul, M. J., Reljic, R., Resende Co, T., Rodriguez, A., et al. (2019). *Mucosal delivery of tuberculosis vaccines: A review of current approaches and challenges.* https://core.ac.uk/download/286270868.pdf (accessed on 16th July 2025).

14. Dube, A. L., Baschieri, A., Cleland, J., Floyd, S., Molesworth, A., Parrott, F., French, N., & Glynn, J. R. (2012). Fertility intentions and use of contraception among monogamous couples in northern Malawi in the context of HIV testing: a cross-sectional analysis. *PloS one*, *7*(12), e51861. https://doi.org/10.1371/journal.pone.0051861(accessed on 16th July 2025).

15. Bentley, S. D., Blanco, M., Buckley, T., Cherevach, I., et al. (2010). *The genome of a pathogenic Rhodococcus: Cooptive virulence underpinned by key gene acquisitions.* https://core.ac.uk/download/19553779.pdf (accessed on 16th July 2025).

16. Floto, R. A., Olivier, K. N., Saiman, L., Daley, C. L., Herrmann, J. L., Nick, J. A., Noone, P. G., Bilton, D., Corris, P., Gibson, R. L., Hempstead, S. E., Koetz, K., Sabadosa, K. A., Sermet-Gaudelus, I., Smyth, A. R., van Ingen, J., Wallace, R. J., Winthrop, K. L., Marshall, B. C., Haworth, C. S., ... US Cystic Fibrosis Foundation and European Cystic Fibrosis Society (2016). US Cystic Fibrosis Foundation and European Cystic Fibrosis Society consensus recommendations for the management of non-tuberculous mycobacteria in individuals with cystic fibrosis. *Thorax*, *71 Suppl 1*(Suppl 1), i1–i22. https://doi.org/10.1136/thoraxjnl-2015-207360 (accessed on 16th July 2025).

17. Hayward, S. E., Dowd, J. B., Fletcher, H., Nellums, L. B., Wurie, F., & Boccia, D. (2019). A systematic review of the impact of psychosocial factors on immunity: Implications for enhancing BCG response against tuberculosis. *SSM - population health*, *10*, 100522. https://doi.org/10.1016/j.ssmph.2019.100522(accessed on 16th July 2025).

18. Crump, J. A., Morrissey, A. B., Nicholson, W. L., Massung, R. F., Stoddard, R. A., Galloway, R. L., Ooi, E. E., Maro, V. P., Saganda, W., Kinabo, G. D., Muiruri, C., & Bartlett, J. A. (2013). Etiology of severe non-malaria febrile illness in Northern Tanzania: a prospective cohort study. *PLoS neglected tropical diseases*, *7*(7), e2324. https://doi.org/10.1371/journal.pntd.0002324(accessed on 16th July 2025).

19. Drummond, R. A., & Brown, G. D. (2013). Signalling C-type lectins in antimicrobial immunity. *PLoS pathogens*, *9*(7), e1003417. https://doi.org/10.1371/journal.ppat.1003417(accessed on 16th July 2025).

20. Chen, T. X., Tian, Z. Q., Wang, L. L., Wang, H., et al. (2014). *Clinical features and genetic analysis of 20 Chinese patients with X-linked hyper-IgM syndrome.* https://core.ac.uk/download/79821686.pdf (accessed on 16th July 2025).

21. Chindelevitch, L., Cohen, T., Colijn, C., Moodley, P., et al. (2015). *ClassTR: Classifying within-host heterogeneity based on tandem repeats with application to Mycobacterium tuberculosis infections.* https://core.ac.uk/download/77008538.pdf (accessed on 16th July 2025).

22. Tweyongyere, R., Mawa, P. A., Kihembo, M., Jones, F. M., Webb, E. L., Cose, S., Dunne, D. W., Vennervald, B. J., & Elliott, A. M. (2011). Effect of praziquantel treatment of Schistosoma mansoni during pregnancy on immune responses to schistosome antigens among the offspring: results of a randomised, placebo-controlled trial. *BMC infectious diseases*, *11*, 234. https://doi.org/10.1186/1471-2334-11-234 (accessed on 16th July 2025).

23. Scorzolini, L., Mengoni, F., Mastroianni, C. M., Baldan, R., Cirillo, D. M., De Giusti, M., Marinelli, L., Cottarelli, A., Fattorini, L., & Vullo, V. (2016). Pseudo-outbreak of Mycobacterium gordonae in a teaching hospital: importance of strictly following decontamination procedures and emerging issues concerning sterilization. *The new microbiologica*, *39*(1), 25–34.(accessed on 16th July 2025).

24. Monin, L., Mehta, S., Elsegeiny, W., Gopal, R., McAleer, J. P., Oury, T. D., Kolls, J., & Khader, S. A. (2018). Aspergillus fumigatus Preexposure Worsens Pathology and Improves Control of Mycobacterium abscessus Pulmonary Infection in Mice. *Infection and immunity*, *86*(3), e00859-17. https://doi.org/10.1128/IAI.00859-17(accessed on 16th July 2025).

25. Rue-Albrecht, K., Magee, D. A., Killick, K. E., Nalpas, N. C., Gordon, S. V., & MacHugh, D. E. (2014). Comparative functional genomics and the bovine macrophage response to strains of the mycobacterium genus. *Frontiers in immunology*, *5*, 536. https://doi.org/10.3389/fimmu.2014.00536 (accessed on 16th July 2025).

26. Gorvetzian, S., Pacheco, A. G., Anderson, E., Ray, S. M., & Schechter, M. (2023). 1877. Post-tuberculosis treatment mortality in Georgia (2009–2018). *Open Forum Infectious Diseases, 10.* https://www.semanticscholar.org/paper/4dfc48c0fca2238f725fbc9a2cb6f350c3323dd5 (accessed on 16th July 2025).

27. Jacobs, J. M., & Ottinger, C. A. (2006). *USGS/NOAA Workshop on Mycobacteriosis in Striped Bass, May 7–10, 2006, Annapolis, Maryland.* https://core.ac.uk/download/11017969.pdf (accessed on 16th July 2025).

28. Szewczyk, R., Kowalski, K., Janiszewska-Drobinska, B., & Druszczyńska, M. (2013). Rapid method for Mycobacterium tuberculosis identification using electrospray ionization tandem mass spectrometry analysis of mycolic acids. *Diagnostic microbiology and infectious disease*, *76*(3), 298–305. https://doi.org/10.1016/j.diagmicrobio.2013.03.025 (accessed on 16th July 2025).

29. Kumar, R., Singh, A. K., Singla, M., Gupta, A., El-Kenawy, E. M., & Alharbi, A. H. (2025). Advancements in cancer care by exploring multimodality imaging techniques and their applications. *Current Medical Imaging*. https://www.semanticscholar.org/paper/b2bafacce265fbeccab335404ba20108472cc104 (accessed on 16th July 2025).

30. Finan, C., Ota, M. O., Marchant, A., & Newport, M. J. (2008). Natural variation in immune responses to neonatal Mycobacterium bovis Bacillus Calmette-Guerin (BCG) Vaccination in a Cohort of Gambian infants. *PloS one*, *3*(10), e3485. https://doi.org/10.1371/journal.pone.0003485 (accessed on 16th July 2025).

31. Moreira-Teixeira, L., Mayer-Barber, K., Sher, A., & O'Garra, A. (2018). Type I interferons in tuberculosis: Foe and occasionally friend. *The Journal of experimental medicine*, *215*(5), 1273–1285. https://doi.org/10.1084/jem.20180325(accessed on 16th July 2025).

32. Nicolle, D., Ganz, J., & Mohr, M. (2024). A case of zoonotic domestically acquired Hansen disease (leprosy) in the state of Georgia. *SKIN The Journal of Cutaneous Medicine*. https://www.semanticscholar.org/paper/f9a73eab434575b8cdc3872e427af08437093dbb (accessed on 16th July 2025).

33. O. N. J. (2025). Cancer prevention programs and public policy initiatives in Nigeria. *Newport International Journal of Public Health and Pharmacy*. https://www.semanticscholar.org/paper/d123b3dbfce002ed1838ad7ef5f48f9123ebb282 (accessed on 16th July 2025).

34. Pawar, Y. P., Shimpi, H., Shrivastav, A., Awasare, S. U., Rakshit, S., Karpe, M., Damle, A. A., et al. (2024). Role of advanced nuclear medicine imaging techniques in preclinical drug development and three R's in animal research. *Journal of Laboratory Animal Science*. https://www.semanticscholar.org/paper/872cfab68fb460e6cccc2938a232921c5865a79c (accessed on 16th July 2025).

35. Shree, S., Joshi, S., Kumar, R., & Biswas, D. (2025). Developing strategies to combat hospital-acquired infections: Innovations in prevention and management. *Asian Journal of Medicine and Health*. https://www.semanticscholar.org/paper/ebac8ab1fa69f6d3c7371b9130092f947bee06ac (accessed on 16th July 2025).

36. Srivastav, Y., Prajapati, A., Jaiswal, A., Yadav, S., Prajapati, A., & Madhaw, K. (2023). Overview of leprosy, including the diagnosis and current available treatments. *Journal of Innovations in Applied Pharmaceutical Science (JIAPS)*. https://www.semanticscholar.org/paper/3196f5ee36b5ebb5552c4c09b4f98c04de4b6826 (accessed on 16th July 2025).

37. Yusti, G., Heres, M., González, A., Fielli, M., Ceccato, A., & Zapata, A. (2018). *Mycobacterium kansasii* as the primary etiology of pulmonary infections due to non-tuberculous mycobacterium (NTM) in patients without human immunodeficiency virus (HIV): Experience from a center in Buenos Aires, Argentina. *Journal of Respiratory Infections*. https://www.semanticscholar.org/paper/0d5082fb6ce4d609f2178afb9c66f061023c04d3 (accessed on 16th July 2025).

38. Zelazny, A., & Olivier, K. (2015). "You can't always get what you want..." the *Mycobacterium abscessus* issue. Name versus function. *Annals of the American Thoracic Society, 12*(3), 300–302. https://www.semanticscholar.org/paper/a430fe1a5369bed6b962fa1899506cd388f023d5 (accessed on 16th July 2025).

39. Zhdan, D. V., Leonova, O. N., Rassokhin, V., Tulinova, I. A., & Muha, T. A. (2025). Analysis of lethal cases in patients with HIV infection based on the experience of Voronezh Regional AIDS Clinical Center. *HIV Infection and Immunosuppressive Disorders*. https://www.semanticscholar.org/paper/7e37262665182d0afa0f8ac87cbec668db6d7b7e (accessed on 16th July 2025).

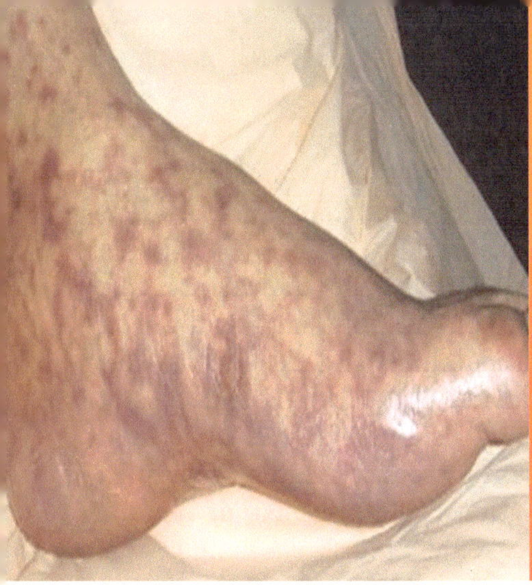

Chapter 10

SPIROCHETES AND RICKETTSIAL INFECTIONS

Contents

Introduction

The investigation of spirochetes and rickettsial diseases has garnered increasing relevance due to the escalating incidence of tick-borne diseases globally. Spirochetes constitute a distinct bacterial group characterised by their corkscrew morphology, with *Borrelia* species such as *Borrelia burgdorferi* being notable etiological agents of Lyme disease. Rickettsial diseases, predominantly caused by bacteria of the order *Rickettsiales,* including *Rickettsia* and *Anaplasma*, pose significant public health challenges. These pathogens are primarily transmitted through the bites of infected ticks, underscoring the importance of examining their ecology and epidemiology. As climatic conditions evolve and human interactions with natural habitats expand, the risk of exposure to these pathogens increases, necessitating focused research on their transmission mechanisms and potential health impacts. Understanding these parameters is vital for the development of effective surveillance, prevention, and control strategies. The rising occurrence of Lyme borreliosis cases in regions previously considered non-endemic emphasises the need for enhanced surveillance and research initiatives. Recent discoveries suggest that species such as *Borrelia bissettii*, which may share pathogenic characteristics with *B. burgdorferi*, could pose emerging health threats, particularly in areas formerly deemed non-endemic. Furthermore, it is imperative to pay particular attention to the broader spectrum of rickettsial infections, given their diverse clinical presentations and the potential for severe health consequences. Studies have documented the presence of *Borrelia* species and rickettsial agents in both rural and urban environments, highlighting the significant ecological roles of small mammals and ticks in disease transmission dynamics. The increasing complexity of pathogen prevalence underscores the necessity for public health advocacy and policy initiatives to mitigate associated risks (Leydet, 2014; Rizzoli et al., 2014). The interplay among human, animal, and environmental factors creates a complex system facilitating the emergence and dissemination of these infections. The presence of various tick populations as vectors in both rural and urban settings presents unique challenges and opportunities for research. Surveillance data reveal a notable prevalence of infected ticks within human residences, posing considerable risks for potential disease transmission. A comprehensive understanding of tick ecology and host interactions is fundamental to formulating effective public health interventions. Moreover, as urban environments increasingly serve as reservoirs for tick-borne diseases, awareness of their significance becomes critically pertinent. Accordingly, an integrated approach combining ecology, epidemiology, and clinical science is essential to effectively address the threats posed by spirochetes and rickettsial infections.

Definition of Spirochetes

Spirochetes constitute a distinctive group of bacteria characterised by a helical structure and an elastic cell wall that confer high motility.

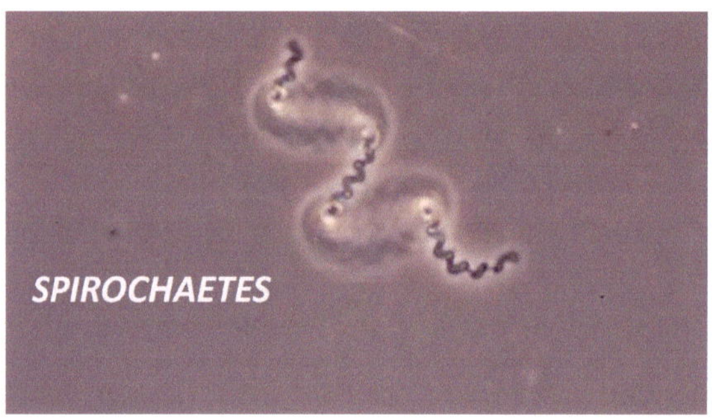

Figure 10.1. Spirochetes.

Source: https://external-content.duckduckgo.com/iu/?u=https%3A%2F%2Fi.ytimg.com%2Fvi%2FcXYfT5hSLoQ%2Fmaxresdefault.jpg&f=1&nofb=1&ipt=a17cc1948dc6b4c7dfa81963d62dfc5282208d259a74a9de2b90d3a70a6fefba.

They are typically described as exhibiting a corkscrew-like motion, moving in and out. Belonging to the phylum *Spirochaetes*, this group includes prominent genera such as *Borrelia*, *Treponema*, and *Leptospira*. These microorganisms inhabit diverse environments, including soil, water, and the gastrointestinal tracts of animals as commensals. Their complex morphology, featuring an internal flagellum within the cell envelope and outer membrane, facilitates their movement through viscous environments. This specialized structure is essential for their mobility within host tissues and for maintaining their pathogenic potential, thereby enhancing the virulence of spirochetal infections, particularly those affecting humans, such as Lyme disease and syphilis. Spirochetes are of significant importance to human health, especially as pathogenic organisms. For instance, Lyme disease is caused by the pathogen *Borrelia burgdorferi*, which constitutes a notable public health concern globally. The intricate life cycle of spirochetes, often involving multiple hosts and vector species, presents a complex challenge for understanding and controlling these infections. Recent discoveries of additional *Borrelia* species, such as *Borrelia bissettii*, underscore the ongoing threat posed by these organisms, indicating that spirochetes are implicated in a broader spectrum of human diseases than previously recognised (Leydet, 2014) (Figure 10.1).

Their capacity to evade the immune system through antigenic variation introduces an additional complex aspect to the infection paradigm, thereby necessitating ongoing research into both diagnostic and therapeutic methods. Simultaneously, spirochetes possess a compelling eco-epidemiological dimension that highlights their associations with the environment and hosts. For example, a study conducted in Portugal demonstrated that ticks, which serve as primary vectors for the majority of spirochetal infections, are infested with multiple species of *Borrelia*, some of which are implicated in symptomatic human infections (Carvalho, 2010).

Furthermore, the presence of co-infections in various host species, ranging from small mammals to lizards, raises fundamental questions regarding spirochetal transmission dynamics. It is essential to comprehend these ecological interactions to develop effective public health interventions, especially as patterns of spirochetal infection continually evolve with changing environmental conditions. Collectively, the definition and investigation of spirochetes underscore their significance in infectious diseases, prompting enhanced surveillance and more comprehensive research initiatives.

Definition of Rickettsial Infections

Rickettsial infections constitute a category of illnesses caused by intracellular bacteria within the genus *Rickettsia*. These infections are predominantly transmitted to humans via arthropod vectors such as ticks, fleas, and lice. *Rickettsiae* exhibit distinctive biological characteristics, including the ability to infect endothelial cells, induce inflammation, and invade blood vessels.

The clinical spectrum of rickettsial infections is broad, ranging from mild influenza-like symptoms to severe diseases that may result in mortality. Early detection and prompt treatment are imperative, as untreated infections can progress rapidly; hence, awareness of these pathogens is crucial (Leydet, 2014). The etiological agents responsible for rickettsial diseases include several species, notably *Rickettsia rickettsii*, which causes Rocky Mountain spotted fever, and *Rickettsia prowazekii*, the causative agent of epidemic typhus.

The clinical presentation of these infections is often nonspecific and mimics other febrile illnesses, complicating diagnosis. Common symptoms include fever, headache, rash, and various systemic manifestations. If not treated promptly with appropriate antibiotics, rickettsial infections can lead to severe vascular and multiorgan complications. Therefore, further development of diagnostic techniques and the formulation of effective vaccines are essential, especially considering the increasing geographical distribution of these pathogens attributable to ecological and human behavioral changes (Carvalho, 2010) (Figure 10.2).

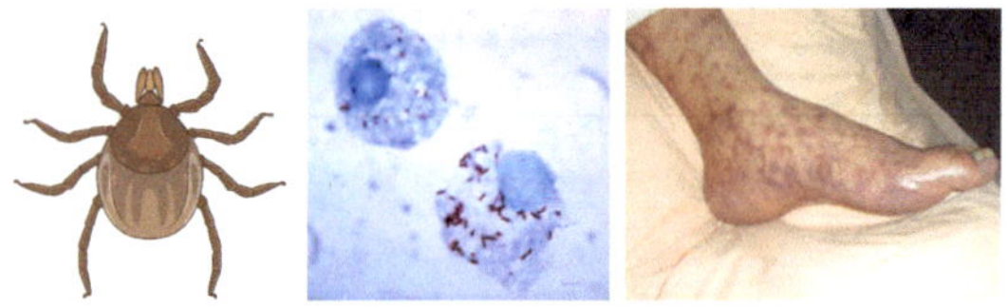

Figure 10.2. *Rickettsia* infection.

Source: https://external-content.duckduckgo.com/iu/?u=https%3A%2F%2Fmicrobenotes.com%2Fwp-content%2Fuploads%2F2022%2F05%2F*Rickettsia*-Infection-Tick-Borne-Rickettsioses-And-Spotted-Fever.jpeg&f=1&nofb=1&ipt=d2076c115b3916a81d7e9238c2d0e76d6e2911ffdd7970cf8aac2a4ef2847f6a.

One of the significant aspects of rickettsial infections is their manifestation in non-endemic areas, posing new public health challenges. Some literature indicates that various environmental, ecological, and societal factors contribute to shifts in the incidence rates of rickettsial diseases. For example, the rising incidence of Lyme disease and other tick-borne pathogens exemplifies the complexity and interconnectedness of arthropod-borne illnesses. A comprehensive understanding of the interactions between *Rickettsia* species, their vectors, and ecological environments is essential for developing effective surveillance and control strategies. This evolving epidemiological landscape necessitates increased awareness and rigorous research to mitigate the impact of rickettsial diseases on public health and safety (Leyde, 2014).

10.1. Characteristics of Spirochetes

Phylum *Spirochaetes* encompasses a diverse group of bacteria distinguished by their characteristic helical shape and remarkable motility, primarily facilitated by their specialized flagellar apparatus. These microorganisms feature cells with a peptidoglycan cell wall covered by a thin outer membrane, essential for maintaining cellular integrity. Unlike most bacteria, spirochetes possess periplasmic flagella situated between the cell wall and the outer membrane, enabling them to move in a corkscrew manner. This distinctive motility allows them to navigate viscous environments, such as mucosal surfaces and connective tissues, thereby enhancing their pathogenic potential in humans. Their ability to thrive in various habitats — including anaerobic and microaerophilic conditions — demonstrates their ecological versatility and evolutionary success within the bacterial domain. The pathogenicity exhibited by the majority of spirochete species significantly impacts human health, with *Borrelia burgdorferi*, the etiological agent of Lyme disease, exemplifying complex host and ecological interactions that pose challenges to disease management. Recent research highlights an increasing recognition of *Borrelia* species responsible for human disease, emphasising the importance of enhanced surveillance and awareness, particularly in non-endemic regions (Leydet, 2014) (Figure 10.3).

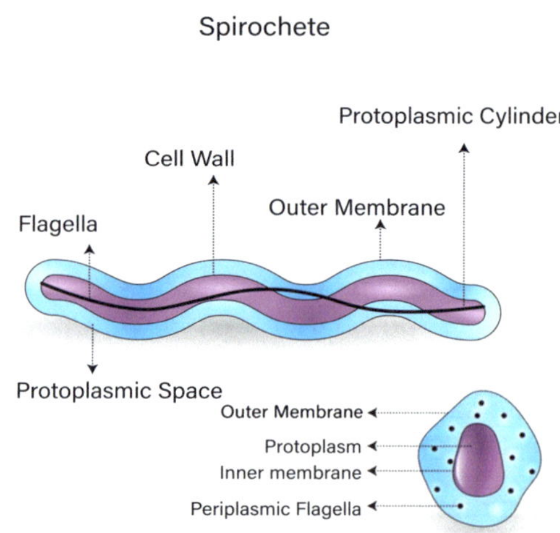

Figure 10.3. Structure of spirochete.

Source: https://external-content.duckduckgo.com/iu/?u=https%3A%2F%2Fas2.ftcdn.net%2Fv2%2Fjpg%2F03%2F85%2F39%2F07%2F1000_F_385390728_ndmjnyMLbNQ1RczP0AiLIxu0RF2LkMRN.jpg&f=1&nofb=1&ipt=5137899fd794f294c8d3ac31fc4ff4b4c4eabe3494f5a51e8e740784755f48e9.

Furthermore, the ecological dynamics involved in the transmission of spirochetes by their arthropod vectors, including ticks, underscore their role as vectors within the ecological framework of zoonotic infections. These properties not only facilitate the dissemination of infections but also complicate the accurate diagnosis of spirochete infections, as many species possess similar antigenic characteristics, rendering serological diagnosis more challenging. Beyond their morphological and pathogenic traits, the genomic attributes of spirochetes provide valuable insights into their evolutionary strategies and host interactions. The genetic diversity among these bacteria enables them to exhibit varying levels of virulence and environmental tolerance. Recent studies have demonstrated that certain species of spirochetes, such as *Borrelia bissettii*, possess unique pathogenic potentials, and novel mechanisms of pathogenicity have been proposed that warrant further investigation (Carvalho, 2010). This genetic heterogeneity serves as a foundational basis for understanding the ecological functions of spirochetes, their potential for co-infection, and their interactions with other tick-borne diseases. Consequently, a comprehensive assessment of spirochete characteristics, including their genetic diversity, is essential for the development of public health strategies aimed at reducing the burden of spirochetal infections among human populations.

10.1.1. Morphological features

The morphological features of rickettsial species and spirochetes reveal their diversity and complexity. Spirochetes, characterised by their corkscrew shape, exhibit distinct motility thanks to flagella located in the periplasmic space, which allows them to effectively navigate viscous environments. This adaptable morphology not only supports survival but also boosts pathogenicity by promoting tissue invasion. In contrast, rickettsial bacteria are typically small, coccoid or rod-shaped, and lack flagella, making them well-adapted for intracellular existence within host cells and functioning as effective intracellular pathogens. Recognising these morphological differences is crucial for developing precise diagnostics and treatments.

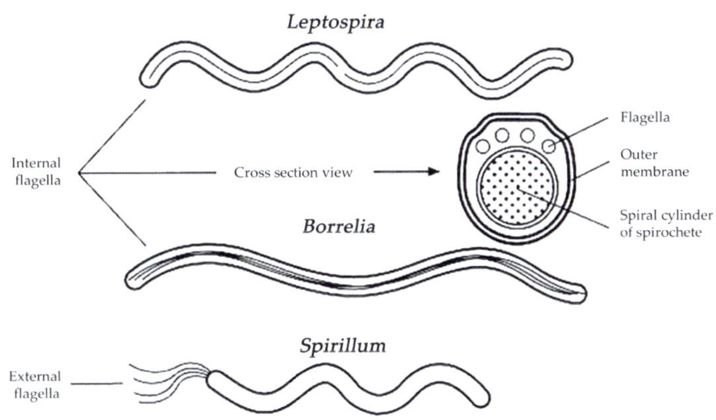

Figure 10.4. Comparative morphology of spirochetes.

Source: https://external-content.duckduckgo.com/iu/?u=https%3A%2F%2Fimage.slidesharecdn.com%2F17-spirochetes-150727151009-lva1-app6891%2F95%2F17-spirochetes-6-1024.jpg%3Fcb%3D1438014206&f=1&nofb=1&ipt=debc498499b12897a8520704a0aa3445b9d647f85cc7053c7c700069de5ea355.

Morphology also involves internal structural distinctions that influence bacterial behaviour and virulence. For example, rickettsiae lack an intact cell wall — unlike typical Gram-negative bacteria — providing resistance to certain antibiotics that target cell wall synthesis. This feature enables rickettsiae to grow inside endothelial cells and evade host immunity. Spirochete morphology includes complex elements like the extracellular sheath, which offers protection from the environment and aids in immune evasion and pathogenicity. The link between form and function is key to understanding how both spirochetes and rickettsiae cause disease. Recent studies highlight detailed morphological variations in these bacteria across different hosts. For instance, a study identified various forms of a rickettsia-like bacterium in the hepatopancreatic cells of Pacific white shrimp, indicating adaptation to crustacean hosts (Krol et al., 1991) (Figure 10.4).

Furthermore, spirochetes such as *Borrelia spp.* exhibit morphological variations in response to environmental factors and host interactions, which influence their infectivity and transmission efficiency. As observed in Lyme borreliosis, morphological convergence among *Borrelia* species raises concerns regarding identification and potential health implications (Leydet, 2014). Consequently, the complex relationship between morphology and pathogenicity necessitates ongoing research. This study not only elucidates the morphological diversity of these organisms but also underscores the challenges in devising effective public health strategies to control spirochete and rickettsial diseases.

10.1.2. Genetic structure

In the examination of the genomic organization and infections caused by spirochetes and Rickettsial organisms, the understanding of their genomic characteristics is of significant importance. For instance, spirochetes, including those responsible for Lyme disease, exhibit considerable genetic versatility. This versatility is largely attributed to mechanisms such as horizontal gene transfer and genetic recombination, which are crucial for their adaptation to a variety of hosts and environments. Recent evidence has identified new *Borrelia* species, such as *Borrelia bissettii*, which complicate existing diagnostic and therapeutic approaches to Lyme borreliosis. The genetic composition of these species is homologous to *Borrelia burgdorferi* sensu stricto. The ongoing research into their pathogenicity and transmission dynamics is vital, as these species not only occupy similar ecological niches but also share genetic features that enable their survival within complex host environments (Leydet, 2014). Additionally, understanding the genetic makeup of Rickettsial species is essential, given their role as zoonotic agents. These bacteria possess relatively small genomes, reflecting their obligate intracellular lifestyle and dependence on host cells for survival and replication. The genomes of *Rickettsia spp.* have been shaped by various evolutionary pressures, including interactions with diverse hosts and vectors such as ticks. Emerging evidence indicates that urban environments are increasingly serving as reservoirs for Rickettsial species, with these pathogens being detected among tick populations in such areas. Consequently, there is a need for further genetic studies to investigate the adaptability and competitive fitness of Rickettsial pathogens, especially considering their capacity to acquire new virulence factors in response to changing ecological conditions (Rizzoli et al., 2014) (Figure 10.5).

Furthermore, the integration of genetic studies into public health surveillance systems is of paramount importance in controlling spirochetes and rickettsial infections. Genetic markers serve as valuable tools for monitoring the epidemiology of these microorganisms, particularly in light of increasing cases of diseases such as Lyme borreliosis in non-endemic regions. Genetic surveillance that includes genetic typing of spirochetes and Rickettsial species can yield insights into population dynamics, transmission pathways, and potential reservoirs. For instance, the detection of several *Borrelia spp.* in urban areas underscores the necessity for enhanced surveillance in such regions, where human-animal encounters with infected ticks are likely to rise. An understanding of these genetic frameworks not only facilitates the identification of at-risk populations but also informs the development of effective control and prevention strategies against tick-borne illnesses (Leydet, 2014; Rizzoli et al., 2014).

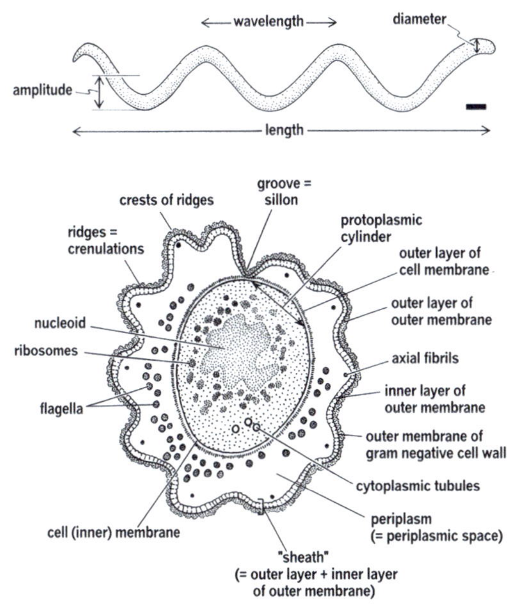

Figure 10.5. Spirochete structure as a basis for morphometric analysis. This drawing of a transverse section of a large, structurally complex spirochete, *Pillotina* sp., is based on many electron micrographs.

Source: https://www.researchgate.net/profile/James-Macallister/publication/225584681/figure/fig3/AS:667774850449428@1536221339840/Spirochete-structure-as-basis-for-morphometric-analysis-Margulis-2000-This-drawing-of.ppm.

10.1.3. Metabolic capabilities

The metabolic capabilities of spirochetes and rickettsial species are complex and vary according to their specialized ecological niches and evolutionary history. For example, *Treponema pallidum* has a relatively limited metabolic repertoire and depends heavily on its host for nutrients, especially as it cannot synthesize some essential amino acids, relying on the host environment for survival and replication. Rickettsial species also show minimal metabolic independence and depend on their hosts, with *Rickettsia prowazekii* being unable to perform glycolysis and needing to acquire ATP directly from eukaryotic hosts. This metabolic dependency highlights the intricacies of their life cycles and the evolutionary pressures that shape these bacteria into resource-dependent pathogens. Genomic analyses reveal significant reductions in metabolic pathways compared to their free-living relatives. A notable example is Wolbachia, an obligate endosymbiont of the human filarial nematode *Brugia malayi*. Despite a degenerate genome, *Wolbachia* retains a reduced yet functional set of metabolic pathways, including the ability to produce vital nutrients like riboflavin and nucleotides, which are essential for the host's survival. These metabolic capabilities underscore the mutualistic relationship between Wolbachia and its nematode host, reflecting evolutionary adaptations to specific ecological niches. The retention of certain pathways in *Wolbachia*, contrasted with the broader genomic loss in Rickettsias, suggests survival mechanisms employed by these closely related bacteria, highlighting their complex metabolic interdependencies. Moreover, the metabolic activity of these intracellular pathogens demonstrates their resourcefulness and adaptability despite host immune defences. As both spirochetes and rickettsial bacteria have evolved mechanisms to evade host defences while satisfying their metabolic needs, their small genomes and reliance on host-derived metabolites enable successful replication within host cells. These survival strategies not only enhance their pathogenicity but also present potential targets for therapeutic intervention. Ongoing research into their metabolic interactions with hosts may reveal new ways to combat infections caused by these bacteria and underscore the importance of their metabolic processes in managing infectious diseases (Charrel et al., 2017).

10.2. Major Spirochetal Diseases

The significance of spirochetal infections in public health is heightened by the broad spectrum of diseases they cause, driven by various species of spirochetes. One of the most well-known is Lyme disease, caused by *Borrelia burgdorferi*, now recognised as one of the leading vector-borne diseases in the United States. The Centers for Disease Control and Prevention estimates that around 300,000 cases of Lyme disease are diagnosed each year, indicating a concerning increase in cases, especially in non-traditional regions such as Louisiana. The complexity of Lyme borreliosis has been further increased by the discovery of other species of Borrelia, such as *Borrelia bissettii*, which may also play a role in human disease. With the ongoing evolution and adaptation of spirochetal pathogens, widespread surveillance and innovative diagnostic methods are becoming increasingly vital to combat emerging threats to human health (Leydet, 2014).

Syphilis, caused by *Treponema pallidum*, is another significant spirochetal disease. As a sexually transmitted infection, syphilis has experienced a resurgence in recent years, with rising infection rates reported among certain groups. It is notorious for its complex phases, each presenting diverse clinical features, from asymptomatic to widespread systemic illness. Its unpredictable presentation hampers diagnosis but also increases the likelihood of transmission, highlighting the urgent need for public health education as a key control strategy. Moreover, the treatment of syphilitic patients is hindered by social stigmatisation and limited access to healthcare, further complicating efforts to control the infection. Addressing these challenges requires a multi-faceted approach, including awareness campaigns, regular screening programmes, and improved healthcare services for at-risk populations (Leydet, 2014).

Further complicating the ecosystem of spirochetal diseases is leptospirosis, a zoonotic disease caused by *Leptospira* bacteria. Typically linked to waterborne exposure, leptospirosis can range from asymptomatic or mild flu-like symptoms to severe illness involving jaundice, renal failure, and haemorrhages. Its close association with occupational and agricultural exposures, especially among high-risk groups such as farmers and animal handlers, necessitates targeted occupational health interventions. Workplace infections, particularly in high-risk environments, are often underreported and insufficiently managed, thereby concealing the true burden of disease. Since spirochetal infections remain a health concern across diverse settings, it is essential to ensure that effective prevention and control measures are implemented to protect public health and reduce the incidence of these disabling illnesses (Chung et al., 2010).

10.2.1. Lyme disease

Lyme disease, primarily caused by the spirochete *Borrelia burgdorferi*, has emerged as a significant public health concern, particularly in the northeastern and north-central regions of the United States. The infection is transmitted through the bite of an infected *Ixodes* tick, commonly known as the deer tick. The epidemiology of Lyme disease has evolved, with evidence demonstrating a remarkable increase in annual diagnoses to approximately 300,000 cases. Additionally, cases have been reported in areas previously not recognised as endemic for the disease, indicating a widening of its geographical distribution. Recent findings also identify other *Borrelia* species, such as *Borrelia bissettii*, as potential threats, underscoring the necessity for enhanced surveillance and research — especially in regions traditionally not associated with Lyme disease, such as Louisiana. This situation calls for a reconsideration of regional health policies to appropriately address the shifting risks posed by various *Borrelia* species (Leydet, 2014). Beyond its rising incidence, Lyme disease presents diagnostic and therapeutic challenges. Its manifestations are highly variable, and initial symptoms often resemble those of other viral infections. Common symptoms include fever, malaise, and erythema migrans, or the characteristic bull's-eye rash. Early symptoms can be subtle and frequently overlooked, leading to delayed diagnosis and treatment. Diagnosis predominantly relies on serological tests designed to detect anti-Borrelia antibodies. However, comparative studies with other tick-borne diseases reveal that the accuracy of such tests is inconsistent, particularly in differentiating between *Borrelia* species. Current diagnostic kits may not distinguish among various *Borrelia* species, complicating clinical decision-making. This diagnostic uncertainty highlights the urgent need for technological advancements to improve the specificity and reliability of Lyme disease detection (Wong et al., 2011) (Figure 10.6).

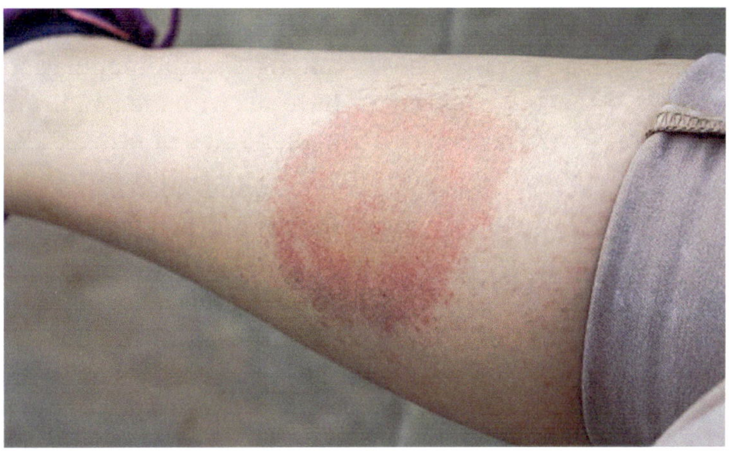

Figure 10.6. Lyme disease.

Source: https://post.medicalnewstoday.com/wp-content/uploads/sites/3/2020/05/shutterstock_537518422_header-1024x575.jpg.

Furthermore, the impact of Lyme disease extends to broader environmental and economic concerns. Climate change, land use patterns, and evolving wildlife populations have contributed to an increase in tick populations, which in turn has led to more frequent human-tick interactions. This issue not only poses a significant public health concern but also has substantial economic implications due to the costs associated with healthcare, treatment, and management of Lyme disease. Moreover, symptoms of chronic Lyme disease can persist despite treatment, resulting in long-term disability and diminished quality of life for affected individuals. These nuances highlight the importance of ongoing research into Lyme disease and other spirochetal infections, which can inform preventive strategies, improve patient outcomes, and ultimately reduce the societal burden of these tickborne diseases. Proactive measures and comprehensive information are essential to effectively address the challenges presented by Lyme disease (Leydet, 2014).

10.2.2. Syphilis

Syphilis has been a significant public health concern throughout history, especially during times of war and social upheaval. This venereal disease, caused by the spirochete *Treponema pallidum*, occurs in several stages, with primary lesions that are sometimes asymptomatic. Secondary syphilis presents with systemic features, including rashes and mucous membrane lesions, which can be severe if left untreated. The pathogen's ability to evade the host's immune response makes it persistent and can lead to latent infections.

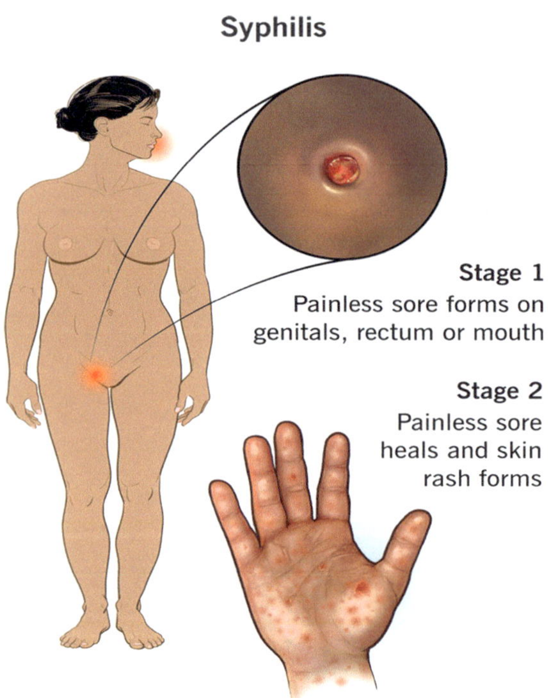

Figure 10.7. Syphilis is a sexually transmitted infection (STI) that causes sores and a skin rash. It can be life-threatening without treatment.

Source: https://pharmaceutical-journal.com/wp-content/uploads/2021/01/secondary-syphilis-rash-spl-18.png.

Moreover, unsuspected syphilis can progress to tertiary syphilis, where serious complications such as cardiovascular and neurological diseases may develop decades after the initial infection. Understanding the clinical features and natural history of syphilis is crucial for early diagnosis and treatment, emphasising the importance of ongoing research and public health programmes to control this spirochetal disease. The transmission dynamics of syphilis highlight the need for comprehensive sexual health education. While primarily transmitted sexually, syphilis can also be passed from an infected mother to her unborn baby during pregnancy, potentially resulting in congenital syphilis, a condition that can cause severe neonatal illness or stillbirth. Recently, there has been a rise in syphilis infections, particularly among specific populations such as men who have sex with men, indicating a correlation with higher rates of other STIs.

Public health initiatives must therefore focus on targeted interventions such as routine screening and affordable treatment for high-risk groups. Education programmes aimed at demystifying syphilis screening and raising awareness have the potential to reduce transmission rates and improve health outcomes. Syphilis remains a significant global health challenge, and its diagnostic and treatment strategies require regular reassessment. Advances in molecular techniques, including real-time PCR, have improved detection capabilities with faster and more accurate diagnoses compared to traditional serological tests. These breakthroughs are crucial in controlling outbreaks and reducing the disease's impact on public health. Additionally, the emergence of new strains and co-infections with other pathogens presents further challenges in effective treatment. Continued research into spirochete biology will not only guide therapeutic approaches but also yield important insights into the evolving landscape of infectious diseases. Ongoing collaboration between public health authorities, healthcare providers, and researchers is essential to effectively combat syphilis and its complications, reminding us of the persistent threat this ancient disease poses.

10.2.3. Leptospirosis

Leptospirosis, caused by the spirochete *Leptospira*, constitutes a significant zoonosis with substantial public health implications, especially in tropical regions. The infection typically occurs through contact with contaminated water, soil, or environments and can manifest as a spectrum of clinical syndromes, ranging from mild influenza-like illness to severe, life-threatening complications. Notably, reproductive lesions in farm animals such as pigs have been extensively documented. Research indicates that in the Mekong Delta of Vietnam, high seroprevalence rates among sows reflect serious issues related to farm production and animal health. Furthermore, as a zoonotic disease, leptospirosis also poses health risks to humans, particularly those in close contact with animals, underscoring the necessity for enhanced preventive measures to effectively mitigate this risk (Boqvist, 2002) (Figure 10.8).

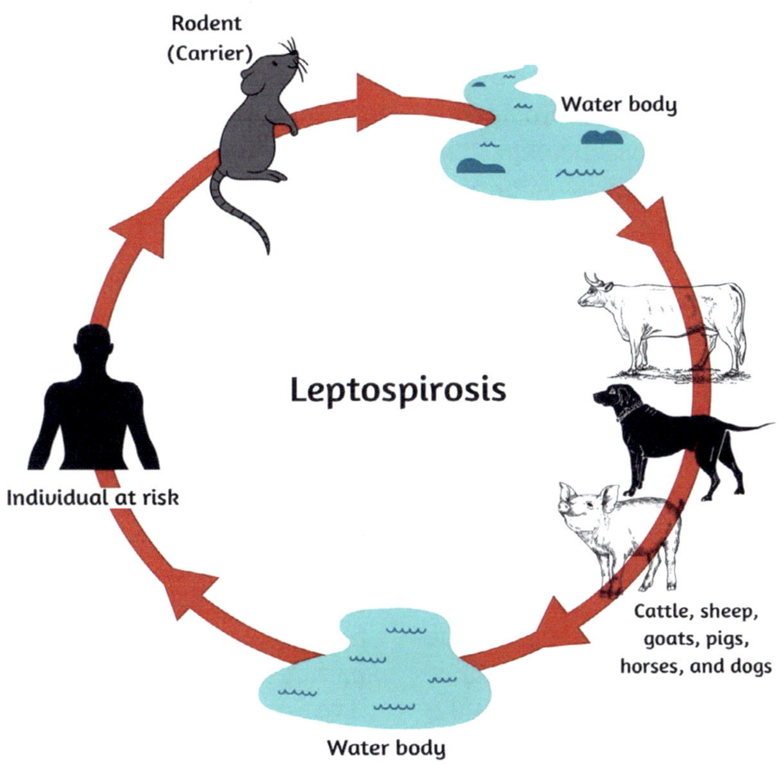

Figure 10.8. Leptospirosis.

Source: https://www.keeptalkinggreece.com/2023/10/13/leptospirosis-disease-infections-flooded-thessaly-greece/.

The epidemiological pattern of leptospirosis is influenced by various socio-economic and environmental determinants. Highly populated areas with inadequate sanitation standards and extensive animal husbandry activities create an environment conducive to the transmission and persistence of *Leptospira* among animal reservoirs and the human population. The tropical climate exacerbates this issue by further supporting the survival and proliferation of the bacteria in the environment, resulting in increased incidence rates of infection in both animals and humans. In Latin America, South, and Southeast Asia, as well as other regions worldwide, populations are already burdened by healthcare disparities alongside the disease burden, which amplifies the risk of community-acquired acute kidney injury (AKI) secondary to infections such as leptospirosis. This confluence of factors underscores the need for a specialized public health response addressing both the immediate impacts of the disease and the broader socioeconomic determinants of health (Burdmann & Jha, 2017). Prevention and control of leptospirosis rely on a comprehensive approach encompassing education, awareness, and improvements in infrastructure. Public health strategies must aim to reduce exposure to contaminated water sources, especially in areas affected by flooding, which increases disease incidence. Vaccination of animals plays a critical role in interrupting animal-to-human transmission. Additionally, implementing surveillance systems with rapid response capabilities can facilitate early detection and management of outbreaks. As ongoing research advances understanding of the epidemiology and incidence of leptospirosis, there is a growing recognition of the importance of interdisciplinary collaboration to enhance knowledge and disease control (Boqvist, 2002; Burdmann & Jha, 2017).

10.3. Characteristics of Rickettsial Infections

Infections with Rickettsia, obligate intracellular bacteria of the genus *Rickettsia*, are mainly transmitted by arthropod vectors such as ticks, fleas, and lice. Infection of endothelial cells by the causative agent results in acute fever and various systemic symptoms, which can range from mild to severe. Common signs include rashes, eschar, and in some cases, complications like vasculitis or organ impairment. Due to their mode of transmission, rickettsial infections are zoonotic, with wildlife reservoir hosts — particularly rodents — serving as sources of bacteria that can be transmitted to humans. Understanding these aspects is important because early diagnosis and treatment are key to improving patient outcomes in regions where these infections are endemic. Another intriguing aspect of rickettsial infections is their geographic distribution and the environmental factors that influence their prevalence. These pathogens interact complexly with vector populations, reservoir hosts, and human activities, leading to their appearance in new areas. Many studies have shown that climate change alters tick habitats and expands the range of diseases like Rocky Mountain spotted fever and Endemic Typhus. For example, as climate shifts modify tick and mammal ecology, areas with traditionally low incidence are now experiencing more cases, challenging public health efforts. This changing ecology not only helps map the risk of rickettsial infection but also aids in developing preventive strategies to meet emerging challenges effectively. Studying rickettsial infections also offers crucial insights into host-pathogen interactions, including immune responses. Similar to other tick-borne pathogens, rickettsial agents display varying levels of pathogenicity and virulence, influenced by their genetic diversity and environmental niches. Notably, some *Rickettsia* strains, like *Borrelia* agents, have specialized to specific vectors and hosts, eliciting different clinical reactions. These host-specific associations are important for understanding the risk of spillover events when pathogens transfer from wildlife to humans, highlighting the interconnectedness of ecosystem health. Further research in this area not only clarifies the features of rickettsial infections but also underscores the importance of monitoring *Rickettsia* and *Borrelia* species to prevent future outbreaks (Leydet, 2014; Stephenson & Foley, 2016) (Figure 10.9).

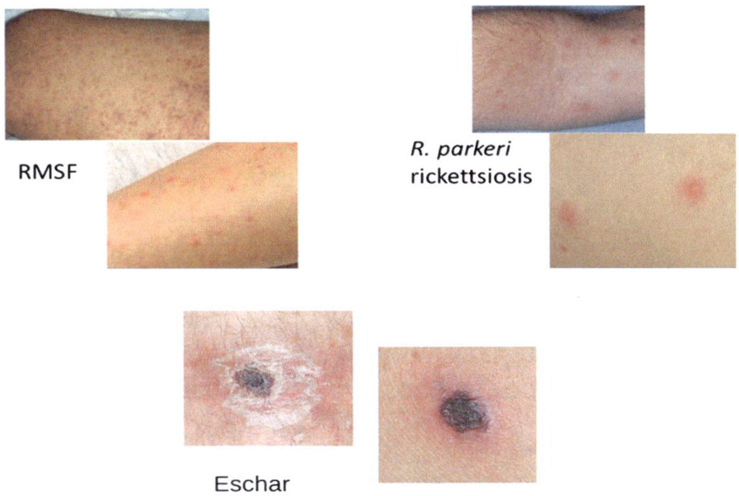

Figure 10.9. Distinctive rashes of *rickettsial* diseases.

Source: https://www.lymedisease.org/images/distinctive-rashes-of-rikettsial-diseases.jpg.

10.3.1. Morphological features

The morphological characters provide significant insights into the classification and pathogenicity of spirochetes and rickettsial bacteria. Spirochetes, characterised by their traditional helical form, are elongated, slender bacteria with a specialized motility mechanism rooted in axial filaments, or periplasmic flagella. These flagella are embedded within the periplasmic space and facilitate a corkscrew motion, which is particularly advantageous in viscous environments such as host tissues. The structural intricacies of these organisms, including the arrangement of their outer membrane and cell walls, distinguish spirochetes from other bacterial taxa. This unique morphology not only aids in ecological adaptation but also plays a role in pathogenicity, as their shape and motility enable them to evade the host immune response and penetrate tissues, thereby influencing the infection process and host health. Conversely, rickettsial bacteria exhibit a morphology indicative of their intracellular parasitic lifestyle. *Rickettsiae* are typically rod- or coccoid-shaped and possess both a plasma membrane and peptidoglycan cell wall, aligning with their affinity to Gram-negative bacteria. Recent research has revealed that rickettsiae reside within host cells, where they reproduce and induce pathological alterations, including granuloma formation in affected tissues. For example, in cultured Pacific white shrimp, researchers identified rickettsia-like bacteria from cytoplasmic infections, indicating their potential pathogenicity across various hosts and environments (Krol et al., 1991) (Figure 10.10).

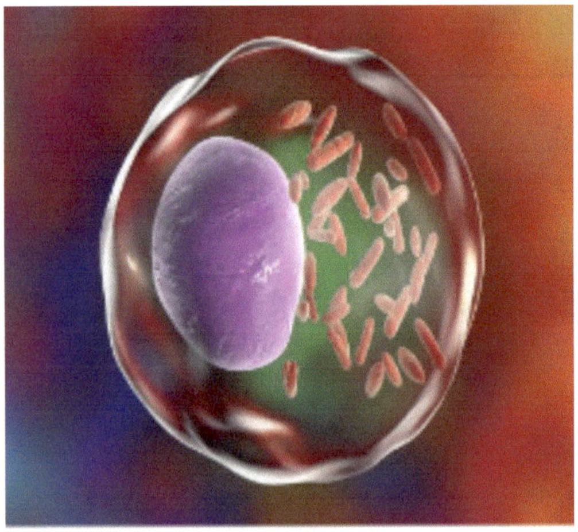

Figure 10.10. Morphology of *rickettsiae.*

Source: https://www.slideshare.net/slideshow/rickettsia-life-cycle-and-diagnostic-methods-pptx/271608272.

The morphological transformations in rickettsiae enable them to survive and replicate within host cells, which contribute to their pathogenic mechanisms and the clinical features of rickettsial diseases. Ongoing research into the morphological characteristics of spirochetes and rickettsial bacteria is vital for understanding their biology and potential to cause disease. Emerging groups, such as new *Borrelia* species associated with Lyme borreliosis, highlight the importance of continued investigation into these organisms, especially in areas where they were previously unknown (Leydet, 2014). The morphological similarities and differences between these bacterial families not only reveal their evolutionary history but also their environmental niches and host adaptations. This knowledge is essential for developing accurate diagnostic tests and effective treatments for infections caused by these morphologically complex pathogens. Further research into their morphology will enhance our understanding of their advanced biology and their risks to public health.

10.3.2. Genetic structure

The genomic structure of spirochetes, particularly the *Borrelia* species, is essential for predicting their pathogenicity, transmission potential, and, ultimately, their role in human disease. Recent research has demonstrated that genetic variation among different *Borrelia* species significantly influences infectivity and disease manifestation. For example, *Borrelia burgdorferi* sensu stricto is the primary causative agent of Lyme disease in North America, whereas other species, such as *Borrelia bissettii,* complicate disease surveillance and management. These genetic disparities can cause varied host responses, thereby complicating public health efforts. Studies conducted in non-endemic regions, such as Louisiana, highlight the importance of investigating both prominent and minor species, thereby unveiling a complex genetic landscape that underpins spirochetal infections (Leydet, 2014). The genetic makeup of Rickettsial bacteria also provides insights into their pathogenic mechanisms and evolutionary adaptations. Members of the *Rickettsiales* order display diverse genetic profiles that enable adaptation to various environments, including urban landscapes where interactions between human and animal hosts are common. These bacteria typically engage in intricate relationships with their ectoparasite vectors, such as ticks, which function as reservoirs and transmission agents. For instance, research indicates that urban green spaces can harbour dense populations of *Ixodes ricinus* ticks, which act as vectors for multiple Rickettsial species. Understanding the genetic foundations of both the ticks and the pathogens they carry is crucial, as this knowledge directly influences the emergence of new diseases and informs public health interventions (Rizzoli et al., 2014). Analysing the gene architecture of spirochetes and Rickettsial pathogens is vital not only for identifying emerging health threats but also for developing effective diagnostic tools. Genetic similarities and differences across species may pose challenges to diagnostic accuracy, as exemplified by the difficulty in distinguishing *Borrelia bissettii* from *Borrelia burgdorferi* in certain cases. Such uncertainties may result in delayed treatment or misdiagnosis, adversely affecting patient outcomes. Furthermore, given the ongoing suitability of urban environments for tick proliferation, understanding the genetic profiles of vectors and pathogens is essential for designing targeted surveillance and control strategies. Ultimately, adopting a comprehensive genetic approach will enhance capacities to monitor, predict, and combat spirochetal and Rickettsial diseases more effectively (Leydet, 2014; Rizzoli et al., 2014).

10.3.3. Transmission methods

The dissemination of spirochetes and rickettsial diseases is typically facilitated by specific environmental vectors, with ticks being the most prominent agents of transmission. Notably, ticks belonging to the *Ixodes* genus serve as vectors for *Borrelia* species, such as *Borrelia burgdorferi*, which is responsible for Lyme disease. The infectious cycle commences when an infected host s blood is ingested by a tick, thereby acquiring the spirochetes. Subsequent feeding periods enable the transmission of these agents to other mammalian hosts, thereby completing the cycle of infection. The ability of these pathogens to persist within such vectors underscores the critical link between tick-borne disease prevalence and environmental factors, thereby emphasising the importance of vector control measures to mitigate infection risks associated with spirochetes. Rickettsial infections are primarily transmitted via arthropod vectors, including ticks, fleas, and mites, all of which play substantial roles in the epidemiology of these infections. For example, a tick bite infected with *Rickettsia* species can introduce the pathogen into the bloodstream of humans and animals, eliciting diverse clinical manifestations. Transmission of rickettsiae may occur through direct inoculation via saliva during feeding or through scratching of bite sites. An illustrative case is the transmission of *Rickettsia rickettsii*, the etiological agent of Rocky Mountain spotted fever, which exhibits a particular affinity for certain wildlife reservoirs. A comprehensive understanding of the ecological processes governing tick populations is essential for predicting outbreak patterns and protecting vulnerable populations from exposure to rickettsial infections. Overall, the transmission of spirochetes and rickettsiae exemplifies the intricate interactions between vectors and hosts. Recent studies have revealed the presence of various Borrelia species beyond the well-characterised pathogens, suggesting emerging threats to human health. Evidence indicates that although *Ixodes* scapularis effectively transmits *Borrelia burgdorferi*, other *Borrelia* species, such as *Borrelia bissettii*, may utilize secondary vectors, as observed in research conducted in regions such as Louisiana. These findings highlight the necessity for ongoing research into vector ecology and pathogen surveillance, particularly in regions not traditionally considered endemic, to preemptively address future health risks posed by spirochete and rickettsial diseases (Krol et al., 1991; Leydet, 2014).

10.4. Major Rickettsial Diseases

Rickettsial diseases constitute a significant group of illnesses caused by pathogens belonging to the genus *Rickettsia*, primarily transmitted through arthropod vectors such as ticks, fleas, and lice. Among these, typhus fever, Rocky Mountain spotted fever (RMSF), and ehrlichiosis are of particular significance due to their clinical manifestations and public health implications. Typhus fever, resulting from *Rickettsia prowazekii* infection, has been frequently associated with crowded living conditions and inadequate hygiene; consequently, outbreaks are commonly observed in refugee camps and urban areas where body lice proliferate. The capability of these organisms to exploit human hosts during times of social upheaval underscores the importance of environmental and vector control measures in preventing transmission. Similarly, RMSF, primarily transmitted by the American dog tick, presents with a distinctive rash and can lead to severe complications if not diagnosed and treated promptly, emphasising the necessity of early diagnosis and intervention. Another noteworthy rickettsial infection is relapsing fever of the louse-borne variety, caused by *Rickettsia* species transmitted through infestations of body lice. Literature in public health underscores that such infestations remain relevant in contemporary American settings, particularly in institutions such as schools and nursing homes where large populations are susceptible to lice infestation (Pratt & Littig, 1973).

Moreover, the relationship between rickettsial infection and environmental factors highlights the importance of robust public health interventions. For instance, controlling louse infestations can significantly reduce the incidence of lice-borne diseases. Comprehending these processes is crucial for preventing outbreaks and safeguarding vulnerable populations, especially in environments with high infestation rates and limited healthcare resources. Additionally, chronic Fatigue Syndrome (CFS) has been suggested to have a possible association with rickettsial infections, although this relationship remains complex. Research has demonstrated that infection may contribute to immune dysregulation and subsequent symptoms similar to those observed in CFS. A prevalence study examining tick exposure- borne pathogens in CFS patients found that a considerable proportion exhibited evidence of infection compared to healthy controls, representing a noteworthy correlation (Kelly, 2014). This observation opens avenues for further investigation into the long-term health impacts of rickettsial diseases. Understanding how rickettsial bacteria influence immune function may enhance our comprehension of rickettsial diseases and inform treatment strategies for chronic illnesses associated with infectious agents.

10.4.1. Rocky Mountain spotted fever

Rocky Mountain spotted fever (RMSF) is a severe rickettsial disease most often caused by the bacterium *Rickettsia rickettsii*. It results from the bite of an infected tick, particularly the American dog tick, *Dermacentor variabilis*.

The disease can develop suddenly and typically presents with fever, headache, and rash a few days after initial infection. The case fatality rate for untreated cases may vary from 25%, highlighting the importance of early diagnosis and treatment with appropriate antibiotics. Additionally, the disease can lead to life-threatening complications involving vital organs, emphasising the need for awareness of vector control and prompt clinical recognition among at-risk populations, especially those in endemic areas. The epidemiology of RMSF is notable for its geographic distribution patterns. Despite its name referencing the Rocky Mountain region of the United States, cases have been reported across many parts of the country, notably the Southeast and Atlantic coast. The disease peaks during warmer months when ticks are most active. Therefore, public health initiatives that educate communities on the prevention of tick bites are crucial. While general awareness typically involves checking for ticks after outdoor activities and using insecticides, epidemiological data from studies such as "Tickborne Diseases in Massachusetts: A Physician's Reference Manual" offer healthcare professionals valuable tools for informing patients and reducing infection risks (Figure 10.11).

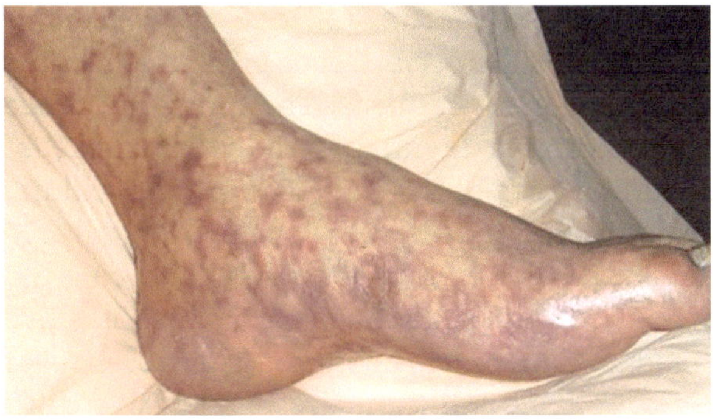

Figure 10.11. Rocky Mountain spotted fever.

Source: https://www.cdc.gov/rocky-mountain-spotted-fever/media/images/rmsffoot.jpg.

The prevention of Rocky Mountain Spotted Fever (RMSF) constitutes a comprehensive, multi-faceted approach that encompasses individual protection measures and community education initiatives. It is recommended that individuals wear protective clothing that fully covers the skin surface and utilize insect repellents containing DEET or permethrin when operating in areas infested with ticks. Environmental management strategies, such as maintaining clean yards and reducing brush where ticks commonly breed, are also effective in preventing RMSF. Additionally, public awareness campaigns play a crucial role in educating communities about the risks associated with RMSF and in promoting best practices for avoiding tick exposure. Early detection of RMSF symptoms significantly improves treatment outcomes, underscoring the importance of initiating doxycycline therapy before the development of severe illness. Therefore, a combination of public education and personal protective measures is essential to mitigate the impact of Rocky Mountain Spotted Fever within the region.

10.4.2. Typhus

Typhus, a severe infectious disease characterised by high fever and systemic manifestations, possesses a historical significance that underscores its impact on human health. It is primarily caused by *Rickettsia*, with various species responsible for distinct forms of typhus; for instance, epidemic typhus is caused by *Rickettsia prowazekii*, and murine typhus by *Rickettsia typhi*. Louse-borne epidemic typhus has garnered particular notoriety during periods of war and social upheaval, leading to devastating epidemics. Understanding the transmission dynamics and clinical epidemiology of typhus is imperative for effective public health interventions and disease control, especially in environments conducive to outbreaks — such as areas with overcrowding and inadequate sanitation — where lice infestations tend to proliferate.

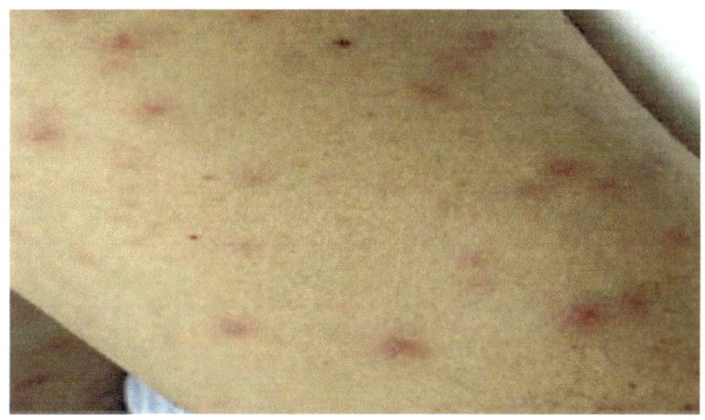

Figure 10.12. Typhus.

Source: https://media.post.rvohealth.io/wp-content/uploads/2020/08/642x361_Typhus.jpg.

The correlation between such social conditions and the incidence of typhus emphasises the necessity of addressing social determinants to mitigate outbreaks effectively. The pathophysiology of typhus involves complex interactions between *Rickettsia* and the host immune system. Once infected, *Rickettsia* target endothelial cells, resulting in vasculitis and accompanying symptoms including fever, rash, and, in severe cases, multi-organ failure. The immune response to Rickettsia infection is multifaceted, involving both innate and adaptive mechanisms. Early diagnosis and prompt antibiotic treatment are vital, as the disease's non-specific symptoms can delay detection and lead to serious complications. Recent research suggests a potential association between chronic infections, such as typhus, and chronic conditions like chronic fatigue syndrome (CFS). Persistent *Rickettsia* presence has been hypothesised to contribute to long-term fatigue and immune dysregulation, complicating recovery from acute infections (Kelly, 2014) (Figure 10.12).

The historical and contemporary significance of typhus in epidemiological studies warrants attention. Advancements in scientific research have enhanced prevention and control strategies for typhus outbreaks, leading to improved surveillance and immunisation measures. Despite these progressions, typhus remains a significant public health concern in many regions worldwide. Ongoing research continues to investigate the genetic diversity of Rickettsial species, their ecological reservoirs, and their interactions with vectors, primarily fleas and lice. These studies are essential for developing effective control strategies. Additionally, understanding the causal relationship between typhus and large-scale epidemiological patterns highlights the influence of socioeconomic and environmental factors on rickettsial diseases, thereby underscoring the critical connection between infectious diseases and public health policy (Ruiz, 2014).

10.4.3. Ehrlichiosis

Ehrlichiosis consists of a group of emerging infectious diseases caused by bacteria of the genus *Ehrlichia*, which are obligate intracellular, tick-transmitted organisms. It manifests in various clinical forms, from mild to severe, and is mainly associated with animal hosts like domestic dogs and some wild ruminants. The bacteria infect white blood cells, disrupting immune function and potentially leading to systemic complications if untreated. Notably, the disease exists in forms linked to *Ehrlichia canis* and *Ehrlichia chaffeensis*, each exhibiting distinct epidemiological patterns. The rising incidence of ehrlichiosis highlights the importance of understanding ecological factors that facilitate transmission and prevention, especially in regions with high tick populations bearing the pathogen. Diagnostic challenges hinder effective management of ehrlichiosis. The absence of rapid, reliable point-of-care tests delays early detection, which can result in severe outcomes, particularly in immunocompromised patients. Recent studies have shown variable agreement between serological tests and molecular methods such as polymerase chain reaction (PCR), indicating that factors like testing timing may affect accuracy. For example, a study comparing an immunochromatographic test to a comprehensive PCR panel found notable discrepancies, especially with *Ehrlichia canis*. These findings stress the need to develop diagnostic approaches that better determine infection status and enable earlier treatment, thereby reducing the risks associated with untreated ehrlichiosis (Wong et al., 2011) (Figure 10.13).

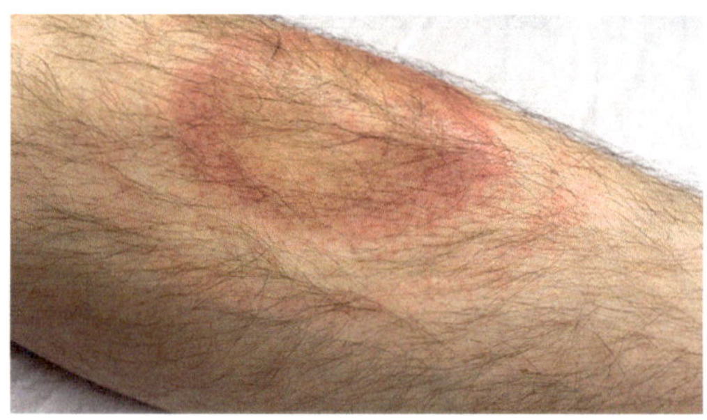

Figure 10.13. Ehrlichiosis.

Source: https://images-prod.healthline.com/hlcmsresource/images/Image-Galleries/ehrilichiosis/1203-Ehrilichiosis-642x361-slide3.jpg.

Epidemiological studies of Ehrlichiosis have highlighted its significance not only in veterinary medicine but also in human health. The zoonotic nature of *Ehrlichia phagocytophila*, which infects various vertebrate hosts, indicates a complex relationship among wildlife, domestic animals, and human populations. Evidence suggests that domesticated animals such as dogs, cats, and feral deer can serve as reservoirs for the disease, thereby increasing the risk of transmission. Additionally, seroepidemiologic surveys have shown high exposure rates in rural dogs and certain wildlife populations, justifying ongoing surveillance and investigation. Information on the genetic diversity of these agents across different geographic regions will be essential for developing effective prevention strategies and vaccines. Further genomic analysis will enable a clearer understanding of their phylogenetic relationships and environmental interactions, ultimately aiding in the management of ehrlichiosis and other rickettsial diseases (Kelly, 2014).

10.5. Diagnosis of Spirochetes and Rickettsial Infections

Spirochetal and rickettsial infections pose significant diagnostic challenges due to their broad spectrum of pathogenic characteristics and clinical manifestations. For instance, spirochetes such as those from the *Borrelia* species, transmitted primarily via tick bites, are responsible for diseases such as Lyme disease and borreliosis. These infections often present with non-specific symptoms that can be easily mistaken for other conditions. Serological testing is predominantly employed to measure antibodies specific to spirochetes; however, the specificity and sensitivity of these tests can vary substantially. Recent studies have increasingly recognised the discovery of new *Borrelia* species, which are not consistently diagnosed by conventional methods. Consequently, there is a suggestion for the adoption of improved diagnostic protocols, particularly in regions where these infections are emerging (Krol et al., 1991). Rickettsial diseases encompass a wide array of pathogens requiring diverse diagnostic approaches. Well-documented rickettsial illnesses such as Rocky Mountain spotted fever and typhus manifest with high fever, rash, and systemic symptoms. Diagnosis primarily relies on serological assays or PCR techniques, which facilitate rapid and precise detection of the pathogen's genetic material. Recent research indicates that these infections may co-occur with other bacterial populations, complicating clinical presentations and necessitating comprehensive diagnostic evaluations to achieve accurate identification. Specifically, co-infections involving rickettsial and spirochetal agents have been associated with severe morbidity; therefore, clinicians must remain vigilant to these possibilities during diagnostic assessments (Krol et al., 1991). Molecular diagnostic methods, including real-time PCR and next-generation sequencing, have markedly improved the sensitivity and specificity of detecting spirochete and rickettsial infections. These techniques provide immediate results and can identify low microbial loads within patient specimens, proving especially valuable when traditional serological tests are inconclusive due to prior antibiotic administration or cross-reactivity between pathogens. The identification of novel *Borrelia* species, such as *B. bisher*, underscores the importance of incorporating comprehensive diagnostic strategies. Ongoing surveillance and research into tick-borne pathogens, including spirochetes and rickettsiae, enhance our understanding of their epidemiology and support the development of effective diagnostic tools tailored to emerging clinical needs (Leydet, 2014).

10.5.1. Laboratory techniques

The pathobiology of rickettsial and spirochetal diseases necessitates the use of advanced laboratory techniques that are vital for accurate diagnosis and effective research. Molecular methods such as the polymerase chain reaction (PCR) have transformed the detection of these organisms. Not only does PCR improve sensitivity and enable scientists to diagnose infections from tiny samples, but it also allows for the identification of specific species, such as *Borrelia burgdorferi* and *Rickettsia spp*. This specificity is crucial, as new evidence now suggests that several novel strains of *Borrelia*, such as *Borrelia bissettii*, may cause human disease, especially in areas previously considered non-endemic (Leydet, 2014). Consequently, rigorous laboratory techniques are essential to track the epidemiological patterns of these infections and assess their potential public health impact. In addition, serological examinations are highly valuable for diagnosing rickettsial infections and detecting antibody responses to such pathogens.

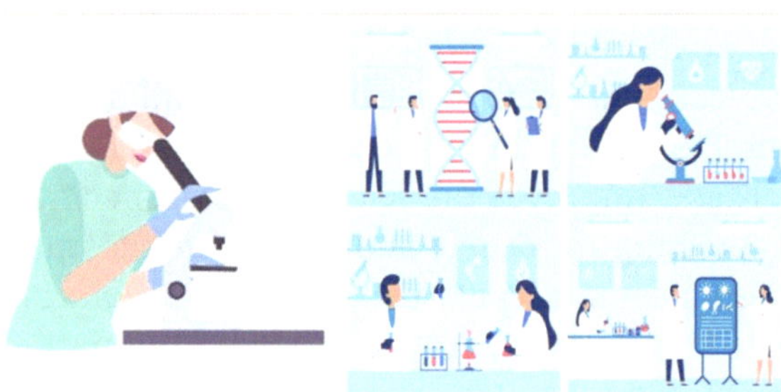

Figure 10.14. Laboratory diagnosis of spirochetes and *rickettsial* infections.

Source: https://external-content.duckduckgo.com/iu/?u=https%3A%2F%2Fmicrobiologynotes.org%2Fwp-content%2Fuploads%2F2021%2F12%2FMethods-for-Laboratory-diagnosis-of-viral-infections-1024x576.jpg&f=1&nofb=1&ipt=e858fc0f85de47eb7a115db3164ebdde1fac278764d90a9173cd0a274acff9cb.

Enzyme-linked immunosorbent assays (ELISA), for instance, are commonly used to measure antibody titres against rickettsial antigens, revealing both past and current infections. Given the complexity of the immune response to spirochetes, these approaches should be used carefully and often alongside molecular diagnostic tests to acquire comprehensive information regarding the host's immune status. Current research on the pathogenic potential of uncharacterised species underscores the need to utilize diverse laboratory methods. Accurate differential diagnosis depends on such detailed techniques to ensure appropriate clinical management and guide public health measures for vector-borne diseases, especially in regions where these infections have previously been underdiagnosed (Charrel et al., 2017) (Figure 10.14).

In addition to molecular and serological techniques, culture procedures continue to be the cornerstone of laboratory investigations into spirochetes and rickettsial diseases. Although contemporary techniques have gained prominence, traditional culture methods remain in use, particularly for specific rickettsial organisms that are less amenable to molecular detection. Cultivating these pathogens can yield valuable insights into their growth patterns and virulence, thereby advancing understanding of host-pathogen interactions. Furthermore, the identification of new species, as observed in the non-endemic regions of the United States, underscores the necessity for ongoing surveillance and research utilising these conventional methodologies. By integrating traditional culture techniques with modern molecular and serological approaches, researchers are able to develop a more comprehensive understanding of spirochete and rickettsial infections, which, in turn, facilitates improvements in diagnostic and therapeutic strategies (Leydet, 2014).

10.5.2. Clinical symptoms

The clinical presentation of spirochetal infections, particularly Lyme disease, is multifaceted and dynamic, posing diagnostic challenges. Early in the disease course, patients may exhibit the characteristic erythema migrans, a bull's-eye rash occurring at the site of a tick bite, which may signify localised *Borrelia burgdorferi* infection. As the disease progresses, systemic manifestations such as fever, fatigue, headache, and myalgia are frequently observed, reflecting the dissemination of the spirochetes throughout the body. These symptoms contribute to the complex clinical picture of Lyme borreliosis and, if untreated, may lead to additional complications.

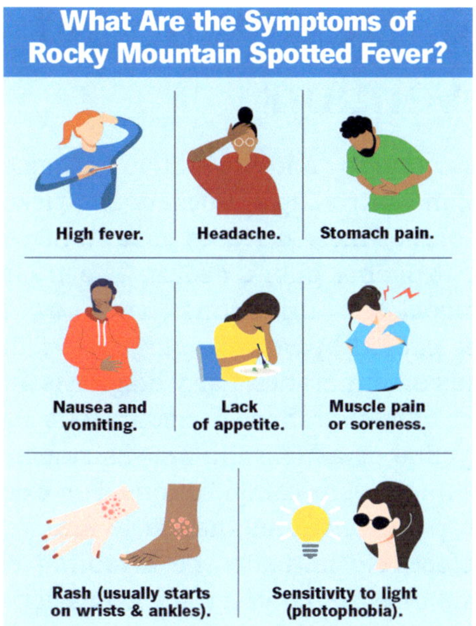
What Are the Symptoms of Rocky Mountain Spotted Fever?
High fever.
Headache.
Stomach pain.
Nausea and vomiting.
Lack of appetite.
Muscle pain or soreness.
Rash (usually starts on wrists & ankles).
Sensitivity to light (photophobia).

Figure 10.15. Symptoms of Rocky Mountain spotted fever.

Source: https://my.clevelandclinic.org/-/scassets/images/org/health/articles/17838-rocky-mountain-spotted-fever.

The complexity of such presentations underscores the necessity for increased awareness among healthcare professionals and underscores the importance of precise diagnostic procedures to distinguish among various tick-borne illnesses and their associated symptoms, as highlighted in recent epidemiological research (Leydet, 2014). Further complicating the clinical profile are findings that other *Borrelia* species, such as *B. bissettii*, can induce similar yet distinct clinical symptoms. Research indicates that although *Borrelia burgdorferi* remains the most recognised causative agent of Lyme disease, the pathogenic potential of other genospecies is increasingly acknowledged. Notably, the immune response triggered by *B. bissettii* can display overlapping signs with those caused by *B. burgdorferi*, thereby complicating diagnosis and treatment. A recent study on these alternative *Borrelia* strains reveals that *Ixodes scapularis* ticks can harbour and transmit *B. bissettii*, posing a threat by causing cases of disease in humans that remain unrecognised.

Therefore, increased vigilance in non-endemic areas, where awareness of Lyme disease is lower, is crucial for effective public health responses. Rickettsial infections typically present with acute fever and rash; in severe cases, they can cause vasculitis or organ failure. The range of symptoms linked to various *Rickettsia* species reflects their ability to invade and impact different body systems, especially if untreated. For example, infections like Rocky Mountain spotted fever, caused by *Rickettsia rickettsii*, often show fever, rash, and an eschar at the infection site. The severity of symptoms usually correlates with how quickly treatment begins, emphasising the importance of early diagnosis and intervention by healthcare providers. Ongoing clinical research into Rickettsial and spirochetal diseases aims to improve diagnostic accuracy and treatment approaches (Leydet, 2014).

10.5.3. Differential diagnosis

Differential diagnosis holds paramount importance in the identification of rickettsial infections and spirochete-related illnesses, given that numerous infections manifest with analogous clinical features. For instance, Lyme borreliosis may present with symptoms that are also observed in other conditions, such as viral infections, arthritis, or even multiple sclerosis, owing to its multisystemic presentation (Leydet, 2014). Patients may exhibit erythema migrans along with musculoskeletal and neurological symptoms, necessitating meticulous evaluation to exclude various etiologies. Similarly, diseases caused by *Rickettsia* species, such as Rocky Mountain spotted fever, can exhibit symptoms including fever, rash, and potentially respiratory distress, which may lead to misdiagnosis unless clinicians consider the possibility of a tick-borne pathogen. This underscores the importance of comprehensive patient history collection, emphasising exposure risk and symptom chronology as initial steps toward refining differential diagnoses. For patients presenting with symptoms indicative of spirochete or rickettsial infections, it is essential to employ serological testing and other diagnostic procedures to confirm or exclude differential diagnoses. Tests such as enzyme-linked immunosorbent assays (ELISA) for detecting antibodies to specific Borrelia species, alongside PCR (polymerase chain reaction) assays to identify rickettsial DNA in clinical specimens, are instrumental (Carvalho, 2010). Since the pathogenesis and therapeutic approaches for these infections substantially depend on accurate diagnosis, it is critically important to exclude other bacterial, viral, or autoimmune diseases. Co-infections involving rickettsiae and spirochetes further complicate diagnosis by potentially exacerbating or attenuating symptoms, thereby necessitating a multi-step diagnostic process that considers other infectious agents endemic to particular regions. Furthermore, the application of differential diagnosis is indispensable for guiding effective treatment strategies for spirochete and rickettsial infections, as misdiagnosis could result in inappropriate therapy, chronic complications, and increased morbidity. Therefore, healthcare practitioners must exercise diligence in recognising the overlap of symptomatology associated with these diseases, employing the latest diagnostic techniques, and maintaining vigilance regarding evolving epidemiological data. This includes understanding the geographic distribution of tick-borne diseases and their associated pathogens, which can inform clinical suspicion even in non-endemic regions experiencing cases of Lyme disease and related illnesses. Continued education and collaborative research are vital to advancing knowledge and ensuring effective management of these complex infections.

10.6. Treatment and Prevention

Effective therapy and preventive strategies are crucial in controlling spirochete and rickettsial infections, as these diseases pose an increasing threat to global public health. The treatment of spirochetal infections, such as Lyme disease caused by *Borrelia burgdorferi*, largely depends on antibiotics. Early diagnosis and the prompt administration of medications such as doxycycline or amoxicillin are instrumental in preventing severe complications. For example, research demonstrates that early intervention can effectively mitigate the disabling effects of Lyme disease; however, it also underscores the importance of heightened awareness and education among healthcare providers and the public regarding disease symptoms and transmission, especially in non-endemic regions (Leydet, 2014). This highlights the need for caution in diagnostic procedures to ensure early detection and treatment of infections. Preventive measures are equally vital in the prevention of spirochete and rickettsial infections. Public health initiatives should prioritise community education about the risks associated with exposure to ticks and mites, as these arthropods serve as incidental vectors. The implementation of integrated pest management strategies- such as acaricide application, habitat modification, and personal protective measures like wearing long sleeves and using repellents- can significantly reduce tick exposure. Moreover, the establishment of surveillance programs in developing regions can facilitate early identification of endemic areas, thereby preventing outbreaks of infections such as Lyme disease (Carvalho, 2010). The combination of these strategies can substantially reduce the burden of spirochete-related diseases on public health systems. Furthermore, ongoing research should aim to improve vaccines targeting spirochetes and rickettsial diseases. Efforts are underway to develop vaccines against various *Borrelia* species, which will be increasingly valuable as new strains are identified and disseminate into non-traditional areas. Equally important is the advancement of diagnostic kits that allow for the precise detection of infections, thereby enhancing treatment efficacy and surveillance capabilities. The coexistence of multiple pathogens within vectors complicates disease dynamics, emphasising the need to consider potential co-infections that could hinder treatment effectiveness (Leydet, 2014). Consequently, a comprehensive approach encompassing education, research, and innovative public health policies is imperative to effectively mitigate the impact of these infections and support the overall well-being of the population.

10.6.1. Antibiotic therapies

The management of spirochetal and rickettsial infections relies heavily on effective antibiotic therapy, which is vital in preventing severe complications associated with these infections. Agents such as doxycycline are frequently employed in the treatment of infections like Lyme disease, caused by *Borrelia burgdorferi*, whereas classes of agents such as tetracyclines and macrolides are essential for managing Rickettsial infections. The early initiation of these treatments is not only advantageous but also crucial, as delays can result in severe symptoms and increased incidence of chronic disease. In the context of chronic fatigue syndrome (CFS), research indicates a potential link between underlying infectious etiologies and the development of malaise and chronic fatigue; consequently, antibiotic-targeted therapies are considered viable options for recovery and symptom management, as supported by current studies (Kelly, 2014). The efficacy of antibiotic therapy extends beyond the eradication of pathogenic organisms; it also plays a significant role in modulating inflammatory responses associated with infection. In severe cases, prompt administration of antibiotics has been shown to significantly reduce morbidity and mortality, particularly in infections such as sepsis, where Rickettsial infections may progress to advanced stages. This underscores the importance of understanding pharmacokinetics and pharmacodynamics in antibiotic treatment, enabling healthcare professionals to optimize treatment protocols for critically ill patients. Moreover, given the escalating concerns regarding antibiotic resistance, practitioners must adopt prudent prescribing practices that are not only effective against infections but also help preserve the efficacy of these vital medications. Initiatives such as antibiotic stewardship are indispensable in ensuring the judicious use of antibiotics and in mitigating the threat of resistance (Chan et al., 2017). In addition to selecting appropriate antibiotic agents, vigilant monitoring of therapeutic response is imperative for the effective management of spirochetal and rickettsial diseases. Clinicians must remain attentive to both clinical outcomes and potential adverse effects of antibiotic regimens. Recognising the heterogeneity of patient responses necessitates a personalized approach, often involving dosage adjustments or tailoring antibiotic choice based on tolerance and efficacy. As preliminary evidence suggests an interaction between chronic infections and conditions such as CFS, it is essential to thoroughly understand the effects of prolonged antibiotic therapy on recovery patterns. Further investigation into this interaction may facilitate the optimisation of treatment regimens and ultimately improve patient outcomes, thereby providing more effective management for individuals adversely affected by these challenging infections (Kelly, 2014).

10.6.2. Vaccination efforts

The critical necessity for effective vaccination against spirochetal and rickettsial infections has become increasingly evident amidst the rising incidence of bacterial tick-borne infections (BTBDs). These infections, which encompass Lyme disease, anaplasmosis, and rickettsiosis, pose significant public health concerns due to their intricate life cycles within vector-tick and vertebrate host reservoirs. To develop effective countermeasures, immunisation strategies must consider the complexity of disease vectors and their interactions across diverse ecosystems. The urgency of this matter pertains not only to human disease prevention but also to the protection of livestock and the preservation of animal health, thereby necessitating a One Health approach to disease management (Kirkan et al., 2017). The field of vaccination has undergone substantial evolution, particularly through advances in molecular biology and immunology. Researchers have concentrated on utilising recombinant antigens and tick saliva toxins to create vaccines that ensure safety and efficacy. These advancements provide a foundation for targeted immunisation strategies aimed at eliciting specific immune responses to combat tick infestation and, concomitantly, the transmission of tick-borne pathogens. Furthermore, current research emphasises exploring the potential application of multi-target vaccines designed to disrupt the enzootic cycle of ticks by incorporating protein antigens derived from both tick salivary glands and midguts. An integrated approach is deemed essential for enhancing the overall effectiveness of vaccines against spirochetal and rickettsial pathogens (Yadav & Upadhyay, 2022) (Figure 10.16).

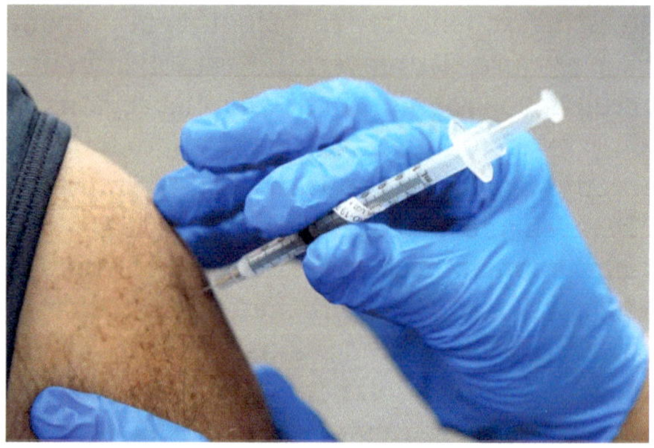

Figure 10.16. Routine vaccination or therapeutic treatment procedures.

Source: https://www.aljazeera.com/wp-content/uploads/2021/03/AP_21008627936484.jpg?resize=770%2C513&quality=80.

Despite positive developments in vaccination campaigns, significant challenges still exist in effectively implementing and disseminating these vaccines across diverse populations. Public hesitation to receive vaccines, combined with difficulties in reaching rural or underserved communities, can considerably slow their broad adoption. Additionally, ongoing education and sustained contact with at-risk populations are essential to raise awareness of the benefits of vaccinating against spirochetal and rickettsial diseases. Overcoming these barriers is vital for the success of vaccination programmes, as they not only provide individual protection but also enhance herd immunity and reduce disease burden at the population level. Therefore, establishing strong vaccination programmes is crucial for the long-term control of BTBDs and the safeguarding of human and animal health.

10.6.3. Public health measures

The emergence of spirochetal and rickettsial diseases has mandated the implementation of rigorous public health measures aimed at reducing transmission risks. Such interventions are particularly crucial as reports of diseases such as Lyme borreliosis become increasingly frequent. Surveillance programs serve as the cornerstone of these efforts; they enable health authorities to identify high-risk areas and monitor the prevalence of causative agents. Moreover, public education regarding the dangers posed by ticks and other vectors is vital for controlling disease dissemination. A unified initiative to inform communities about personal protective strategies — including appropriate clothing and the use of insect repellents — is essential for reducing human exposure to infected ticks. This educational effort plays a critical role in shaping public attitudes toward preventative actions and in responding effectively to health threats posed by tick-borne illnesses (Vozmediano et al., 2021). Managing tick-borne infections involves not only diligent surveillance but also underscores the importance of interdisciplinary research aimed at improving preventive measures. Public health initiatives should facilitate collaboration among entomologists, epidemiologists, and community health institutions to deepen understanding of spirochete and rickettsial infections across various ecosystems. Research has identified several *Borrelia* species in new geographic regions, underscoring the expanding scope of contagious diseases within the United States (Leydet, 2014). Consequently, continuous education and public awareness campaigns are imperative, especially in unconventional environments where awareness of tick-borne diseases remains limited. By integrating research findings into public health policy, communities can enhance their preparedness and response capacity, thereby mitigating the impact of emerging threats and safeguarding public health. Additionally, public health officials must evaluate and adapt their strategies according to risk perceptions among populations. Evidence indicates that many individuals tend to underestimate the threat posed by ticks, even in areas with rising incidences of tick-borne diseases. Education campaigns should thus aim to close this knowledge gap by emphasising personal experiences and local statistics related to Lyme disease and other tick-borne illnesses to ensure efficacy. Furthermore, establishing partnerships with local organisations such as recreation centres and parks can expand outreach initiatives, promoting responsible engagement with natural environments. These collaborations also facilitate resource distribution during peak tick activity seasons, thus enhancing community awareness and knowledge (Vozmediano et al., 2021). Ultimately, proactive public health strategies that are tailored to local realities and responsive to community needs are essential for preventing the emergence and spread of spirochetes and rickettsial infections.

SUMMARY

In synthesising the issues of spirochetal and rickettsial diseases, the complex interactions between pathogens and vectors emphasise the importance of targeted epidemiological surveillance. The evidence demonstrates that geographic distribution and environmental factors significantly influence infection prevalence. Recent studies in regions such as the Northern Apennines record the presence of several *Borrelia* species and *Rickettsia spp.* in immature ticks infesting local lizards, which clearly show no host-pathogen interaction dynamics. These findings highlight that lizards play a crucial role in tick-borne pathogen transmission cycles and, therefore, warrant ongoing research to assess their epidemiological significance (Ceballos et al., 2017). Public health initiatives must develop strategies to address multiple reservoirs and vectors, enhancing tick-borne disease prevention and control efforts. The expanding range of spirochetes — particularly *Borrelia burgdorferi* — has made Lyme disease a growing public health concern in the United States and beyond. Annually, approximately 300,000 cases are diagnosed, prompting further investigation into the epidemiology and ecology of these pathogens. The discovery of new species like *Borrelia bissettii* raises concerns about unrecognised human diseases, especially in non-endemic areas. In Louisiana, efforts to screen regional fauna and insect populations for *Borrelia* species uncovered complex enzootic cycles among various ticks and animals, underlining the need for vigilance in previously less-affected localities (Leydet, 2014). Through increased awareness and integrating findings from recent research into public health policies, stakeholders can better address the escalating threat posed by these pathogens. Ultimately, understanding spirochetal and rickettsial infections requires an interdisciplinary model incorporating ecology, microbiology, and public health. As further research uncovers new vectors and pathogens, healthcare systems must maintain a broad surveillance approach across diverse geographical areas. This will facilitate early detection and response to emerging threats. Public education campaigns emphasising preventive measures — such as tick control and personal protective practices — can bolster community resilience against these infections. As the knowledge base advances, it will be vital for health professionals to stay informed of the latest discoveries and adapt their strategies accordingly, optimally protecting populations at risk from spirochetes and rickettsial diseases.

Research into spirochetal and rickettsial infections provides valuable insights into the escalating public health threats posed by these pathogens, especially concerning Lyme disease and other tick-borne illnesses. Notably, Lyme borreliosis has become a significant health concern, with an estimated 300 300,000 diagnosed cases annually in the United States alone. This statistic underscores the necessity for continuous surveillance and research, particularly in non-endemic regions where novel *Borrelia* species are routinely identified. For example, studies in Louisiana have documented the presence of an enzootic cycle of *Borrelia burgdorferi* sensu stricto, with potential implications from *Borrelia bissettii*, emphasising the critical importance of understanding these lesser-studied species for human health and underscoring the urgent need for comprehensive research in this domain (Leydet, 2014). Beyond *Borrelia*, the interactions between wildlife and tick-borne diseases offer further insights into the epidemiology of rickettsial infections. Species such as wild boars and roe deer serve as key hosts for ticks, influencing both tick population dynamics and pathogen transmission. A study conducted in southern Germany examined the prevalence of tick and pathogen infestation in these wildlife hosts and elucidated their roles within the life cycle of tick-borne diseases. The findings highlight the intricate ecosystem relationships that facilitate the transmission of spirochetes and rickettsiae, advocating for a holistic approach to sustainable tick-borne disease management that incorporates wildlife health (Muders, 2015). Furthermore, the rising incidence of spirochetal and rickettsial diseases necessitates the development of more advanced diagnostic techniques and public awareness initiatives. The cross-reactivity among various *Borrelia* species, combined with the challenges in differentiating these conditions using current diagnostic tools, presents significant clinical difficulties. As evidenced in Louisiana, *Borrelia bissettii* may pose health risks even in regions where *Borrelia burgdorferi* is less prevalent, indicating gaps in existing knowledge. The relative stagnation of research in this area underscores the importance of further investigations into the pathogenic potential of lesser-studied organisms and vectors. As the prevalence of Lyme disease and other related illnesses continues to rise in new regions, vigilant surveillance and educational efforts will be vital in mitigating the public health impact of these emerging diseases, ensuring that communities remain informed and prepared as the epidemiological landscape evolves.

CLOSER LOOK

ANTIGENIC VARIATION IN LYME DISEASE AND RELAPSING FEVER

Antigenic variation is a sophisticated mechanism by which the pathogens alter the surface antigens to escape the host immune system detection and destruction. Antigenic variation is crucial in the pathogenesis of *Borrelia* species infections, particularly Lyme disease and relapsing fever. The two diseases are caused by spirochete bacteria of the genus *Borrelia*, but they differ according to the transmission vectors, clinical expression, and mechanisms of antigenic variation.

Lyme disease, primarily transmitted in North America by *Borrelia burgdorferi*, is transmitted by *Ixodes ticks*. The primary mechanism of antigenic variation in *B. burgdorferi* is offered by the *VlsE* (variable major protein-like sequence, expressed) lipoprotein. The *vlsE* gene resides on a linear plasmid (lp28-1) and is bounded by a series of silent vls cassettes. Upon infection, there is gene conversion between the expression site and these silent cassettes that creates modified *VlsE* proteins with different amino acid sequences. This process is non-reciprocal and one-way. It is not a transcriptional switch wherein rather, it forms a new mosaic variant of the *VlsE* protein through segmental recombination.

This antigenic variation allows *B. burgdorferi* to escape antibody-mediated clearance by constantly exposing the host immune system to new surface antigens. It allows the bacterium to be sustained in many tissues, such as the joints, skin, heart, and nervous system and also induces chronic manifestations such as Lyme arthritis and neuroborreliosis. The variation occurs only during infection of the mammalian host and not during *in vitro* growth or within the tick vector, indicating a host-dependent regulatory process.

Relapsing fever, on the other hand, is caused by different *Borrelia* species such as *Borrelia hermsii* (tick-borne) and *Borrelia recurrentis* (louse-borne). The defining symptom of the disease is relapsing fevers that are associated with waves of bacteremia. Antigenic variation for relapsing fever is more virulent and has a higher speed compared to Lyme disease and comprises Variable Major Proteins (Vmps) classified as Variable Large Proteins (Vlps) and Variable Small Proteins (Vsps). Each bacterium synthesizes only one Vmp simultaneously from a single site of expression.

Vmps are switched by gene conversion or site-specific recombination, replacing the expressed gene with a silent copy from a *vmp* gene pool. When the host mounts an immune response against the expressed Vmp in current expression, the switched bacteria evade the immune system, increase in number, and trigger a new bout of fever, thus accounting for the disease's relapsing nature. The process recurs until effective immunological clearance or therapy.

REFERENCES

1. Chung, Y. K., Ahn, Y. S., & Jeong, J. S. (2010). Occupational infection in Korea. *Journal of Korean medical science, 25*(Suppl), S53–S61. https://doi.org/10.3346/jkms.2010.25.S.S53(accessed on 16th July 2025).
2. Foster, J., Ganatra, M., Kamal, I., Ware, J., Makarova, K., Ivanova, N., Bhattacharyya, A., Kapatral, V., Kumar, S., Posfai, J., Vincze, T., Ingram, J., Moran, L., Lapidus, A., Omelchenko, M., Kyrpides, N., Ghedin, E., Wang, S., Goltsman, E., Joukov, V., ... Slatko, B. (2005). The Wolbachia genome of Brugia malayi: endosymbiont evolution within a human pathogenic nematode. *PLoS biology, 3*(4), e121. https://doi.org/10.1371/journal.pbio.0030121Alberdi Vélez, M. P. (2000). *Epidemiology and molecular characterization of Ehrlichia phagocytophila in relation to emerging ehrlichie.* https://core.ac.uk/download/429718070.pdf (accessed on 16th July 2025).
3. Rizzoli, A., Silaghi, C., Obiegala, A., Rudolf, I., Hubálek, Z., Földvári, G., Plantard, O., Vayssier-Taussat, M., Bonnet, S., Spitalská, E., & Kazimírová, M. (2014). Ixodes ricinus and Its Transmitted Pathogens in Urban and Peri-Urban Areas in Europe: New Hazards and Relevance for Public Health. *Frontiers in public health, 2*, 251. https://doi.org/10.3389/fpubh.2014.00251(accessed on 16th July 2025).
4. Boqvist, S. (2002). *Leptospira Infection among Pigs in Southern Vietnam.* https://core.ac.uk/download/11694568.pdf (accessed on 16th July 2025).
5. Burdmann, E. A., & Jha, V. (2017). Acute kidney injury due to tropical infectious diseases and animal venoms: a tale of 2 continents. *Kidney international, 91*(5), 1033–1046. https://doi.org/10.1016/j.kint.2016.09.051(accessed on 16th July 2025).
6. Ceballos, L. A., de Sousa, R., Mannelli, A., Martello, E., et al. (2017). *Importance of common wall lizards in the transmission dynamics of tick-borne pathogens in the Northern Apennine Mountains, Italy.* https://core.ac.uk/download/154161016.pdf (accessed on 16th July 2025).
7. Wong, S. S., Teng, J. L., Poon, R. W., Choi, G. K., Chan, K. H., Yeung, M. L., Hui, J. J., & Yuen, K. Y. (2011). Comparative evaluation of a point-of-care immunochromatographic test SNAP 4Dx with molecular detection tests for vector-borne canine pathogens in Hong Kong. *Vector borne and zoonotic diseases (Larchmont, N.Y.), 11*(9), 1269–1277. https://doi.org/10.1089/vbz.2010.0265(accessed on 16th July 2025).
8. Chan, L., Ibrahim, N. A., Mat Nor, M. B., Tai, N. S. M., et al. (2017). *Guide to Antimicrobial Therapy 2017.* https://core.ac.uk/download/300453506.pdf (accessed on 16th July 2025).
9. Charrel, R. N., Lempereur, L., Mihalca, A. D., Vayssier-Taussat, M., et al. (2017). European Network for Neglected Vectors and Vector-Borne Infections COST Action guidelines: What is this about and what is this for? https://orbi.ulg.ac.be/bitstream/2268/206106/1/VBZD.pdf (accessed on 16th July 2025).
10. Kirkan, S., Erbas, G., & Parin, U. (2017). Bacterial Tick-Borne Diseases of Livestock Animals. InTech. doi: 10.5772/66122(accessed on 16th July 2025).
11. Stephenson, N., & Foley, J. (2016). Parallelisms and Contrasts in the Diverse Ecologies of the Anaplasma phagocytophilum and Borrelia burgdorferi Complexes of Bacteria in the Far Western United States. *Veterinary sciences, 3*(4), 26. https://doi.org/10.3390/vetsci3040026(accessed on 16th July 2025).

12. Garcia Vozmediano, A., Giglio, G., Nobili, F., Ramassa, E., et al. (2021). *Low risk perception about ticks and tick-borne diseases in an area recently invaded by ticks in northwestern Italy.* https://core.ac.uk/download/482676113.pdf (accessed on 16th July 2025).

13. Krol, Rena M.; Hawkins, William E.; and Overstreet, Robin M., "Rickettsial and Mollicute Infections in Hepatopancreatic Cells of Cultured Pacific White Shrimp (Penaeus vannamei)" (1991). Faculty Publications from the Harold W. Manter Laboratory of Parasitology. 880. https://digitalcommons.unl.edu/parasitologyfacpubs/880(accessed on 16th July 2025).

14. Kelly, T. (2014). *Do certain microbiological pathogens cause or have a role in the aetiology of the disease entity known as chronic fatigue syndrome?* https://core.ac.uk/download/41238184.pdf (accessed on 16th July 2025).

15. Leydet Jr, Brian Francis, "North American Lyme Borreliae: New Distributions and an Insight Into Borrelia bissettii Infection, Immune Response and Transmission in a Murine Model" (2014). *LSU Doctoral Dissertations.* 1985. https://repository.lsu.edu/gradschool_dissertations/1985(accessed on 16th July 2025).

16. Harry D. Pratt and Kent S. Littig (1973). *Lice of Public Health Importance and Their Control.* DHEW Publication No. (CDC) 74-8265 https://core.ac.uk/download/610528477.pdf (accessed on 16th July 2025).

17. Lopes De Carvalho, I. (2010). *Borrelia lusitaniae and Lyme borreliosis in Portugal: A contribution to the study of an emerging bacterial zoonosis with an impact on public health.* http://hdl.handle.net/10400.18/4676 (accessed on 16th July 2025).

18. Molina Ruiz, A. M. (2014*). Immunohistochemistry in the Diagnosis of Cutaneous Viral and Bacterial Infections.* https://repositorio.uam.es/bitstream/10486/662932/1/molina_ruiz_ana_maria.pdf (accessed on 16th July 2025).

19. Muders, S. V. (2015). *The role of European big game (Capreolus capreolus and Sus scrofa) as hosts for ticks and in the epidemiological life cycle of tick-borne diseases.* https://core.ac.uk/download/197533708.pdf (accessed on 16th July 2025).

20. Nidhi Yadav & Ravi Kant Upadhyay

21. (2022). *Tick Saliva Antigen-Based Vaccines, Disease Protection and Prophylaxis.* ISSN 2449-8955 (Online) Publisher TMKarpinski Publisher, Tomasz M. Karpiński, https://core.ac.uk/download/523087599.pdf (accessed on 16th July 2025).

INDEX

C

D

E

F

G

H

N

O

P

Q

R

S